STUDY GUIDE TO
PSYCHOSOMATIC MEDICINE

A Companion to
The American Psychiatric Publishing Textbook of Psychosomatic Medicine,
Second Edition

D1205545

STUDY GUIDE TO
PSYCHOSOMATIC MEDICINE

A Companion to
The American Psychiatric Publishing Textbook of Psychosomatic Medicine,
Second Edition

James A. Bourgeois, O.D., M.D.
Professor and Vice-Chair of Education
Department of Psychiatry and Behavioural Neurosciences
McMaster University
Hamilton, Ontario, Canada

Robert E. Hales, M.D., M.B.A.
Joe P. Tupin Chair and Professor and Chair
Department of Psychiatry and Behavioral Sciences
University of California, Davis School of Medicine
Sacramento, California

Narriman C. Shahrokh
Chief Administrative Officer
Department of Psychiatry and Behavioral Sciences
University of California, Davis School of Medicine
Sacramento, California

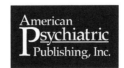

American
Psychiatric
Publishing, Inc.

Washington, DC
London, England

If you would like to buy between 25 and 99 copies of this or any other APPI title, you are eligible for a 20% discount; please contact APPI Customer Service at appi@psych.org or 800-368-5777. If you wish to buy 100 or more copies of the same title, please email us at bulksales@psych.org for a price quote.

Copyright © 2011 American Psychiatric Publishing, Inc.
ALL RIGHTS RESERVED

Manufactured in the United States of America on acid-free paper
15 14 13 12 11   5 4 3 2 1

ISBN 978-1-58562-403-4
First Edition

Typeset in Revival BT and Adobe's The Mix

American Psychiatric Publishing, Inc.
1000 Wilson Boulevard
Arlington, VA 22209-3901
www.appi.org

Contents

Preface xi

Questions

CHAPTER 1
Psychiatric Assessment and Consultation 1

CHAPTER 2
Legal Issues 3

CHAPTER 3
Ethical Issues 5

CHAPTER 4
Psychological Responses to Illness 7

CHAPTER 5
Delirium 9

CHAPTER 6
Dementia 11

CHAPTER 7
Aggression and Violence 13

CHAPTER 8
Depression 15

CHAPTER 9
Suicidality 17

CHAPTER 10
Psychosis, Mania, and Catatonia 19

CHAPTER 11
Anxiety Disorders 21

CHAPTER 12
Somatization and Somatoform Disorders 23

CHAPTER 13
Deception Syndromes: Factitious Disorders and Malingering 25

CHAPTER 14
Eating Disorders...27

CHAPTER 15
Sleep Disorders..29

CHAPTER 16
Sexual Dysfunction..31

CHAPTER 17
Substance-Related Disorders..33

CHAPTER 18
Heart Disease..35

CHAPTER 19
Lung Disease...37

CHAPTER 20
Gastrointestinal Disorders..39

CHAPTER 21
Renal Disease..41

CHAPTER 22
Endocrine and Metabolic Disorders....................................43

CHAPTER 23
Oncology...45

CHAPTER 24
Hematology...47

CHAPTER 25
Rheumatology..49

CHAPTER 26
Chronic Fatigue and Fibromyalgia Syndromes.....................51

CHAPTER 27
Infectious Diseases..53

CHAPTER 28
HIV/AIDS...55

CHAPTER 29
Dermatology..57

CHAPTER 30
Surgery 59

CHAPTER 31
Organ Transplantation. 61

CHAPTER 32
Neurology and Neurosurgery. 63

CHAPTER 33
Obstetrics and Gynecology 65

CHAPTER 34
Pediatrics 67

CHAPTER 35
Physical Medicine and Rehabilitation 68

CHAPTER 36
Pain 70

CHAPTER 37
Medical Toxicology 72

CHAPTER 38
Psychopharmacology 74

CHAPTER 39
Psychotherapy. 76

CHAPTER 40
Electroconvulsive Therapy. 78

CHAPTER 41
Palliative Care 80

Answer Guide

CHAPTER 1
Psychiatric Assessment and Consultation 82

CHAPTER 2
Legal Issues 86

CHAPTER 3
Ethical Issues 90

CHAPTER 4
Psychological Responses to Illness 95

CHAPTER 5
Delirium 100

CHAPTER 6
Dementia 104

CHAPTER 7
Aggression and Violence 107

CHAPTER 8
Depression 111

CHAPTER 9
Suicidality 116

CHAPTER 10
Psychosis, Mania, and Catatonia 119

CHAPTER 11
Anxiety Disorders 123

CHAPTER 12
Somatization and Somatoform Disorders 127

CHAPTER 13
Deception Syndromes: Factitious Disorders and Malingering 132

CHAPTER 14
Eating Disorders 135

CHAPTER 15
Sleep Disorders 139

CHAPTER 16
Sexual Dysfunction 142

CHAPTER 17
Substance-Related Disorders 145

CHAPTER 18
Heart Disease 149

CHAPTER 19
Lung Disease 155

CHAPTER 20
Gastrointestinal Disorders 158

CHAPTER 21
Renal Disease.. 164

CHAPTER 22
Endocrine and Metabolic Disorders 168

CHAPTER 23
Oncology... 172

CHAPTER 24
Hematology... 175

CHAPTER 25
Rheumatology... 179

CHAPTER 26
Chronic Fatigue and Fibromyalgia Syndromes 183

CHAPTER 27
Infectious Diseases 187

CHAPTER 28
HIV/AIDS.. 191

CHAPTER 29
Dermatology 197

CHAPTER 30
Surgery 201

CHAPTER 31
Organ Transplantation.. 206

CHAPTER 32
Neurology and Neurosurgery... 211

CHAPTER 33
Obstetrics and Gynecology 216

CHAPTER 34
Pediatrics 221

CHAPTER 35
Physical Medicine and Rehabilitation 224

CHAPTER 36
Pain 228

CHAPTER 37
Medical Toxicology 233

CHAPTER 38
Psychopharmacology 237

CHAPTER 39
Psychotherapy. 241

CHAPTER 40
Electroconvulsive Therapy. 245

CHAPTER 41
Palliative Care 249

Preface

The purpose of this study guide is to provide individuals who have purchased the Second Edition of *The American Psychiatric Publishing Textbook of Psychosomatic Medicine: Psychiatric Care of the Medically Ill* an opportunity to evaluate their understanding of the material contained in the textbook. Whenever possible, the selected questions emphasize the major points of each chapter. In addition, every effort is made to select those questions of most relevance to psychiatrists who see patients in a variety of clinical practice settings.

We encourage the readers of the textbook to answer the questions after reading each chapter. The format for the questions is similar to what candidates would expect to encounter when taking Part I of the American Board of Psychiatry and Neurology initial certification examination or the maintenance-of-certification examination in psychiatry that is required every 10 years. At the end of the study guide, the questions are repeated along with detailed answers. The answer section includes an explanation of the correct response for each question, as well as an explanation, in most cases, for why the other responses were incorrect.

An online version is available in addition to the printed study guide. Psychiatrists who wish to earn continuing medical education credits may purchase the online version and obtain CME credit by completing it.

We hope you will find the study guide a useful addition to *The American Psychiatric Publishing Textbook of Psychosomatic Medicine*, Second Edition. Our goal is to have an assessment instrument that is helpful for your understanding of the material and for clarification of important concepts. Although the questions are reviewed numerous times, both by the authors and by editors at American Psychiatric Publishing, Inc., occasionally an incorrect response may be included. If this is the case, we would appreciate your notifying the publisher of the error so it can be corrected in the online version of the self-assessment examination. If you have other suggestions concerning this study guide, please e-mail Dr. Hales at rehales@ucdavis.edu.

Best of luck with your self-examination.

James A. Bourgeois, O.D., M.D.
Robert E. Hales, M.D., M.B.A.
Narriman C. Shahrokh

Page numbers in the Answer Guide refer to
The American Psychiatric Publishing Textbook of
Psychosomatic Medicine, Second Edition.
Visit **www.appi.org** for more information about this textbook.

| | | |

Purchase the online version of this Study Guide at
www.psychiatryonline.com; click "Subscribe/Renew"
and receive instant scoring and CME credits.

Chapter 1

Psychiatric Assessment and Consultation

Select the single best response for each question.

1.1 To function most effectively in a psychosomatic medicine clinical environment, the psychiatrist is advised to modify the style used to interview outpatients. Which of the following would *not* be a recommended interview style in the inpatient psychosomatic medicine environment?

    A. Assume an active, open, and "spontaneous" interpersonal stance to establish rapport efficiently.
    B. Do not allow long silences, as psychosomatic medicine patients may have limited stamina for the interview and essential data could be missed.
    C. Immediately and in depth, seek to explore the experience and meaning of major trauma early in the therapeutic relationship.
    D. Attempt to strike a pragmatic balance between a "biological" and a "psychodynamic" approach to clinical problems.
    E. Elicit the patient's belief system about the presenting systemic illness.

1.2 The clinical examination in psychosomatic medicine differs from other clinical interviews by the needed focus on cognitive disorders and cognitive examination. Executive function, localized behaviorally to the frontal lobes, is tested by a series of useful bedside tests. Which of the following is *not* a test of executive function?

    A. Naming of visually recognized common objects.
    B. Listing as many animals as possible in 1 minute.
    C. Replicating three hand positions.
    D. The go/no-go task.
    E. Tests of abstraction.

1.3 Language disorders, or aphasias, are common in neurologically impaired patients and are associated with a high degree of comorbid psychiatric illness. A stroke patient presents with fluent speech that is largely sensible, and he appears to respond to examination instructions. He can name objects readily and accurately but shows a focal deficit in repetition; however, with rehearsal he can learn new material. This presentation is characteristic of which type of aphasia?

    A. Receptive.
    B. Expressive.
    C. Global.
    D. Anomic.
    E. Conduction.

1.4   Advancements in neuroimaging have been part of the revolution in the clinical practice of psychosomatic medicine. The physician must be aware of the relative indications of various neuroimaging techniques for specific illnesses. Which of the following neurological lesions is better imaged by computed tomography (CT) than by magnetic resonance imaging (MRI)?

    A. Acute intracranial hemorrhage.
    B. Basal ganglia disease.
    C. Brain stem glioma.
    D. White matter disease.
    E. Tumor of the posterior fossa.

1.5   Which of the following clinical scenarios would *not* routinely prompt early use of neuroimaging for evaluation?

    A. Acute onset of psychotic illness, without delirium, in a previously healthy patient.
    B. First presentation of apparent dementia.
    C. Pretreatment workup for electroconvulsive therapy (ECT) in a patient with psychotic depression.
    D. Mental status changes associated with lateralizing neurological signs.
    E. Delirium following documented overdose with anticholinergic medication with normal motor examination.

1.6   The Folstein Mini-Mental State Examination (MMSE) is a well-known instrument for rapid screening of cognitive impairment at the bedside. In assessment of temporoparietal and frontal lobe function, the MMSE may be usefully supplemented with the Mini-Cog, a convenient test that combines the Clock Drawing Test with which portion of the MMSE?

    A. Immediate memory (repeat three objects).
    B. Concentration (serial 100–7 or spell "world" backwards).
    C. Follow the three-step motor command.
    D. The five elements of place orientation.
    E. Three-minute recall of three objects.

1.7   The Patient Health Questionnaire (PHQ) is a self-administered questionnaire that can be useful in screening for psychiatric disorders in the primary care environment. This instrument reliably assesses all of the following psychiatric disorders *except*

    A. Cognitive disorders.
    B. Mood disorders.
    C. Anxiety disorders.
    D. Eating disorders.
    E. Somatoform disorders.

Chapter 2

Legal Issues

Select the single best response for each question.

2.1 What effect did the Health Insurance Portability and Accountability Act of 1996 (HIPAA) have on confidentiality?

    A. It reinforced the concept of absolute confidentiality between physician and patient.
    B. It limited doctor–patient confidentiality if confidentiality is determined to be counter to public safety.
    C. It did not address the issue of confidentiality, but focused on other important issues.
    D. It recognized that the efficiency and effectiveness of the health care system need to be balanced against the safeguarding of protected health information.
    E. It reemphasized the concept of confidentiality as stated in the Hippocratic oath.

2.2 Every U.S. jurisdiction identifies physicians as mandated reporters of suspected cases of *elder abuse and neglect*, which most states define as encompassing five categories of harm or risk of harm to an elderly person. Which of the following is *not* one of these categories?

    A. Refusal of medical care by an adult older than 65 years.
    B. Infliction of pain.
    C. Sexual assault.
    D. Financial exploitation.
    E. Infliction of emotional distress.

2.3 A 28-year-old man whom you have been treating confides that he intends to kill his ex-wife by shooting her next week, upon her return from a vacation. He has already revealed to you that the court has imposed a restraining order against him for previous assaults. He also has an unregistered handgun. In assessing whether you have a duty to warn the ex-wife of this patient, relevant considerations include all of the following *except*

    A. The patient has stated a specific threat.
    B. The patient has a past history of violence.
    C. The patient has identified the victim.
    D. The patient has a mental disorder.
    E. You have a basis for anticipatory violence if the wife is not warned.

2.4 You are called by the surgical team to evaluate a patient's capacity to reject a surgical treatment for colon cancer that may prolong his life. In assessing this patient's decisional capacity, you elect to follow the four-pronged approach developed by Appelbaum and Grisso. Which of the following is *not* one of the four factors requiring consideration in this model?

    A. Rational manipulation of information.
    B. Absence of a serious mental disorder.
    C. Preference.
    D. Appreciation of the facts presented.
    E. Factual understanding of the procedure.

2.5 An oncologist believes that a bone marrow transplant will benefit his patient with pancreatic cancer. In the course of the informed consent process, the physician summarizes the patient's diagnosis, outlines the expected benefits and risks of the procedure to the patient, and explains that the results of the treatment cannot be precisely predicted. Finally, he reviews the risks and benefits of alternative or no treatment. What important information did he forget to provide the patient?

    A. What he (the oncologist) would do if he were the patient.
    B. The cost of the treatment.
    C. The potential irreversibility of the treatment.
    D. An explanation of the procedure to the patient's wife.
    E. A discussion of recent journal articles published concerning the procedure.

2.6 Advance directives are a legal means by which patients may make their treatment preferences known in case they later experience incapacity for decision making. Which of the following statements concerning advance directives is *true?*

    A. An advance directive may be prepared and executed by a patient even if he or she is incompetent.
    B. Once executed, an advance directive is considered active regardless of whether the patient is competent.
    C. Hospitals are encouraged, but not legally required, to ask patients whether they have an advance directive when they are admitted.
    D. Even if a patient regains capacity, the advance directive takes precedence when a medical decision needs to be made.
    E. If a patient does not have an advance directive, some states allow the use of a surrogate decision maker.

Chapter 3

Ethical Issues

Select the single best response for each question.

3.1 Psychosomatic medicine psychiatrists who also serve as hospital ethics consultants are obliged to master two separate clinical roles, each requiring a different orientation and approach. In regard to these separate roles, which of the following statements is *false?*

    A. Ethics consultants should avoid identifying unaddressed clinical problems, as doing so represents a violation of professional boundaries.

    B. A psychiatric consultation follows the medical model of providing specific advice on diagnosis and treatment.

    C. Health care professionals frequently expect ethics consultants to provide the same type of specific direction provided by medical specialty consultants.

    D. The ethics community favors a more process-oriented type of consultation, as opposed to the traditional medical model.

    E. A common result of an ethics consultation is the generation of a list of permissible options rather than a single "right answer."

3.2 Ethics consultations benefit from an organizational framework to define the various domains of clinical ethics. Ethics discussions are organized around the major "principles of biomedical ethics" that may all be present in a particular case. Which of the following ethical principles covers the issue of informed consent?

    A. Nonmaleficence.

    B. Justice.

    C. Respect for patient autonomy.

    D. Beneficence.

    E. Altruism.

3.3 Psychiatrists are frequently consulted in ethically problematic cases regarding decision-making capacity (DMC). Whereas some clinical psychiatric syndromes are associated with fluctuating DMC, others characteristically involve stable DMC, and consulting clinicians must take this degree of clinical (hence capacity) stability into account in their assessments of DMC. In which of the following conditions is DMC more likely to be stable?

    A. Mania from steroids.

    B. Traumatic brain injury.

    C. Delirium.

    D. Depression.

    E. Dementia.

3.4 Determination of decision-making capacity (DMC) requires the assessment of multiple domains of mental functioning. To date, the bulk of clinical research on DMC has focused on which of the following functional domains?

    A. Social functioning.

    B. Mood.

C. Trust.

D. Motivation.

E. Cognitive function.

3.5 In recent years, the clinical and ethical appropriateness of the use of physical restraints in the medical setting has come under increasing scrutiny, leading to an evolution in medical and nursing practice regarding the use of restraints. In regard to the ethics of restraint use for an acutely agitated and confused medical patient, which of the following statements is *true*?

A. Agitated and confused patients should never be restrained.

B. Agitated and confused patients may be restrained only after a formal determination of decision-making capacity.

C. Immediate safety concerns transcend ethics discussions and allow for restraint as the unequivocal standard of care in acute agitation and confusion.

D. Restraints may be legally permissible but are always unethical.

E. Refusal of care by an agitated and confused patient should be treated no differently from refusal of care by a competent and informed patient.

3.6 Research on the use of advance directives and the behavior of substitute decision makers has found that

A. Most patients welcome the opportunity to put into writing the kind of medical care they would like to receive if they were to become gravely ill and incompetent.

B. Substitute decision makers tend to follow patients' stated preferences in their decisions.

C. Substitute decision makers generally employ a *substituted judgment standard*, basing their decisions on what is in the best interests of the patient.

D. Substitute decision makers do not base their decisions on what they would want for themselves.

E. Only a minority of patients execute advance directives.

3.7 A medically ill patient's mood symptoms may be of importance in a decision-making capacity (DMC) evaluation given the often "cognitive" presentation of mood disorders, especially in ill and geriatric patients. Depression in the medically ill is typically associated with all of the following *except*

A. Reduced ability to tolerate discomfort.

B. Difficulty maintaining hope.

C. Poor adherence with medical care.

D. Impaired DMC.

E. Greater likelihood of considering physician-assisted suicide.

3.8 Ethics methodology pertinent to the conduct of research with human participants takes pains to ensure that research design and consent procedures afford protection to participants considered to be "vulnerable to coercion or undue influence," including the "mentally disabled." Which of the following psychiatric illnesses is specifically included in the "mentally disabled" category?

A. Dementia.

B. Delirium.

C. Schizophrenia.

D. Mental retardation.

E. None of the above.

Chapter 4

Psychological Responses to Illness

Select the single best response for each question.

4.1 Which of the following is an example of stresses that a patient may experience when hospitalized?

    A. Lack of privacy.
    B. Bodily invasion.
    C. Pain.
    D. Separation from family.
    E. All of the above.

4.2 Attachment theory provides fruitful way of examining patients' interactions with the health care setting and their physicians. Among the four predominant attachment styles described by Bartholomew and Horowitz (1991), which attachment style is believed to derive from early experiences with unresponsive caregivers, leading individuals to excessively value self-reliance and to have difficulty trusting others?

    A. Fearful attachment style.
    B. Dismissing attachment style.
    C. Secure attachment style.
    D. Preoccupied attachment style.
    E. Histrionic attachment style.

4.3 Kahana and Bibring's (1964) seven personality types can provide a useful framework for understanding a patient's response to medical illness. Which of the following is *not* one of these seven personality types?

    A. Dependent.
    B. Paranoid.
    C. Antisocial.
    D. Obsessional.
    E. Schizoid.

4.4 The personality type of a hospitalized patient may elicit various countertransferance responses from the treating physician. A physician notices that she feels little connection with a patient and finds the patient difficult to engage. Which of the following personality types might elicit this countertransference response?

    A. Masochistic.
    B. Histrionic.
    C. Paranoid.
    D. Narcissistic.
    E. Schizoid.

4.5   Folkman et al. (1986) identified various categories of coping styles used by people faced with stressful situations. A patient who appears to expend considerable effort on harnessing his feelings and trying to keep his family members from knowing how ill he is might be exhibiting which of the following coping styles?

      A. Escape-avoidance.
      B. Distancing.
      C. Positive reappraisal.
      D. Self-controlling.
      E. Planful problem solving.

4.6   Vaillant (1993) proposed a hierarchy of defense mechanisms based on how much each defense distorts reality and how effectively it allows expression of the individual's wishes or needs without causing untoward external consequences. Patients with personality disorders, especially the Cluster B disorders, usually employ which of the following types of defenses?

      A. Neurotic defenses.
      B. Immature defenses.
      C. Psychotic defenses.
      D. Mature defenses.
      E. Adaptive defenses.

4.7   An oncologist asks you to evaluate a patient with terminal cancer because he is concerned that her calm acceptance of treatment, courageous good humor, and lack of expressed fears indicate that she is "in denial." What type of defense mechanism might this patient be exhibiting?

      A. Suppression.
      B. Psychotic denial.
      C. Repression.
      D. Intermediate denial.
      E. Intellectualization.

C h a p t e r   5

Delirium

Select the single best response for each question.

5.1 In the diagnosis of delirium, it is phenomenologically important to distinguish delirium from similar neuropsychiatric disorders with which delirium can merge in clinical practice. A condition in which the patient has an intact level of arousal, a normal sleep–wake cycle, but a complete absence of apparent "awareness" both of the self and of the environment is considered to be

    A. Hypoactive delirium.
    B. Hyperactive delirium.
    C. Coma.
    D. Minimally conscious state.
    E. Vegetative state.

5.2 Delirium is associated with increased medical and surgical morbidity and greater medical resource consumption. In the review of delirium risk by Saravay and Strain (1994) which of the following patient groups had the *lowest* increase in hospital length of stay as a result of delirium?

    A. General medical patients.
    B. Elderly patients.
    C. Stroke patients.
    D. Cardiac surgery patients.
    E. Hip fracture patients.

5.3 Dementia is a well established risk factor for delirium. Which of the following dementia subtypes is considered to have a particularly high risk for the development of delirium?

    A. Alzheimer's disease of early onset.
    B. Alzheimer's disease of late onset.
    C. Dementia due to head trauma.
    D. Dementia due to hypothyroidism.
    E. Dementia due to Parkinson's disease.

5.4 A clinically useful model for understanding and modifying delirium risk was described by Inouye and Charpentier (1996). This predictive model addresses both predisposing and precipitating factors in the development of delirium. According to this model, which of the following items is considered to be a *precipitating* factor?

    A. More than three medications added.
    B. Cognitive impairment before the development of delirium.
    C. Severe systemic illness.
    D. Dehydration.
    E. Visual impairment.

5.5 While not routinely used in the majority of delirium cases, the electroencephalogram (EEG) is typically abnormal in delirium. Furthermore, the type of delirium may be associated with specific EEG findings. Which EEG pattern is suggestive of delirium tremens due to alcohol withdrawal?

    A. Bilateral diffuse slowing.
    B. Frontocentral spikes and polyspikes.
    C. Left or bilateral slowing or delta bursts.
    D. Generalized epileptiform activity.
    E. Low-voltage fast activity.

5.6 The distinction between delirium and dementia is an important clinical decision, often made more complex by the high rates of comorbidity and the overlapping symptom profiles of these disorders of cognition. Which dementia type, characterized by fluctuations in symptoms, visual hallucinations, attention deficits, altered levels of consciousness, and delusions, can be particularly challenging to distinguish from delirium?

    A. Vascular dementia.
    B. Dementia due to Parkinson's disease.
    C. Dementia due to multiple sclerosis.
    D. Alzheimer's disease.
    E. Lewy body dementia.

5.7 Management of delirium routinely includes the use of antipsychotic medications. A serious side effect of many of these medications (particularly intravenous haloperidol) is prolonged QTc interval and torsade des pointes. Risk factors for antipsychotic-induced torsade des pointes include all of the following *except*

    A. Male gender.
    B. Heart disease.
    C. Hypokalemia.
    D. Higher antipsychotic doses.
    E. History of long QT syndrome.

Chapter 6

Dementia

Select the single best response for each question.

6.1   Which of the following statements regarding the epidemiology of dementia in the United States is *false?*

    A. The estimated prevalence rate for all dementias in the U.S. population older than 65 years is 19.8%.

    B. The incidence of dementia of the Alzheimer's type (DAT) is 56.1 per 1,000 person-years in the population older than 90 years.

    C. In one large-scale study, approximately 9.1% of patients 55 years and older who were admitted to a teaching hospital medical service had dementia.

    D. The prevalence of minor cognitive impairment in individuals 65 years or older ranges between 3% and 19%.

    E. Approximately one-third of patients referred to memory clinics have minor cognitive impairment.

6.2   Which of the following is a confirmed protective factor for dementia of the Alzheimer's type (DAT)?

    A. Low cholesterol level.

    B. Aspirin use.

    C. Diet high in vitamin E and antioxidants.

    D. Apolipoprotein ε2 allele.

    E. Moderate alcohol consumption.

6.3   A number of clinical characteristics differentiate cortical and subcortical dementia syndromes. Which of the following is indicative of subcortical dementia as opposed to cortical dementia?

    A. Aphasia.

    B. Agnosia.

    C. Apathy.

    D. Alexia.

    E. Apraxia.

6.4   A 70-year-old male patient presents with parkinsonian features, fluctuating cognitive performance, hallucinations, and delusions. He also has a history of frequent falls and transient, unexplained episodes of loss of consciousness. Which of the following is the most likely diagnosis?

    A. Frontotemporal dementia.

    B. Parkinson's disease.

    C. Wilson's disease.

    D. Normal-pressure hydrocephalus.

    E. Dementia with Lewy bodies.

6.5   Clinical characteristics suggestive of vascular dementia include all of the following *except*

A. Gradual onset with a slow decline.
B. Emotional lability.
C. Uneven cognitive deterioration.
D. Focal neurological signs and symptoms.
E. Relative preservation of insight and judgment.

Chapter 7

Aggression and Violence

Select the single best response for each question.

7.1   The association of violence and psychiatric disorders has been the subject of various studies. However, not all psychiatric disorders confer the same risk of violence. In the study by Swanson et al. (1990), which of the following psychiatric disorders was associated with the *lowest* risk of violence?

    A. Anxiety disorders.
    B. Substance abuse.
    C. Substance dependence.
    D. Mood disorders.
    E. Schizophrenia.

7.2   Aggressive behavior can be viewed as the product of an interaction between a *host* with a baseline propensity for aggression and specific provocations (*agents*) in particular contexts (*circumstances*). Within this framework, which of the following would be a *circumstance* associated with violence, rather than an *agent*?

    A. Threats by others.
    B. Misperceptions.
    C. Conflicts.
    D. Physical discomfort.
    E. Hospitalization for serious illness.

7.3   The prefrontal cortex is functionally implicated in the control of aggression and the maintenance of self-control and prosocial behavior. Patients with which of the following types of dementia characteristically exhibit disinhibited behavior, including impulsivity and aggressive outbursts?

    A. Parkinson's dementia.
    B. Vascular dementia.
    C. Lewy body dementia.
    D. Alzheimer's dementia.
    E. Frontotemporal dementia.

7.4   Violence associated with personality disorders is best understood as being consistent with the patient's habitual range of behaviors. Which of the following personality disorders is most frequently associated with habitual aggression?

    A. Narcissistic personality disorder.
    B. Borderline personality disorder.
    C. Antisocial personality disorder.
    D. Schizoid personality disorder.
    E. Paranoid personality disorder.

7.5 Various substances of abuse are associated with violent behavior, with the effects usually mediated by the psychoactive properties of the particular substance. Which of the following substances is the *least* associated with violent behavior?

A. LSD.
B. Alcohol.
C. Cocaine.
D. Amphetamine.
E. Phencyclidine.

7.6 A phenomenon that may link seizure disorder with violent behavior is postictal psychosis, which although usually transient may become persistent. Which of the following statements regarding postictal psychosis is *false*?

A. Symptoms of postictal psychosis may include mania or depression with mood-congruent psychosis.
B. Patients with postictal psychosis may manifest a formal thought disorder.
C. Patients with postictal psychosis may experience hallucinations.
D. Delusions in postictal psychosis are commonly of a paranoid nature.
E. Violence is less likely in postictal psychosis than in interictal psychosis or postictal confusion.

7.7 Dementia in elderly patients is unfortunately associated with aggressive behavior, which can complicate clinical management and may require changes in the care model and living arrangements. Which of the following aggressive behaviors is *less* common in elderly people with dementia?

A. Throwing objects.
B. Pushing and shoving.
C. Kicking.
D. Scratching.
E. Goal-directed destruction of property.

7.8 The psychosomatic medicine consultant is often called upon to offer psychopharmacological interventions for patients with a history of violent behavior. In the Citrome et al. (2001) randomized study comparing the anti-aggressive effects of various antipsychotics, which of the following agents was found to be most effective?

A. Clozapine.
B. Olanzapine.
C. Risperidone.
D. Haloperidol.
E. Aripiprazole.

Chapter 8

Depression

Select the single best response for each question.

8.1 It has been hypothesized that the prevalence of major depressive disorder (MDD) in medical settings increases progressively with the severity of the medical disease. What is the prevalence of MDD in patients hospitalized on an inpatient medical unit?

    A. 2%–4%.
    B. 6%–14%.
    C. 15%–20%.
    D. 21%–25%.
    E. 26%–31%.

8.2 Various approaches have been proposed to diminish the confounding effect of medical symptoms in the diagnosis of major depressive disorder (MDD). In one approach, symptoms that are more likely to be confused with medical illness, such as loss of energy, weight loss, and impaired concentration, are replaced by symptoms more likely to be affective in origin, such as irritability, tearfulness, social withdrawal, and feeling punished. What is this approach called?

    A. Exclusive.
    B. Etiological.
    C. Dimensional.
    D. Substitutive.
    E. Categorical.

8.3 Various rating scales have been developed to measure depressive symptoms in medically ill patients. One widely used self-report screening instrument was originally developed as a measure of symptom severity in psychiatric patients but has been used and found to be accurate in numerous studies of depression in the medically ill. What is the name of this instrument?

    A. Hospital Anxiety and Depression Scale (HADS).
    B. Patient Health Questionnaire Depression Module (PHQ-9).
    C. Center for Epidemiologic Studies Depression Scale (CES-D).
    D. Primary Care Evaluation of Mental Disorders (PRIME-MD).
    E. Beck Depression Inventory–II (BDI-II).

8.4　The association of depression with specific medical diseases is of concern because of its impact on the treatment, course, and outcome of these conditions. Which of the following statements concerning depression and its treatment in patients with serious and chronic medical illnesses is *false*?

　　A. Antidepressants and psychotherapeutic treatment of depression in cancer patients improve survival.
　　B. The majority of trials of antidepressants and psychotherapeutic interventions have failed to demonstrate beneficial effects on cardiac outcomes.
　　C. Depression in individuals with diabetes mellitus has been associated with poorer adherence to diabetic dietary and medication regimens.
　　D. Depressive disorders in patients with Parkinson's disease are associated with increased impairment of cognitive function and lower perceived quality of life.
　　E. Depressive symptoms in older adults have been associated with an increased risk for the development of mild cognitive impairment.

8.5　Which of the following medications or medication classes have been shown in randomized controlled trials to be effective in treating depression in patients with medical illnesses such as cardiac disease, stroke, and cancer?

　　A. Venlafaxine.
　　B. Mirtazapine.
　　C. Selective serotonin reuptake inhibitors (SSRIs).
　　D. Bupropion.
　　E. Duloxetine.

Chapter 9

Suicidality

Select the single best response for each question.

9.1 Mann's (1998) diathesis–stress model of suicidal behavior is a useful clinical construct, wherein diathesis represents more long-standing components, while stress relates to more momentary circumstances. Suicidality is felt to result when an acute stress is "superimposed" on a suicide diathesis. Which of the following components would be considered a *stress* rather than a *diathesis* component of suicidal behavior?

    A. Genetic predisposition.
    B. Early life experiences.
    C. Chronic substance abuse.
    D. Family and social dynamics.
    E. Chronic illness.

9.2 Serotonin hypofunction has been correlated with suicidal behavior and has been proposed as a biological marker for suicide risk. Factors associated with lower serotonergic activity and greater suicide risk include all of the following *except*

    A. History of childhood abuse.
    B. Family history of depression.
    C. Substance abuse.
    D. High serum cholesterol.
    E. Traumatic brain injury.

9.3 Kishi and Kathol (2002) described four "pragmatic reasons" for suicidal acts. Which of the following is *not* one of these four reasons?

    A. Despair at losing cognitive function in early dementia.
    B. Psychosis.
    C. Depression.
    D. Poor impulse control.
    E. Philosophical reasons.

9.4 An understanding of the epidemiology of suicide can be useful in clinical decision making. Which of the following statements regarding suicide rates is *true*?

    A. The known suicide rate today is at least 1.5 times the rate in 1900.
    B. Between 1990 and 2001, the suicide rate increased in every age category.
    C. The current suicide rate in the United States is approximately 20 per 100,000 population.
    D. Suicide is the third leading cause of death in 15- to 24-year-olds in the United States.
    E. Nonwhite Americans have twice the rate of suicide of white Americans.

9.5   Findings from the Misono et al. (2008) study of suicide risk in cancer patients included all of the following *except*

A. The standardized mortality ratio of suicide in cancer patients was 1.9 relative to the general population.
B. The highest suicide rate reported was for cancers of the larynx (5.75).
C. Older white male cancer patients were at especially high risk for suicide.
D. Suicide risk was highest in the first 5 years after diagnosis of cancer.
E. Cancer patients continued to have an elevated suicide risk 15 years after their diagnosis.

9.6   In a recent survey by Ganzini et al. (2009) of patients' motivations for seeking physician-assisted death (PAD), the reason most commonly cited was

A. Desire to control timing of death and to avoid loss of independence.
B. Concerns about future unbearable pain.
C. Worry about compromised quality of life.
D. Limited social support.
E. Current physical and mental symptoms.

Chapter 10

Psychosis, Mania, and Catatonia

Select the single best response for each question.

10.1 Hallucinations are a hallmark of a psychotic disorder due to a medical condition. A visually impaired patient who remains aware of the abnormal nature of his hallucinations, and as a result is hesitant to divulge information about them, is likely experiencing which of the following?

   A. Hypnopompic hallucinations.
   B. Peduncular hallucinosis.
   C. Pseudohallucinations.
   D. Functional hallucinations.
   E. Hypnagogic hallucinations.

10.2 Delusions are often classified by their content and style. A syndrome in which the patient believes that a family member or close friend has been replaced by an exact double is called

   A. Othello syndrome.
   B. Ganser syndrome.
   C. Charles Bonnet syndrome.
   D. Capgras' delusion.
   E. Cotard's syndrome.

10.3 A form of catatonia characterized by fever, autonomic dysfunction with tachycardia and elevated blood pressure, rigidity, mutism, and stupor is called

   A. Catatonic withdrawal.
   B. Neuroleptic malignant syndrome (NMS).
   C. Catatonic excitement.
   D. Lethal catatonia.
   E. Malignant catatonia.

10.4 The modified Bush-Francis Catatonia Rating Scale (BFCRS) is commonly used to evaluate the signs and symptoms of catatonia. According to symptom definitions provided in this instrument, motor activity that is perseverative, non-goal-directed, and not inherently abnormal, such as playing with fingers, is called

   A. Stereotypy.
   B. Mannerisms.
   C. Negativism.
   D. *Mitgehen.*
   E. Excitement.

10.5   Which of the following medications has been found to be most effective in the treatment of catatonia?

    A. Selective serotonin reuptake inhibitors.
    B. Beta-blockers.
    C. Second-generation antipsychotics.
    D. Mood stabilizers.
    E. Benzodiazepines.

Chapter 11

Anxiety Disorders

Select the single best response for each question.

11.1 Anxiety symptoms are common in medical patients; for this reason, it is a good clinical practice to use validated screening instruments to assist in the identification of anxiety disorder cases. The Generalized Anxiety Disorder–7 (GAD-7) scale is an effective screen for all of the following anxiety disorders *except*

    A. Generalized anxiety disorder (GAD).
    B. Panic disorder.
    C. Posttraumatic stress disorder (PTSD).
    D. Obsessive-compulsive disorder (OCD).
    E. Social phobia.

11.2 Posttraumatic stress disorder (PTSD) has a higher prevalence in medical/surgical settings than in the general population. Findings from studies of PTSD in medical settings have included all of the following *except*

    A. PTSD has been reported in 20%–45% of burn patients.
    B. Approximately one-third of motor vehicle accident victims reported PTSD symptoms.
    C. Patients with stimulant intoxication reported higher PTSD symptom levels.
    D. Female trauma patients had more PTSD symptoms than male patients.
    E. In patients with implanted cardioverter defibrillators, PTSD was associated with greater morbidity but not greater mortality.

11.3 Given the often life-threatening nature of the illness, it is not surprising that posttraumatic stress disorder (PTSD) has been reported in patients being treated for cancer. In this context, which of the following variables is *not* associated with a greater risk of PTSD?

    A. Past psychological trauma.
    B. Severity of the cancer.
    C. Prior psychiatric illness.
    D. Lower levels of social support.
    E. Other recent psychosocial stressors.

11.4 One of the prototypical models in psychosomatic medicine is the relationship between thyroid disease and many psychiatric disorders, notably anxiety disorders. In regard to this relationship, which of the following statements is *false?*

    A. Anxiety due to hyperthyroidism is accompanied by persistent tachycardia.
    B. Anxiety due to hyperthyroidism is associated with cold, "clammy" palms.
    C. Complaints of fatigue are associated with a desire to be active.
    D. Hyperthyroidism is associated with cognitive impairment as well as anxiety.
    E. Anxiety treatment should be instituted while hyperthyroidism is treated medically.

11.5 Yalom (1980) has written on the phenomenon of death anxiety in the context of life-threatening and/or terminal illness. Which of the following statements regarding the management of death anxiety is *false*?

A. Open, frank discussions about death should be avoided, as they increase anxiety and distress.
B. Maintenance of hope is important in managing death anxiety.
C. Therapy goals for death anxiety may target accomplishment of specific short-term goals rather than attainment of full recovery.
D. Helping patients find meaning despite their suffering is an important therapy goal.
E. Placing emphasis on the importance of patients to their families may decrease anxiety.

11.6 The pharmacological management of anxiety is an important intervention in psychosomatic medicine. However, pharmacological agents delivered in the context of systemic illness need to be chosen carefully. Which benzodiazepine has the advantages of oral, intravenous, or intramuscular administration; a conjugation metabolism; and no active metabolite?

A. Alprazolam.
B. Oxazepam.
C. Lorazepam.
D. Temazepam.
E. Midazolam.

Chapter 12

Somatization and Somatoform Disorders

Select the single best response for each question.

12.1 Etiological factors posited to contribute to the development of somatization and somatoform disorders include all of the following *except*

    A. Childhood exposure to parental chronic illness.
    B. Negative affectivity.
    C. Alexithymia.
    D. Sexual or physical abuse.
    E. Anger or hostility.

12.2 Which of the following statements concerning the epidemiology of somatization disorder is *true*?

    A. The disorder usually develops when patients are in their 40s.
    B. There is no cultural variability in the presentation of somatization disorder.
    C. The prevalence of somatization disorder is higher in medical settings.
    D. The disorder is more common in men than in women.
    E. Patients with somatization disorder are excellent historians who provide detailed and precise descriptions of their medical history.

12.3 Which of the following statements regarding the epidemiology of conversion disorder is *true*?

    A. The prevalence is higher in men than in women.
    B. Conversion symptoms usually begin slowly and innocuously.
    C. The disorder has been reported to occur in 1%–4.5% of hospitalized neurological and medical patients.
    D. Symptoms, if unilateral, usually occur on the right side of the body.
    E. The disorder is typically diagnosed when patients are in their 30s.

12.4 Which of the following statements regarding the epidemiology of hypochondriasis is *false*?

    A. Patients have a high rate of psychiatric comorbidity.
    B. Primary hypochondriasis is an acute condition that responds readily to treatment.
    C. High medical utilization is common.
    D. Patients often have compromised occupational functioning.
    E. Interpersonal relationships are usually impaired.

12.5   The psychiatric disorder most frequently comorbid with body dysmorphic disorder (BDD) is

     A. Major depressive disorder.
     B. Social phobia.
     C. Obsessive-compulsive disorder.
     D. Substance use disorder.
     E. Panic disorder.

12.6   Which of the following has been found to be most effective in treating somatoform disorders?

     A. Interpersonal psychotherapy.
     B. Motivational therapy.
     C. Brief psychodynamic psychotherapy.
     D. Hypnosis.
     E. Cognitive-behavioral therapy.

Chapter 13

Deception Syndromes

Factitious Disorders and Malingering

Select the single best response for each question.

13.1 Factitious disorder, the conscious, surreptitious fraudulent production of symptoms or signs for the purpose of assuming the sick role and to obtain medical care, is commonly classified as either common factitious disorder or Munchausen syndrome. These subtypes can be quite different in terms of clinical appearance and contributory risk factors. Characteristic features of common factitious disorder include all of the following *except*

 A. Female gender.
 B. Unmarried status.
 C. Age in the 30s.
 D. Employment (current or past) in a health care occupation.
 E. Use of alias identity and frequent travel to seek medical care.

13.2 Munchausen syndrome patients may present in classic ways to the health care system, and their behavior while in patient status may help the physician to make the diagnosis. Characteristic features of Munchausen syndrome include all of the following *except*

 A. Travel among many hospitals.
 B. Use of alias identity and possible multiple medical records.
 C. Frequent emergency department presentation.
 D. Presentation with dramatic symptoms of multiple apparently serious disease states.
 E. Refusal to undergo diagnostic studies for presenting symptoms.

13.3 Ganser's syndrome, a rarely encountered condition that has similarities to and some overlap with factitious disorder, should be considered in the differential diagnosis of cases of apparent factitious disorder. Which of the following characteristics is quite specific to this syndrome?

 A. Amnesia.
 B. Disorientation.
 C. Visual hallucinations.
 D. Approximate answers to questions.
 E. Olfactory hallucinations.

13.4 Which is the most common psychiatric comorbidity in factitious disorder?

 A. Schizophrenia.
 B. Major depression.
 C. Cluster A personality disorder.
 D. Cluster B personality disorder.
 E. Cluster C personality disorder.

13.5 Munchausen syndrome by proxy is a recently appreciated and very disruptive problem seen primarily in child psychosomatic medicine practice. In the review by Sheridan (2003), findings included all of the following *except*

    A. Victims were primarily female.
    B. Most victims were age 4 years or younger.
    C. Most cases involved active production of symptoms rather than mere misrepresentation of them.
    D. The most commonly produced symptom was apnea.
    E. There was an extremely high rate of death in victim's siblings.

13.6 Psychometric testing can be a very helpful adjunct in the diagnosis of malingering. Which of the following assessment instruments, by virtue of its forced-choice format and statistical norming, is a useful test for patients who distort symptoms?

    A. Rorschach.
    B. Minnesota Multiphasic Personality Inventory–2 (MMPI-2).
    C. Beck Depression Inventory (BDI).
    D. Hamilton Rating Scale for Depression (HAM-D).
    E. Hopkins Symptom Checklist–90.

Chapter 14

Eating Disorders

Select the single best response for each question.

14.1 Which of the following statements concerning the diagnosis of anorexia nervosa is *false?*

   A. Patients must manifest a weight markedly (≥15%) lower than expected for gender and height.
   B. Amenorrhea is no longer a requirement for postmenarchal women.
   C. The diagnosis requires an overconcern with weight and shape.
   D. Many patients with anorexia nervosa are compulsive exercisers.
   E. Patients with anorexia nervosa are often rigid and perfectionistic.

14.2 Which of the following points should clinicians keep in mind when evaluating a patient for bulimia nervosa?

   A. Progression from anorexia nervosa to bulimia nervosa is quite rare.
   B. Individuals who simultaneously meet criteria for anorexia nervosa and bulimia nervosa are diagnosed as having anorexia nervosa, binge-eating/purging type.
   C. The diagnosis of bulimia nervosa cannot be made in overweight or obese individuals.
   D. Most individuals who present for treatment of bulimia nervosa are more than 15% below their expected weight.
   E. In more than half of cases, normal-weight individuals with bulimia nervosa progress to anorexia nervosa.

14.3 A parent brings her 10-year-old daughter to your office and states that her daughter will eat only a small number of foods. The child's growth and development are normal. What is the most likely diagnosis?

   A. Food phobia.
   B. Food avoidance emotional disorder.
   C. Functional dysphagia.
   D. Pervasive refusal syndrome.
   E. Selective eating disorder.

14.4 Which of the following statements concerning the course and outcome of anorexia nervosa is *false?*

   A. Mortality rates are as high as 5% per decade of illness.
   B. Among surviving patients, fewer than half recover fully.
   C. Approximately one-fifth of patients remain chronically ill.
   D. Patients treated as adolescents have a worse outcome.
   E. The risk of suicide is pronounced.

14.5   The most serious complication of weight restoration in patients with anorexia nervosa is

   A. Refeeding syndrome.
   B. Hypercholesterolemia.
   C. Hypercortisolism.
   D. Low white blood cell count.
   E. Abnormal thyroid hormone status.

Chapter 15

Sleep Disorders

Select the single best response for each question.

15.1 Patients with disrupted sleep usually spend most of the night

    A. In stage N1 with much rapid eye movement (REM) sleep.
    B. In stage N2 with much REM sleep.
    C. In stage N3 with little REM sleep.
    D. In stages N1 and N2 with little REM sleep.
    E. In stage N3 with much REM sleep.

15.2 The multiple sleep latency test (MSLT) is a useful tool for evaluating patients with excessive daytime sleepiness. Which of the following statements regarding the MSLT is *false?*

    A. The MSLT needs to be completed before an overnight sleep study.
    B. Patients need 6 hours of sleep before the MSLT.
    C. The leads attached to the patient are the electroencephalographic, electromyographic, and electro-oculo-graphic leads.
    D. The test measures initial sleep latency and initial rapid eye movement (REM) latency.
    E. Patients must stay awake between the examined naps.

15.3 Which of the following statements regarding narcolepsy is *false?*

    A. Patients have excessive daytime sleepiness.
    B. Patients have episodic, sudden "sleep attacks."
    C. The majority of patients experience cataplexy.
    D. During cataplexy, consciousness is lost.
    E. Patients commonly experience sleep paralysis.

15.4 Which of the following treatments for narcolepsy was initially approved by the U.S. Food and Drug Administration (FDA) for cataplexy and later approved for all narcolepsy symptoms?

    A. Methylphenidate.
    B. Dextroamphetamine.
    C. Modafinil.
    D. Sodium oxybate.
    E. Armodafinil.

15.5 Which of the following is *not* a characteristic feature of Kleine-Levin syndrome?

    A. Male patient.
    B. Young patient.
    C. Periods of profound anorexia.
    D. Periodic hypersomnia.
    E. Approximately 50% risk of concurrent depressed mood.

15.6 Which neurotransmitter abnormality is associated with restless legs syndrome?

    A. Increased dopamine levels.
    B. Increased serotonin levels.
    C. Decreased gamma-aminobutyric acid levels.
    D. Decreased dopamine levels.
    E. Decreased serotonin levels.

Chapter 16

Sexual Dysfunction

Select the single best response for each question.

16.1 In a retrospective analysis of 32,616 healthy male participants from a 1986 study, erectile dysfunction was found to be associated with a fourfold increase in the risk of developing which disease?

    A. Stroke.
    B. Prostate cancer.
    C. Renal failure.
    D. Parkinson's disease.
    E. Diabetes.

16.2 Sexual dysfunction can occur in individuals following a myocardial infarction (MI), in part because patients are concerned about the risks of resuming sexual activity. In regard to this issue, which of the following statements is *false*?

    A. Energy requirements for sexual intercourse and orgasm are estimated to be similar to climbing a flight of stairs.
    B. The risk of a recurrent MI after sex in a 50-year-old patient is two chances in a thousand per hour.
    C. Exercise will increase tolerance for sexual activity.
    D. The risk of further cardiac damage from sexual activity is low and short-lasting.
    E. Threatening symptoms of a recurrent MI are unlikely to occur during sexual activity if no cardiac symptoms arise during exercise testing to 6 metabolic equivalents (METs).

16.3 Sexual dysfunction after traumatic brain injury is common. Which of the following is the single most sensitive predictor of sexual functioning after traumatic brain injury?

    A. Location of brain injury.
    B. Presence of posttraumatic stress disorder.
    C. Duration of coma.
    D. Presence of psychosis.
    E. Presence of depression.

16.4 Dopamine agonists, especially when combined with L-dopa, have been reported to produce

    A. Compulsive gambling.
    B. Anorgasmia in women.
    C. Depression.
    D. Erectile dysfunction in men.
    E. Lack of sexual desire.

16.5 The most common sexual dysfunction in women with end-stage renal disease is

    A. Dyspareunia.
    B. Vaginal dryness.
    C. Low sexual desire.
    D. Lack of orgasm.
    E. Reduced vaginal sensation.

Chapter 17

Substance-Related Disorders

Select the single best response for each question.

17.1 The benzodiazepine antagonist flumazenil is an emergency treatment for acute benzodiazepine intoxication. Which of the following statements concerning flumazenil's clinical use is *false*?

    A. Nausea and vomiting are common side effects of flumazenil.
    B. Flumazenil may not completely reverse benzodiazepine-associated respiratory depression.
    C. Flumazenil carries some risk of seizure provocation in benzodiazepine-dependent patients.
    D. In mixed overdoses with tricyclic antidepressants (TCAs), flumazenil may precipitate arrhythmias.
    E. Flumazenil should be routinely administered in all comatose patients when it is not known what drugs were ingested.

17.2 Opioid intoxication is a common emergency presentation that may prompt a psychosomatic medicine evaluation. Common physical signs of opioid intoxication include all of the following *except*

    A. Dilated pupils.
    B. Decreased respiration.
    C. Decreased level of consciousness.
    D. Miotic pupils.
    E. Absent bowel sounds.

17.3 Hepatitis C virus (HCV) infection is a common cause of liver failure, leading to the need for transplantation. Because many patients with HCV-induced liver disease are on methadone maintenance or buprenorphine treatment, challenging clinical decisions can ensue. Which of the following statements regarding treatment for opioid dependence and comorbid HCV is *false*?

    A. The rate of HCV among methadone maintenance patients is 70%.
    B. Methadone maintenance should be continued while evaluation for liver transplantation is under way.
    C. Methadone maintenance should be discontinued after liver transplantation.
    D. Methadone maintenance is associated with better outcomes (in terms of relapse to heroin use postoperatively) compared with tapering and discontinuing.
    E. Opioid-dependent patients on buprenorphine should continue taking the drug throughout the transplant evaluation process.

17.4 Drug interactions may be problematic with the clinical use of methadone, due to hepatic metabolism pathways. Which of the following medications has been shown to lower serum methadone levels, producing opioid withdrawal?

    A. Risperidone.
    B. Diazepam.
    C. Fluoxetine.
    D. Erythromycin.
    E. None of the above.

17.5 Which of the following statements regarding buprenorphine is *true*?

A. It is a full opioid agonist at the mu receptor.
B. It is known to commonly increase the QTc interval.
C. It is marketed in a combination product with naltrexone.
D. Buprenorphine does not elevate hepatic transaminases in patients with hepatitis C virus (HCV).
E. It has fewer drug interactions than methadone.

17.6 Eye movements, a subtle neurological sign, can be useful in diagnosis of certain drug-related states based on physical examination. Which of the following drugs is associated with a classic vertical nystagmus?

A. Marijuana.
B. Cocaine.
C. Phencyclidine.
D. Methamphetamine.
E. Heroin.

Chapter 18

Heart Disease

Select the single best response for each question.

18.1   The most common psychiatric disorder found in patients with coronary artery disease (CAD) is

    A. Generalized anxiety disorder.
    B. Posttraumatic stress disorder.
    C. Major depression.
    D. Panic disorder.
    E. Acute stress disorder.

18.2   The proposed association of mitral valve prolapse and panic disorder has been supported by which of the following findings?

    A. Panic occurs at higher-than-expected rates in patients with electrocardiogram (ECG) mitral valve prolapse.
    B. Mitral valve prolapse rarely occurs in populations with other psychiatric disorders.
    C. A systemic review conducted in 2008 found substantial evidence of the association.
    D. Genetic studies have established a possible link between panic disorder and mitral valve prolapse and other medical conditions.
    E. A high percentage (60%–70%) of patients with panic disorder have ECG findings of prolapse.

18.3   Risk factors for experiencing delirium after open-heart surgery include all of the following *except*

    A. Cerebrovascular disease.
    B. Use of dexmedetomidine for postoperative sedation.
    C. Metabolic abnormalities.
    D. Older age.
    E. Prolonged postoperative sedation.

18.4   The cardiologist on the inpatient medical unit asks you to evaluate a post–myocardial infarction patient who is experiencing visual hallucinations manifesting as yellow rings around objects. You review the cardiac medications the patient is receiving and immediately identify an agent capable of producing the side effects that the patient is experiencing. The medication responsible is likely

    A. Amiodarone.
    B. An angiotensin-converting enzyme inhibitor.
    C. A beta-blocker.
    D. An angiotensin II receptor blocker.
    E. Digoxin.

18.5 The combination of tendency to experience negative affects and to inhibit expression of negative emotions in social interactions has been termed

    A. Type A personality.
    B. Type B personality.
    C. Type C personality.
    D. Type D personality.
    E. Type E personality.

18.6 Following cardiac bypass surgery, a patient is placed on a thiazide diuretic, an angiotensin-converting enzyme (ACE) inhibitor, and warfarin by his cardiologist. The patient develops sadness, anhedonia, sleep disturbance, decreased energy, guilty feelings, and concentration difficulties. You diagnose major depression and decide to start the patient on paroxetine. Which of the following side effects due to drug–drug interactions should you be most concerned about?

    A. Increased bleeding risk.
    B. Hypertension.
    C. Prolonged QT interval.
    D. Atrioventricular block.
    E. Hypotension.

18.7 Which of the following antidepressants or antidepressant classes may cause cardiac conduction delay as a side effect and ventricular arrhythmias in overdose?

    A. Monoamine oxidase inhibitors (MAOIs).
    B. Selective serotonin reuptake inhibitors (SSRIs).
    C. Tricyclic antidepressants (TCAs).
    D. Bupropion.
    E. Mirtazapine.

C h a p t e r   1 9

Lung Disease

Select the single best response for each question.

19.1   Asthma is well known to be associated with mood and anxiety symptoms, and diagnosis is complicated by the overlap between anxiety symptoms and the hyperadrenergic symptoms characteristic of an asthma exacerbation. Which of the following features is more suggestive of a diagnosis of panic than of asthma?

    A. Shortness of breath.
    B. Palpitations.
    C. Sweating.
    D. Lightheadedness.
    E. Negative methacholine inhalation challenge test.

19.2   Sarcoidosis, even without direct central nervous system involvement, is associated with psychiatric comorbidity. According to the study by Goracci et al. (2008), which of the following comorbidities was most common in sarcoidosis?

    A. Obsessive-compulsive disorder.
    B. Generalized anxiety disorder.
    C. Major depressive disorder.
    D. Panic disorder.
    E. Bipolar disorder.

19.3   Tuberculosis treatment with isoniazid has been associated with mania and psychosis as a drug side effect. Risk factors for this side effect include all of the following *except*

    A. Rapid acetylation.
    B. Alcoholism.
    C. Diabetes mellitus.
    D. Liver disease.
    E. Pyridoxine deficiency.

19.4   Lung cancer, a leading cause of cancer death and most often the consequence of smoking, is well known to be associated with mood and anxiety symptoms. Which of the following statements regarding psychopathology in lung cancer is *false?*

    A. Depression is more common in lung cancer than in breast cancer.
    B. Anxiety is less common in lung cancer than in breast cancer.
    C. Suicide in lung cancer occurs at twice the rate in the U.S. general population.
    D. Lung cancer has the highest standardized mortality ratio among organ cancers.
    E. Suicide risk peaks in the first 5 years after diagnosis.

19.5 The use of benzodiazepines, with appropriate caution, may be considered for anxiety-spectrum symptoms in chronic obstructive pulmonary disease (COPD). Which of the following benzodiazepines would be safest in elderly and/or debilitated COPD patients?

    A. Chlordiazepoxide.
    B. Diazepam.
    C. Clonazepam.
    D. Lorazepam.
    E. Tranxene.

19.6 Given the risk of cytochrome P450 (CYP) interactions with pulmonary drugs, which of the following selective serotonin reuptake inhibitors (SSRIs) would be preferred for management of mood disorders in pulmonary patients?

    A. Fluvoxamine.
    B. Paroxetine.
    C. Fluoxetine.
    D. Citalopram.
    E. Norfluoxetine.

Chapter 20

Gastrointestinal Disorders

Select the single best response for each question.

20.1 An oropharyngeal disorder characterized by subjective complaint of dry mouth that may be associated with reduced saliva production is

    A. Burning mouth syndrome.
    B. Dysphagia.
    C. Globus hystericus.
    D. Rumination syndrome.
    E. Xerostomia.

20.2 A gastroenterologist evaluates a patient who presents with troublesome symptoms due to the efflux of stomach contents. Endoscopically, no reflux esophagitis is seen, but the patient is still symptomatic. What is the likely diagnosis?

    A. Dysphagia.
    B. Functional heartburn.
    C. Gastroesophageal reflux disorder.
    D. Noncardiac chest pain.
    E. Nonerosive reflux disorder.

20.3 The term *functional nausea and vomiting* refers to chronic nausea and vomiting without apparent cause. Several specific conditions are encompassed in this category. One of these, a condition characterized by recurrent, stereotypical bouts of severe nausea and vomiting, is called

    A. Cyclic vomiting syndrome.
    B. Functional vomiting.
    C. Chronic idiopathic nausea.
    D. Anticipatory nausea and vomiting.
    E. Gastroparesis.

20.4 Which of the following is the most common cause of dyspepsia?

    A. Gastroesophageal reflux disorder.
    B. Functional dyspepsia.
    C. Peptic ulcer disease.
    D. Gastric malignancy.
    E. Nonerosive reflux disorder.

20.5   The psychiatric disorder most commonly found in patients with irritable bowel syndrome (IBS) is

   A. Anxiety.
   B. Personality disorder.
   C. Depression.
   D. Substance use disorder.
   E. Somatization disorder.

20.6   Which of the following is the greatest risk factor for hepatitis C virus (HCV) infection?

   A. Hemodialysis.
   B. Blood transfusion.
   C. Sexual contact.
   D. Intravenous drug use.
   E. Tattooing.

20.7   Standard treatment for hepatitis C virus (HCV) infection involves the use of pegylated interferon-alpha and ribavirin (IFN therapy) for 24–48 weeks. Which of the following drug-induced psychiatric symptoms is most likely to occur with IFN therapy?

   A. Cognitive impairment.
   B. Hypomania/mania.
   C. Psychosis.
   D. Depression.
   E. Delirium.

20.8   Which of the following mood stabilizers is most often associated with cases of drug-induced pancreatitis?

   A. Gabapentin.
   B. Carbamazepine.
   C. Valproic acid.
   D. Lamotrigine.
   E. Topiramate.

Chapter 21

Renal Disease

Select the single best response for each question.

21.1   Psychiatric illness is extremely common in renal disease and is the source of much of the caseload on psychosomatic medicine services. In the study by Kimmel et al. (1998) of psychiatric illness in renal dialysis patients, the most common psychiatric diagnoses were

    A. Mood disorders.
    B. Delirium and dementia.
    C. Anxiety disorders.
    D. Psychotic disorders.
    E. Eating disorders.

21.2   In the study by Cukor et al. (2008a) of anxiety disorders in end-stage renal disease (ESRD) patients, the most common anxiety disorder diagnoses in this population were

    A. Acute stress disorder (ASD) and posttraumatic stress disorder (PTSD).
    B. Generalized anxiety disorder and agoraphobia without panic disorder.
    C. Phobias and panic disorder.
    D. GAD and PTSD.
    E. Anxiety disorder due to a general medical condition and panic disorder.

21.3   Cognitive disorders are common in dialysis patients and may complicate the management of this severe chronic illness. Although uremic symptoms may vary among patients, which of the following is *not* a usual behavioral symptom with progression of uremia?

    A. Mild cognitive dysfunction.
    B. Fatigue.
    C. Hyperactive delirium.
    D. Hypoactive delirium.
    E. Coma.

21.4   The decision to withdraw dialysis and accept hastened death may be a controversial one. Which of the following demographic factors is *not* associated with an increased likelihood of a dialysis withdrawal decision?

    A. Female gender.
    B. Increased age.
    C. Asian ethnicity.
    D. Cognitive impairment.
    E. Caucasian ethnicity.

21.5 Depression in renal disease will often require medication management. Among the selective serotonin reuptake inhibitors (SSRIs) in common use, which of the following is associated with reduced clearance in renal disease?

A. Escitalopram.
B. Citalopram.
C. Fluoxetine.
D. Paroxetine.
E. Sertraline.

21.6 Although antipsychotic medication typically can be maintained in renal failure, which of the following antipsychotics may require dosage reduction in patients with renal disease?

A. Olanzapine.
B. Ziprasidone.
C. Aripiprazole.
D. Quetiapine.
E. Paliperidone.

21.7 Dementia is common in renal disease patients, and many of these patients will be on pharmacotherapy for cognitive enhancement. Which of the following antidementia medications is *not* recommended in severe renal insufficiency?

A. Memantine.
B. Donepezil.
C. Rivastigmine.
D. Galantamine.
E. None of the above.

21.8 Several psychotropic agents are known to cause disorders of sodium metabolism. Among these agents, which of the following medications is more typically associated with *hyper*natremia, as opposed to *hypo*natremia?

A. Carbamazepine.
B. Oxcarbazepine.
C. Selective serotonin reuptake inhibitors (SSRIs).
D. Atypical antipsychotics.
E. Lithium.

Chapter 22

Endocrine and Metabolic Disorders

Select the single best response for each question.

22.1   Female patients with type 1 diabetes

    A. Frequently lose weight when their diabetes is intensively controlled.
    B. May use insulin manipulation as a means of caloric purging.
    C. Are less likely than their nondiabetic peers to have disturbed eating behaviors.
    D. Are less likely than their nondiabetic peers to develop an eating disorder.
    E. Do not develop higher hemoglobin A_{1c} values with intermittent insulin omission.

22.2   The most common cause of hyperthyroidism is

    A. Hashimoto's thyroiditis.
    B. Cushing's syndrome.
    C. Addison's disease.
    D. Pheochromocytomas.
    E. Graves' disease.

22.3   Hypoparathyroidism is common in which of the following disorders?

    A. Autism.
    B. Tourette's syndrome.
    C. Fragile X syndrome.
    D. Velocardiofacial syndrome (22q11.2)
    E. Asperger's syndrome.

22.4   The most common psychiatric symptom in patients with Cushing's syndrome is

    A. Anxiety.
    B. Depression.
    C. Psychosis.
    D. Hypomania.
    E. Cognitive dysfunction.

22.5   Which of the following antipsychotics has most often been associated with cases of sustained hyperprolactinemia?

    A. Aripiprazole.
    B. Clozapine.
    C. Olanzapine.
    D. Quetiapine.
    E. Risperidone.

22.6 The classic symptom triad of dermatitis, dementia, and diarrhea is indicative of which of the following vitamin deficiencies?

    A. Thiamine.
    B. Pyridoxine.
    C. Niacin (among other vitamins and amino acids).
    D. Vitamin E.
    E. None of the above.

Chapter 23

Oncology

Select the single best response for each question.

23.1   Depression is commonly comorbid with cancer, yet the symptomatic overlap between the neurovegetative signs of a mood disorder and the physical symptoms of cancer can create ambiguity. Which of the following symptoms is more specific for a mood disorder, as opposed to a symptom of the comorbid cancer?

   A. Insomnia.
   B. Decreased appetite.
   C. Poor concentration.
   D. Hopelessness.
   E. Psychomotor slowing.

23.2   In the Bardwell et al. (2006) study of depression in women with breast cancer, risk for depression was predicted by all of the following *except*

   A. Cancer diagnosis date and stage.
   B. Stressful life events.
   C. Less optimism.
   D. Ambivalence over expressing negative emotions.
   E. Sleep disturbance.

23.3   Although suicide accounts for a very low number of deaths in cancer patients, an elevated risk has been consistently reported. In the Misono et al. (2008) study of suicide risk in cancer patients, which of the following findings was reported?

   A. The risk of suicide in cancer patients was five times that in the general population.
   B. Female cancer patients had a higher suicide rate than male patients.
   C. Caucasians had a lower rate of suicide than other racial groups.
   D. Young age at cancer diagnosis predicted suicide risk.
   E. Head and neck cancers were associated with a notably high suicide risk.

23.4   Anxiety may be a clinically significant comorbidity in cancer. Which of the following conditions should be considered in the differential diagnosis of anxiety in a cancer patient?

   A. Use of antipsychotics and antiemetics.
   B. Pulmonary emboli.
   C. Hypoxia from primary lung cancers.
   D. Uncontrolled pain.
   E. All of the above.

23.5 Limbic encephalopathy is an autoimmune phenomenon associated with altered mental status, including cognitive impairment in many cases. This syndrome is most commonly associated with which type of malignancy?

    A. Non-small-cell lung carcinoma.
    B. Small-cell lung carcinoma.
    C. Melanoma.
    D. Breast cancer.
    E. Head and neck cancer.

23.6 Melanoma, a dermatological cancer with a propensity for central nervous system involvement, may be treated with interferon-alpha. Which of the following is a rare, rather than common, psychiatric complication of interferon-alpha treatment?

    A. Mania.
    B. Fatigue.
    C. Anxiety.
    D. Insomnia.
    E. Depression.

23.7 The antidepressant mirtazapine has properties that may render it particularly helpful in cancer patients with anorexia-cachexia or insomnia. Which of the following statements regarding mirtazapine is *false*?

    A. It has high affinity for H_1 receptors.
    B. It blocks $5\text{-}HT_2$ receptors.
    C. It blocks $5\text{-}HT_3$ receptors.
    D. Its side effects include constipation and drowsiness.
    E. It is commonly associated with neutropenia.

Chapter 24

Hematology

Select the single best response for each question.

24.1 What is the most common cause of iron deficiency anemia (IDA)?

   A. Malnutrition.
   B. Unsupplemented milk diets.
   C. Blood loss.
   D. Pregnancy.
   E. Intestinal malabsorption of iron.

24.2 A deficiency in which of the following has been associated with neural tube defects (NTDs) in newborns?

   A. Vitamin B_{12}.
   B. Vitamin B_6.
   C. Iron.
   D. Folate.
   E. Thiamine.

24.3 Common clinical and neuropsychiatric symptoms of vitamin B_{12} deficiency include all of the following *except*

   A. Macrocytic anemia.
   B. Symmetrical peripheral neuropathy.
   C. Intestinal metaplasia.
   D. Subacute combined degeneration of the spinal cord.
   E. Vaso-occlusive crisis.

24.4 Which of the following antipsychotics has no reported hematological side effects?

   A. Olanzapine.
   B. Ziprasidone.
   C. Clozapine.
   D. Mellaril.
   E. Chlorpromazine.

24.5 The most common and serious hematological side effect of antipsychotics is

   A. Aplastic anemia.
   B. Neutropenia.
   C. Agranulocytosis.
   D. Eosinophilia.
   E. Thrombocytopenia.

24.6 A patient who has been on an antidepressant for 8 weeks begins to experience bruising and bleeding. She reports that the only other medication she takes is low-dose aspirin to reduce the risk of myocardial infarction. Which of the following classes of antidepressants is most likely responsible for this adverse interaction effect?

   A. Tricyclic antidepressants (TCAs).
   B. Monoamine oxidase inhibitors (MAOIs).
   C. Serotonin–2 receptor antagonists with serotonin reuptake blockade.
   D. Selective serotonin reuptake inhibitors (SSRIs).
   E. Alpha-2 antagonists with serotonin-2 and serotonin-3 antagonism.

Chapter 25

Rheumatology

Select the single best response for each question.

25.1 Rating scales for mood disorders may overestimate the diagnosis of depression in rheumatological patients because of their focus on somatic symptoms. Among the following instruments, which is *least* reliant on somatic content and thus potentially more useful for psychiatric screening in rheumatological populations?

    A. Beck Depression Inventory (BDI).
    B. Center for Epidemiologic Studies Depression Scale (CES-D).
    C. Hamilton Rating Scale for Depression (HAM-D).
    D. Hospital Anxiety and Depression Scale (HADS).
    E. Mini-Mental State Examination (MMSE).

25.2 Psychotherapy is a very helpful treatment for rheumatological patients with comorbid depressive symptoms. Based on reviewed evidence, which of the following psychotherapy models has proven to be the most applicable to rheumatological patients?

    A. Interpersonal therapy (IPT).
    B. Psychodynamic psychotherapy.
    C. Cognitive-behavioral therapy (CBT).
    D. Group psychotherapy.
    E. Supportive psychotherapy.

25.3 Antidepressant medications may be a very helpful adjunctive treatment for painful rheumatological conditions. Which of the following antidepressants has been demonstrated to have analgesic efficacy in rheumatological disorders?

    A. Mirtazapine.
    B. Venlafaxine.
    C. Bupropion.
    D. Selective serotonin reuptake inhibitors (SSRIs).
    E. Tricyclic antidepressants (TCAs).

25.4 Systemic lupus erythematosus (SLE) is a complex rheumatological disease with notably problematic central nervous system involvement. Which of the following is the most common psychiatric comorbidity in SLE?

    A. Cognitive disorders.
    B. Mood disorders.
    C. Anxiety disorders.
    D. Psychotic disorders.
    E. Impulse-control disorders.

25.5 What is the most common cause of mania in systemic lupus erythematosus (SLE)?

      A. Direct central nervous system involvement from SLE.
      B. Strokes in the right hemisphere.
      C. Strokes in the left hemisphere.
      D. Preexisting bipolar disorder.
      E. Corticosteroid treatment.

25.6 Other rheumatological illnesses may mimic some of the clinical features of systemic lupus erythematosus (SLE). Clinical laboratory tests may be helpful in the differential diagnosis of these conditions. Which of the following rheumatological illnesses is associated with a medium to high, rather than a low or negative, antinuclear antibody (ANA) titer?

      A. Polyarteritis nodosa.
      B. Wegener's granulomatosis.
      C. Behçet's syndrome.
      D. Rheumatoid arthritis.
      E. Sjögren's syndrome.

25.7 The most common psychiatric side effect of corticosteroid therapy is

      A. Anxiety.
      B. Anorexia.
      C. Mood disorder, often with psychotic features.
      D. Psychosis without mood symptoms.
      E. Delirium.

C h a p t e r 2 6

Chronic Fatigue and Fibromyalgia Syndromes

Select the single best response for each question.

26.1 Which of the following is a core feature of fibromyalgia?

   A. Peripheral neuropathy.
   B. Headache.
   C. Sore throat.
   D. Postexertional malaise lasting more than 24 hours.
   E. Chronic widespread pain.

26.2 Chronic fatigue syndrome (CFS) and fibromyalgia syndrome (FMS) are more common in

   A. Men.
   B. Individuals between 50 and 65 years of age.
   C. Higher socioeconomic classes.
   D. College-educated individuals.
   E. Western nations.

26.3 Etiological factors reported (and to various degrees documented) to predispose to, precipitate, or perpetuate chronic fatigue syndrome (CFS) include all of the following *except*

   A. Genetic factors.
   B. Abuse.
   C. Immunological factors.
   D. Infections.
   E. Life stress.

26.4 One of the best-supported biological abnormalities reported to be associated with both chronic fatigue syndrome (CFS) and fibromyalgia syndrome (FMS) is

   A. Changes in neuroendocrine stress hormones.
   B. Sleep abnormalities.
   C. Chronic infection.
   D. Abnormalities of muscle metabolism.
   E. Structural brain abnormalities.

26.5 Which of the following medical conditions has been reported to be very common (about 1 per 100) in patients with either chronic fatigue syndrome (CFS) or fibromyalgia syndrome (FMS)?

    A. Systemic lupus erythematosus.
    B. Multiple sclerosis.
    C. Narcolepsy.
    D. Thyroid disorders.
    E. Myopathy.

Chapter 27

Infectious Diseases

Select the single best response for each question.

27.1   Rocky Mountain spotted fever (RMSF) can include neuropsychiatric manifestations that may come to the attention of the psychosomatic medicine consultant. Which of the following statements regarding RMSF is *true*?

    A. Central nervous system (CNS) involvement is seen in more than 50% of cases.
    B. Patients may present with lethargy, confusion, or delirium.
    C. Behavioral changes typically follow the emergence of the characteristic rash.
    D. CNS symptoms are rare in the absence of focal lesions on neuroimaging.
    E. Apathy is seen only in adult cases.

27.2   Lyme disease, a systemic infection due to *Borrelia burgdorferi*, which is transmitted by a tick vector, is well known to be associated with neuropsychiatric symptoms. Which of the following is *not* a symptom of classic Lyme disease encephalopathy?

    A. Poor concentration.
    B. Poor memory performance.
    C. Fatigue.
    D. Depression.
    E. Hypochondriasis.

27.3   Because Epstein-Barr virus (EBV) may persist lifelong in a latent state following acute infection, periodic reactivation may occur. Which of the following is *not* a common symptom in patients with EBV reactivation?

    A. Fatigue.
    B. Malaise.
    C. Depression.
    D. Hypomania with excess energy.
    E. Low-grade fever.

27.4   Patients with acute viral encephalitis commonly present with psychiatric symptoms, even in the absence of neurological symptoms. In the review of this topic by Caroff et al. (2001), which of the following psychiatric presentations was the most common?

    A. Psychosis.
    B. Catatonia.
    C. Depression.
    D. Mania.
    E. Obsessive-compulsive disorder.

27.5 Psychiatric disorders can occur in the aftermath of acute viral encephalitis. Which of the following disorders is most commonly seen in this context?

    A. Psychosis.
    B. Anxiety disorders.
    C. Mood disorders.
    D. Cognitive disorders.
    E. Adjustment disorders.

27.6 Even after recovery from acute herpes simplex virus (HSV) infection, patients may manifest persistent behavioral symptoms attributable to the virus. One well-known complication of HSV is Klüver-Bucy syndrome, symptoms of which include all of the following *except*

    A. Oral touching compulsions.
    B. Hyposexuality.
    C. Hyperphagia.
    D. Amnesia.
    E. Agnosia.

27.7 Standard treatment for hepatitis C virus (HCV) infection involves the use of interferon (IFN), which is known to cause depression. In regard to the association between depression and IFN therapy, which of the following statements is *false*?

    A. IFN causes depression in 20%–40% of patients treated.
    B. Depression is the most common adverse effect leading to discontinuation of IFN.
    C. Depression is associated with reduced adherence to IFN treatment.
    D. IFN-associated depression is responsive to antidepressants.
    E. Major depression is a contraindication to IFN treatment for HCV.

Chapter 28

HIV/AIDS

Select the single best response for each question.

28.1   The single most important factor affecting outcome of human immunodeficiency virus (HIV) treatment is

    A. The source of the viral infection.
    B. The age of the patient.
    C. The patient's ability to adhere to the prescribed medication regimen.
    D. The educational level of the patient.
    E. The patient's gender.

28.2   You are working in a human immunodeficiency virus (HIV) clinic, providing psychiatric care to acquired immunodeficiency syndrome (AIDS) patients. One patient whom you are treating has exhibited a change in his level of alertness, confusion, headache, fever, and focal neurological signs. You obtain a computed tomography (CT) scan, which shows multiple bilateral, ring-enhancing lesions in the basal ganglia. What is the most likely medical diagnosis for this patient?

    A. Cytomegalovirus.
    B. Cryptococcal meningitis.
    C. Progressive multifocal leukoencephalopathy.
    D. Toxoplasmosis.
    E. Central nervous system (CNS) lymphoma.

28.3   Specific risk factors associated with acquired immunodeficiency syndrome (AIDS) dementia include all of the following *except*

    A. Illicit drug abuse.
    B. Male sex.
    C. Older age.
    D. Lower educational level.
    E. Anemia.

28.4   Which of the following statements concerning major depression and its relationship to human immunodeficiency virus (HIV) infection is *false?*

    A. Major depression is a risk factor for developing HIV.
    B. HIV patients with depression rarely exhibit somatic symptoms.
    C. Patients with major depression are at increased risk for HIV disease progression.
    D. Fatigue has been found to be more associated with depression than with HIV disease progression.
    E. Certain HIV central nervous system (CNS) infections, such as toxoplasmosis, cryptococcal meningitis, and lymphoma, can cause depressive symptoms.

28.5 Among medications with demonstrated efficacy in the treatment of mania in human immunodeficiency virus (HIV) infection, which of the following, when used in combination with antiviral medications, may lower serum levels of protease inhibitors, thereby increasing the risk for bone marrow suppression?

    A. Lamotrigine.
    B. Valproic acid.
    C. Risperidone.
    D. Lithium.
    E. Carbamazepine.

28.6 The term *triple diagnosis* refers to the concurrent presence of

    A. A substance use disorder, a psychiatric disorder, and human immunodeficiency virus (HIV) infection.
    B. HIV, AIDS, and depression.
    C. Three psychiatric disorders and HIV.
    D. Two medical disorders and HIV.
    E. Two substance use disorders and HIV.

28.7 People with which of the following personality characteristics have been shown to be at highest risk for human immunodeficiency virus (HIV) infection?

    A. Stable extroverts.
    B. Unstable introverts.
    C. Unstable extroverts.
    D. Stable introverts.
    E. None of the above.

Chapter 29

Dermatology

Select the single best response for each question.

29.1   The pharmacological properties of some psychotropic drugs make them useful not only to treat psychiatric disorders but also to treat comorbid dermatological conditions. Which of the following tricyclic antidepressants has antihistaminic effects and is available in a dermatological cream preparation?

   A. Nortriptyline.
   B. Amitriptyline.
   C. Imipramine.
   D. Desipramine.
   E. Doxepin.

29.2   Patients with delusional parasitosis (a primary psychotic disorder with dermatological manifestations) typically first present to dermatologists rather than to psychiatrists. Which of the following statements regarding this illness is *true*?

   A. The mean age at onset is the 30s.
   B. In patients younger than 50 years, the male-to-female prevalence ratio is 1:3.
   C. In patients older than 50 years, the male-to-female prevalence ratio is 1:1.
   D. Tactile and olfactory hallucinations are not a prominent feature of the disorder.
   E. Patients often complain of formication or various cutaneous sensations.

29.3   Although delusional parasitosis may be idiopathic, some cases are associated with abuse of psychoactive substances. Abuse of which of the following is most specifically associated with delusional parasitosis?

   A. Psychostimulants.
   B. Opioids.
   C. Alcohol.
   D. Marijuana.
   E. Inhalants.

29.4   Trichotillomania—nonscarring alopecia as a result of self-plucking of hair—has been associated with all of the following factors *except*

   A. Low dissociation scores.
   B. Psychological trauma.
   C. Posttraumatic stress disorder (PTSD).
   D. Depression.
   E. Mental retardation.

29.5 Which tricyclic antidepressant has been shown to be superior to placebo in the management of trichotillomania?

    A. Nortriptyline.
    B. Amitriptyline.
    C. Imipramine.
    D. Desipramine.
    E. Clomipramine.

29.6 Atopic dermatitis may be managed, in part, by the judicious use of antidepressant medications. Which of the following antidepressants, due to its anticholinergic properties, would be preferred for this condition?

    A. Paroxetine.
    B. Monoamine oxidase inhibitors.
    C. Trimipramine.
    D. Imipramine.
    E. Duloxetine.

29.7 Although psychiatrists may more routinely see cases of lithium-associated acne, lithium-associated psoriasis can also be a painful complication of lithium therapy. Which of the following statements regarding lithium-associated psoriasis is *true*?

    A. Lithium-associated psoriasis is very responsive to topical antipsoriatic treatment.
    B. Psoriasis usually resolves within 2 weeks of discontinuing lithium.
    C. Inositol supplements may have a beneficial effect on psoriasis.
    D. Recent population-based studies document that beta-blockers confer a significant increased risk of psoriasis when given with lithium.
    E. Psoriasis from lithium commonly occurs within the first 4 weeks of treatment.

29.8 Isotretinoin is used in dermatology for the management of problematic acne vulgaris. Which of the following psychiatric complications is associated with isotretinoin?

    A. Depression.
    B. Psychosis.
    C. Suicide.
    D. Aggression.
    E. All of the above.

29.9 Erythema multiforme, a dangerous dermatological reaction, is associated with which of the following psychotropic agents?

    A. Carbamazepine.
    B. Valproate.
    C. Lamotrigine.
    D. Gabapentin.
    E. All of the above.

C h a p t e r   3 0

Surgery

Select the single best response for each question.

30.1 General surgical units and specialized surgical units have different operational styles. According to systems theory, burn units exemplify which of the following system types?

    A. Closed.
    B. Partial.
    C. Random.
    D. Open.
    E. Incomplete.

30.2 Valid informed surgical consent includes all of the following principles *except*

    A. Capacity for decision making.
    B. Disclosure.
    C. Acceptance of the procedure.
    D. Understanding.
    E. Volunteerism.

30.3 Which of the following psychiatric disorders is viewed as a risk factor for development of chronic postsurgical pain?

    A. Posttraumatic stress disorder.
    B. Schizophrenia.
    C. Bipolar disorder.
    D. Depression.
    E. Dementia.

30.4 Which of the following factors is associated with an increased likelihood of developing posttraumatic stress disorder (PTSD) after trauma?

    A. Concussion.
    B. PTSD symptoms during the acute hospitalization period.
    C. Alcohol intoxication.
    D. Severity of the injury.
    E. Better prior emotional adjustment.

30.5 Which of the following factors is *not* associated with improved functional outcome following surgery?

     A. Appropriate pain management.
     B. Management of postsurgical psychiatric problems.
     C. Preparation of the patient for surgery.
     D. Management of preoperative fears.
     E. Actual severity of the trauma or surgery.

30.6 Which of the following psychiatric disorders is most common and problematic in burn patients?

     A. Depression.
     B. Dementia.
     C. Alcohol abuse or dependence.
     D. Bipolar disorder.
     E. Schizophrenia.

30.7 Which of the following psychiatric disorders has been found to be most prevalent in obese patients being evaluated for bariatric surgery?

     A. Eating disorder.
     B. Mood disorder.
     C. Anxiety disorder.
     D. Alcohol abuse or dependence.
     E. Substance use disorder.

Chapter 31

Organ Transplantation

Select the single best response for each question.

31.1 Which of the following groups of transplant patients currently has the highest rates of long-term survival?

    A. Deceased-donor kidney recipients.
    B. Pancreas recipients.
    C. Living-donor liver recipients.
    D. Heart recipients.
    E. Lung recipients.

31.2 The Psychosocial Assessment of Candidates for Transplantation (PACT) is a clinically useful instrument in the psychiatric assessment of organ transplant candidates. In regard to this instrument, which of the following statements is *false*?

    A. It provides an overall numerical score.
    B. It provides a subscale score for psychological health.
    C. It assesses lifestyle factors.
    D. It addresses patient "educability" regarding transplant expectations.
    E. The final rating is determined by an arithmetic mean of the subscale scores.

31.3 Similar to other medically ill populations, transplant recipients experience a significant amount of psychological distress and are at heightened risk of developing psychiatric disorders. Dew et al. (2001) studied the prevalence and risk of psychiatric disorders in 191 heart transplant recipients. Findings from this study included all of the following *except*

    A. The cumulative prevalence of any psychiatric disorder was 38%.
    B. Women were at higher risk than men for posttransplant psychiatric disorders.
    C. Major depression was the most common psychiatric disorder after transplantation.
    D. The cumulative prevalence of posttraumatic stress disorder (PTSD) was 17%.
    E. The incidence of transplant-associated PTSD was the same in each of the 3 years studied.

31.4 Several studies have suggested an association between psychiatric disorders and transplant health outcomes, although the results have been mixed. Which of the following statements regarding the Singh et al. (1997) study of wait-listed liver transplant candidates is *true*?

    A. Three-fourths of cases had a Beck Depression Inventory (BDI) score higher than 16, consistent with a diagnosis of major depression.
    B. Higher BDI scores were primarily attributable to greater burden of somatic symptoms.
    C. Depressed candidates who later received transplants had poorer postoperative survival than nondepressed organ recipients.
    D. Survival outcomes for depressed patients were highly influenced by social factors.
    E. Candidates who were depressed (based on BDI scores) had a significantly higher likelihood of death while awaiting transplant.

31.5 Postoperative immunosuppressant medication adherence is a critical issue in transplant medicine. In the adherence study by Dew et al. (2007), which organ transplant type was associated with the highest rates of medication noncompliance?

    A. Lung.
    B. Liver.
    C. Pancreas.
    D. Heart.
    E. Kidney.

31.6 Personality disorders are an important psychiatric consideration in the evaluation and management of transplant cases. Which of the following personality disorders is considered to present the highest risk for postoperative nonadherence?

    A. Obsessive-compulsive.
    B. Narcissistic.
    C. Avoidant.
    D. Dependent.
    E. Borderline.

31.7 Patients with psychosis pose a particular challenge in management before, during, and after transplantation. In the study of transplant recipients with psychotic disorders by Coffman and Crone (2002), risk factors for nonadherence included all of the following *except*

    A. Family history of schizophrenia.
    B. Antisocial personality features.
    C. Borderline personality features.
    D. Negative symptoms.
    E. Positive symptoms.

31.8 The immunosuppressant tacrolimus is associated with neuropsychiatric side effects that may limit patients' adherence to posttransplant medication regimens. An uncommon side effect of tacrolimus, seen primarily with high plasma levels, is

    A. Tremulousness.
    B. Headache.
    C. Insomnia.
    D. Anxiety.
    E. Delirium.

Chapter 32

Neurology and Neurosurgery

Select the single best response for each question.

32.1 Partial occlusion of which of the following arteries may produce uni- or bilateral pyramidal signs and ipsilateral cranial nerve palsies?

    A. Middle cerebral artery.
    B. Internal carotid artery.
    C. Basilar artery.
    D. Anterior cerebral artery.
    E. Posterior cerebral artery.

32.2 A number of behavioral changes may occur following a stroke. A behavioral syndrome characterized by partial or complete unawareness of a deficit is termed

    A. Affective dysprosodia.
    B. Anosognosia.
    C. Global aphasia.
    D. Apathy.
    E. Catastrophic reaction.

32.3 In both Parkinson's disease (PD) and multiple sclerosis (MS), approximately 50% of patients have

    A. Bradykinesia.
    B. Optic neuritis.
    C. Tremor.
    D. Sensory loss.
    E. Depression.

32.4 Which of the following neuropsychiatric disorders is dominantly inherited?

    A. Wilson's disease.
    B. Leukodystrophies.
    C. Wernicke-Korsakoff syndrome.
    D. Huntington's disease.
    E. Creutzfeldt-Jakob disease.

32.5 Which of the following neuropsychiatric disorders is a rare complication of childhood measles?

    A. Subacute sclerosing panencephalitis.
    B. Progressive multifocal leukodystrophy.
    C. Limbic encephalitis.
    D. Hashimoto's encephalopathy.
    E. Whipple's disease.

32.6 A patient with history of seizures is referred to you for psychiatric evaluation. The patient describes experiencing an aura at the onset of seizures that involves a dream-like state, flashbacks, and déjà vu. On the basis of this description, your working diagnosis is

    A. Simple partial seizure.
    B. Tonic-clonic seizure.
    C. Complex partial seizure.
    D. Simple absence seizure.
    E. Complex absence seizure.

Chapter 33

Obstetrics and Gynecology

Select the single best response for each question.

33.1 Which of the following medications for bipolar disorder has been associated with polycystic ovarian syndrome?

    A. Lithium.
    B. Lamotrigine.
    C. Olanzapine.
    D. Valproic acid.
    E. Carbamazepine.

33.2 The psychosomatic medicine consultant working with OB/GYN patients must be particularly attentive to the potential for drug–drug interactions between psychiatric medications and contraceptive agents. Due to the inhibition of glucuronidation, oral contraceptives may increase serum levels of which of the following?

    A. Tricyclic antidepressants.
    B. Selective serotonin reuptake inhibitors.
    C. Lithium.
    D. Benzodiazepines.
    E. Valproate and lamotrigine.

33.3 Which of the following statements regarding the behavioral consequences of elective sterilization is *true*?

    A. Postsurgical regret is seen in fewer than 2% of cases.
    B. Women younger than 30 years are less likely than older women to experience postsurgical regret.
    C. Marital conflict over the surgical procedure does not increase the risk of postsurgical regret.
    D. Death of a child has been associated with postsurgical regret.
    E. Sexual satisfaction typically increases postoperatively.

33.4 Endometriosis is a painful and life-limiting condition that often requires comprehensive multidisciplinary management. Gonadotropin-releasing hormone (GnRH) agonists are commonly used to treat endometriosis but are known to cause depression. Which of the following antidepressants appears to be particularly helpful in treatment of GnRH agonist–associated mood symptoms?

    A. Monoamine oxidase inhibitors (MAOIs).
    B. Tricyclic antidepressants (TCAs).
    C. Bupropion.
    D. Trazodone.
    E. Selective serotonin reuptake inhibitors (SSRIs).

33.5   Which of the following statements regarding pseudocyesis is *false*?

       A. In pseudocyesis, the patient ceases to menstruate.
       B. Patients with pseudocyesis show increased abdominal girth.
       C. Classical pseudocyesis occurs in women with schizophrenia-spectrum illness.
       D. Patients with pseudocyesis typically refuse psychiatric care for their symptoms.
       E. In pseudocyesis, the cervix may show physical changes associated with pregnancy.

33.6   Postpartum psychosis may affect women with no prior history of psychiatric illness. Which of the following statements regarding postpartum psychosis is *false*?

       A. The usual period of onset is between 3 and 14 days postpartum.
       B. Because of the risks of suicide and/or infanticide, psychiatric hospitalization for observation is warranted.
       C. Most episodes of postpartum psychosis likely represent bipolar disorder.
       D. The rate of postpartum relapse in bipolar disorder is 30%–50%.
       E. The incidence of postpartum psychosis has tripled in the past 100 years among many cultures.

33.7   Although study findings have not been unanimous, which of the following selective serotonin reuptake inhibitors (SSRIs) has most often been associated with fetal heart defects when used in pregnancy?

       A. Fluoxetine.
       B. Fluvoxamine.
       C. Sertraline.
       D. Paroxetine.
       E. Citalopram.

33.8   According to a recent Cochrane Database meta-analysis of premenstrual dysphoric disorder (PMDD) treatment, which of the following tricyclic antidepressants (TCAs) (along with several selective serotonin reuptake inhibitors [SSRIs]) is effective for PMDD?

       A. Nortriptyline.
       B. Doxepin.
       C. Clomipramine.
       D. Imipramine.
       E. Desipramine.

Chapter 34

Pediatrics

Select the single best response for each question.

34.1 In Piaget's stages of cognitive development, preoperational children are in what age range?

    A. Birth to 2 years.
    B. 2–7 years.
    C. 7–11 years.
    D. 11–14 years.
    E. 14–17 years.

34.2 Which of the following statements concerning the diagnosis and clinical course of delirium in hospitalized children is *false?*

    A. Delirium is less frequently diagnosed in children than in adults.
    B. The Glasgow Coma Scale is less effective in predicting prognosis for children than for adults.
    C. Critically ill children who develop delirium are sometimes misdiagnosed as psychotic.
    D. The Delirium Rating Scale does not appear to be applicable to children.
    E. Unlike the case for adults, Delirium Rating Scale scores for children do not predict length of hospital stay.

34.3 The only literature review to date on children and adolescent patients who falsified illness revealed which of the following?

    A. Most patients were male.
    B. The mean age was 8 years.
    C. The average duration of falsification prior to detection was 5–6 months.
    D. Few children admitted to their deceptions when confronted.
    E. One of the most commonly falsified conditions was fever.

34.4 Autism spectrum disorders

    A. Affect about 1 of every 1,000 children.
    B. Rarely occur in children with fragile X syndrome.
    C. Occur more frequently in males.
    D. Are characterized by impairment in communication.
    E. Occur more frequently in Caucasians.

34.5 The most common comorbid psychiatric disorder among children with asthma is

    A. Depression.
    B. Bipolar disorder.
    C. Hypochondriasis.
    D. An anxiety disorder.
    E. Somatization disorder.

Chapter 35

Physical Medicine and Rehabilitation

Select the single best response for each question.

35.1 According to the definition established by the American Congress of Rehabilitation Medicine, a diagnosis of mild traumatic brain injury (TBI) may be made if an injury acutely manifests one or more of a set of four features. Which of the following is *not* one of these four defining features?

   A. Loss of consciousness of 30 minutes or less.
   B. Posttraumatic amnesia of 24 hours or less.
   C. Altered mental state at the time of trauma.
   D. After 30 minutes, an initial Glasgow Coma Scale (GCS) score of 13–15.
   E. "Mild" abnormalities on neuroimaging.

35.2 In contrast to post–traumatic brain injury (TBI) depression, post-TBI bipolar disorder appears to be a much less frequent complication of TBI. In the study by Jorge et al. (1993), post-TBI mania was associated with which of the following?

   A. Basopolar temporal lesions.
   B. More severe TBI.
   C. More intellectual impairment.
   D. Posttraumatic epilepsy.
   E. Personal history of psychiatric illness.

35.3 In the Hibbard et al. (1998) study of mood, anxiety, and substance use disorders following traumatic brain injury (TBI), which of the following was found to be the most common anxiety disorder, with a rate of 14%?

   A. Posttraumatic stress disorder.
   B. Acute stress disorder.
   C. Panic disorder with agoraphobia.
   D. Panic disorder without agoraphobia.
   E. Obsessive-compulsive disorder.

35.4 Aggressive behavior in individuals with traumatic brain injury (TBI) typically has several characteristic features. Descriptive terms for post-TBI aggression include all of the following *except*

   A. Nonreflective.
   B. Nonpurposeful.
   C. Reactive.
   D. Periodic.
   E. Ego-syntonic.

35.5 Postconcussive syndrome, a somewhat ambiguous and controversial construct, overlaps phenomenologically with several psychiatric disorders, including depression. Which of the following symptoms is characteristic of depression but not of postconcussive syndrome?

    A. Psychomotor changes.
    B. Depressed mood.
    C. Irritability.
    D. Sleep disturbance.
    E. Poor concentration.

35.6 In addition to traumatic brain injury, spinal cord injury (SCI) is associated with much psychiatric comorbidity. Which region of the spinal cord is the most common site of SCI?

    A. High cervical.
    B. Midcervical.
    C. High thoracic.
    D. Low thoracic.
    E. Lumbar.

35.7 Because some symptoms of mood disorder in spinal cord injury (SCI) may actually be due to the SCI itself, diagnosis of depression can be challenging. Which of the following symptoms in an SCI patient is more specific for a mood disorder?

    A. Weight loss.
    B. Altered appetite.
    C. Sleep disturbance.
    D. Reduced energy.
    E. Worthlessness and self-blame.

35.8 Many of the medications used to treat fatigue in spinal cord injury act on the dopamine system via various mechanisms. Which of the following medications has been associated with seizures at usual doses and therefore must be used with caution in seizure-prone patients?

    A. Methylphenidate.
    B. Dextroamphetamine.
    C. Bromocriptine.
    D. Amantadine.
    E. Modafinil.

Chapter 36

Pain

Select the single best response for each question.

36.1   A pain sensation characterized by an increased reaction to a stimulus, especially a repetitive stimulus, is called

    A. Hyperesthesia.
    B. Allodynia.
    C. Hyperpathia.
    D. Nociception.
    E. Paresthesia.

36.2   A strong relationship exists between pain and depression. Which of the following statements concerning this relationship is *false?*

    A. Physical symptoms are common in patients suffering from depression.
    B. Depression in patients with chronic pain is associated with greater pain intensity.
    C. Depression is the strongest predictor of suicidal ideation in patients with chronic pain.
    D. Individuals with chronic physical complaints have higher rates of lifetime major depression.
    E. Pain intensity and duration is a better predictor of disability than depression.

36.3   Which of the following is one of the most significant predictors of failure to return to work in patients with chronic low back pain?

    A. Fear–avoidance beliefs.
    B. Physical therapy.
    C. General fears of physical activity.
    D. Disease status.
    E. Physical impairment.

36.4   You are evaluating a 40-year-old woman for depression. She complains of frequent, unilateral, pulsating headaches with associated nausea and photophobia. She also describes a visual prodromal symptom of scintillating scotoma. You conclude that the probable diagnosis is

    A. Tension headache.
    B. Classic migraine.
    C. Chronic daily headache.
    D. Common migraine.
    E. Complicated migraine.

36.5 In the patient described above, you also diagnose bipolar II disorder. You want to prescribe a medication that will treat her hypomanic and depressive symptoms as well as decrease the frequency of her headaches. Which of the following might be a good choice?

    A. Sertraline.
    B. Aripiprazole.
    C. Lithium.
    D. Valproate.
    E. Bupropion.

36.6 Which of the following synthetic opioid analgesics is highly lipophilic and may be used transdermally?

    A. Morphine.
    B. Oxycodone.
    C. Methadone.
    D. Fentanyl.
    E. Hydrocodone.

36.7 Which of the following antidepressant classes have been shown to be most effective in the treatment of both depression and fibromyalgia?

    A. Monoamine oxidase inhibitors (MAOIs).
    B. Selective serotonin reuptake inhibitors (SSRIs).
    C. Serotonin–norepinephrine reuptake inhibitors (SNRIs).
    D. Tricyclic antidepressants (TCAs).
    E. None of the above.

Chapter 37

Medical Toxicology

Select the single best response for each question.

37.1 Acetaminophen overdose is a common means of attempted (and often completed) suicide. Prompt emergency management of this ingestion can significantly improve clinical outcomes. Which of the following statements regarding the metabolism of acetaminophen is *true*?

    A. Following ingestion, 70% of the drug is metabolized to the glucuronide conjugate.
    B. The glucuronide conjugate is directly hepatotoxic.
    C. *N*-acetyl-*p*-benzoquinone imine (NAPQI) is produced solely through the cytochrome P450 (CYP) 3A4 system.
    D. Glutathione depletion leads to systemic toxicity.
    E. *N*-acetylcysteine (NAC) directly neutralizes NAPQI.

37.2 Neuropsychiatric findings associated with strychnine poisoning include all of the following *except*

    A. Nystagmus.
    B. Hyporeflexia.
    C. Muscle contraction.
    D. Hyperthermia.
    E. *Risus sardonicus.*

37.3 Physical signs of chronic organophosphate toxicity include all of the following *except*

    A. Pupillary mydriasis.
    B. Nausea.
    C. Diaphoresis.
    D. Diarrhea.
    E. Weakness.

37.4 A patient presents with depression, irritability, paranoid ideation, and cognitive impairment accompanied with alopecia, nail dystrophy, chorea, and ophthalmoplegia. Neuroimaging reveals cerebral and brain stem edema. Which metal is implicated in this toxicity state?

    A. Manganese.
    B. Lead.
    C. Thallium.
    D. Mercury.
    E. Arsenic.

37.5 A patient presents with personality changes consisting of shyness and social withdrawal paradoxically accompanied by episodic "flushed face" irritability. He also exhibits anxiety and cognitive impairment. This clinical picture suggests chronic exposure to which of the following?

    A. Manganese.
    B. Lead.
    C. Thallium.
    D. Mercury.
    E. Arsenic.

37.6 A delirium patient exhibits aimless picking movements, vivid visual hallucinations, tachycardia, dry mouth, flushed skin, and mydriasis. Which of the following delirium etiologies is suggested by this presentation?

    A. Anticholinergic toxicity.
    B. Cholinergic toxicity.
    C. Opioid toxicity.
    D. Benzodiazepine withdrawal.
    E. Stimulant overdose.

37.7 Which of the following is contraindicated in the treatment of stimulant toxicity?

    A. Benzodiazepines.
    B. Beta-blockers.
    C. Hydralazine.
    D. Nitroprusside.
    E. Phentolamine.

Chapter 38

Psychopharmacology

Select the single best response for each question.

38.1 Drug–drug interactions are either pharmacodynamic or pharmacokinetic in nature. Examples of pharmacokinetic interactions include all of the following *except*

    A. Altered absorption.
    B. Altered pharmacological response.
    C. Altered distribution.
    D. Altered metabolism.
    E. Altered excretion.

38.2 Which of the following is *not* a clinical feature of serotonin syndrome?

    A. Hypertension.
    B. Tachycardia.
    C. Hypotension.
    D. Bradycardia.
    E. Hyperreflexia.

38.3 Which of the following medications is a serotonin agonist (i.e., stimulates serotonin receptors)?

    A. Venlafaxine.
    B. Tramadol.
    C. Buspirone.
    D. Moclobemide.
    E. Amphetamine.

38.4 The nurse on the psychiatric inpatient unit calls you to evaluate one of your patients who has developed acute symptoms suggestive of either serotonin syndrome or neuroleptic malignant syndrome. The patient was recently started on fluoxetine, olanzapine, trazodone, and as-needed intramuscular haloperidol. Which of the following signs or symptoms is more indicative of serotonin syndrome than of neuroleptic malignant syndrome?

    A. Spontaneous or inducible clonus.
    B. Tachycardia.
    C. Elevated body temperature.
    D. Elevated creatine phosphokinase.
    E. Diaphoresis.

38.5   The most common electrocardiogram finding in patients taking lithium is

    A. PR interval prolongation.
    B. Increased heart rate.
    C. Shortened QT interval.
    D. T wave depression.
    E. Prolonged QRS interval.

38.6   Weight gain is a common and problematic side effect of mood stabilizers. Which of the following mood stabilizers is associated with the *greatest* amount of weight gain?

    A. Gabapentin.
    B. Carbamazepine.
    C. Topiramate.
    D. Lamotrigine.
    E. Valproate.

38.7   Which of the following atypical antipsychotics is associated with the *lowest* risk of extrapyramidal symptoms?

    A. Ziprasidone.
    B. Quetiapine.
    C. Aripiprazole.
    D. Risperidone.
    E. Asenapine.

38.8   You believe that your patient with bipolar disorder would benefit from an atypical antipsychotic medication. Because she has a history of cardiac arrhythmias, you want to select the agent with the lowest mean QTc interval prolongation. Which of the following medications fits this profile?

    A. Quetiapine.
    B. Paliperidone.
    C. Ziprasidone.
    D. Aripiprazole.
    E. Risperidone.

38.9   Which of the following nonbenzodiazepine sedatives is a melatonin agonist?

    A. Eszopiclone.
    B. Zopiclone.
    C. Ramelteon.
    D. Zolidem.
    E. Zaleplon.

C h a p t e r   3 9

Psychotherapy

Select the single best response for each question.

39.1 In a recent systematic review by Jacobsen and Jim (2008), psychosocial interventions for mood and anxiety disorders were shown to be of clinical benefit in patients with cancer. Which of the following statements regarding this study is *false*?

   A. All of the reviewed studies involved adult cancer patients.
   B. Counseling was associated with improved functional ability.
   C. Counseling was associated with enhanced quality of life.
   D. Counseling was associated with fewer symptoms of depression.
   E. The reviewed studies typically had good methodological rigor, allowing for meaningful meta-analysis.

39.2 Interpersonal therapy (IPT) includes several elements that are highly relevant to the general medical setting and to patients who have emotional difficulties secondary to physical illness. During the first phase of IPA treatment, problem areas in the patient's interpersonal relationships are identified and sorted into four groups. Which of the following is *not* one of IPT's four defined problem areas?

   A. Grief.
   B. Role transition.
   C. Role disputes.
   D. Interpersonal deficits.
   E. Effects of childhood relationships.

39.3 Psychodynamic Interpersonal Therapy (PIT) is another psychotherapy model with applicability to psychosomatic medicine practice. Which of the following statements regarding PIT is *false*?

   A. Another term for PIT is "Conversational Model" Therapy.
   B. PIT combines elements of psychodynamic and interpersonal therapies.
   C. PIT places less emphasis on the patient–therapist relationship than does interpersonal therapy (IPT).
   D. PIT makes less use of transference interpretations than does conventional psychodynamic psychotherapy.
   E. In PIT, human existence is regarded as being essentially relational, and man is regarded as a "creature of the between."

39.4 Key features of Psychodynamic Interpersonal Therapy (PIT) include all of the following *except*

   A. The therapist endeavors to know about the patient rather than merely 'getting to know" the patient.
   B. The patient's problems are assumed to arise from relationship disturbances.
   C. The therapist uses a "tentative, encouraging, supportive" approach.
   D. The therapist seeks to link the patient's distress to specific interpersonal problems.
   E. The therapist helps the patient test solutions in the "here and now."

39.5 Cognitive-behavioral therapy (CBT) has applicability to the experience of psychiatric symptoms in systemic illness. Which of the following is *not* one of the components of multidimensional "illness representations" according to Leventhal et al. (1997)?

   A. Identity.
   B. Perceived consequences.
   C. Timeline.
   D. Control/cure.
   E. Symbolism of the specific illness.

39.6 In a recent review of mindfulness-based therapies by Arias et al. (2006), the strongest evidence for efficacy of these therapies was found for which of the following disorders?

   A. Mood disorders.
   B. Anxiety disorders.
   C. Autoimmune illness.
   D. Epilepsy.
   E. Psychiatric symptoms in cancer.

39.7 Although psychological treatments can be offered as stand-alone treatments, they are increasingly delivered as part of a stepped-care model offering five different intensities of treatment, sequentially graded according to the severity of the clinical problem. Which of these five steps involves use of brief psychotherapy (e.g., cognitive-behavioral therapy [CBT], counseling, interpersonal therapy) for 6–8 sessions, with consideration of antidepressants?

   A. Step 1.
   B. Step 2.
   C. Step 3.
   D. Step 4.
   E. Step 5.

Chapter 40

Electroconvulsive Therapy

Select the single best response for each question.

40.1 If the electrical stimulus in electroconvulsive therapy (ECT) is not of sufficient intensity to cause a seizure, there have been reports of prolonged asystole requiring resuscitation. Premedication with which of the following classes of medications is recommended to decrease the likelihood of this occurrence?

    A. Beta-blockers.
    B. Antihypertensive agents.
    C. Antimuscarinic agents.
    D. Alpha-adrenergic agents.
    E. Cholinergic agents.

40.2 The most common dysrhythmia in electroconvulsive therapy (ECT) patients is

    A. Atrial fibrillation.
    B. Ventricular fibrillation.
    C. Ventricular tachycardia.
    D. Atrial tachycardia.
    E. Bundle branch block.

40.3 A blood pressure concern in electroconvulsive therapy (ECT) is the management of blood pressure spikes that occur during treatments. Which of the following medication classes is recommended to reduce these spikes?

    A. Alpha-blocker.
    B. Beta-blocker.
    C. Angiotensin-converting enzyme inhibitor.
    D. Angiotensin II receptor blocker.
    E. Thiazide diuretic.

40.4 You are asked to evaluate a patient with Alzheimer's disease and agitated depression who has failed to respond to medication. You decide to refer the patient for a course of electroconvulsive therapy (ECT). Prudence dictates that you

    A. Use bitemporal electrode placement.
    B. Use thrice-weekly treatments.
    C. Premedicate with a cognitive-enhancing agent.
    D. Use twice-weekly scheduling.
    E. Administer modafinil before each treatment.

40.5 Electroconvulsive therapy (ECT) should be avoided, if possible, in patients with which of the following conditions?

     A. Parkinson's disease.
     B. Chronic obstructive pulmonary disease.
     C. Diabetes.
     D. Chronic pain.
     E. Recent stroke.

Chapter 41

Palliative Care

Select the single best response for each question.

41.1   Which of the following is *not* a typical sign of anxiety in a terminally ill patient?

    A. Tension.
    B. Restlessness.
    C. Excessive somnolence.
    D. Autonomic hyperactivity.
    E. Rumination.

41.2   The differential diagnosis of anxiety disorder versus delirium in a terminally ill patient may be difficult, as many symptoms overlap between the two conditions. Which of the following symptoms is more suggestive of delirium than of anxiety disorder?

    A. Disturbed level of consciousness.
    B. Impaired concentration.
    C. Cognitive impairment.
    D. Fluctuation of symptoms over time.
    E. All of the above.

41.3   Treatment of anxiety disorders in terminally ill patients may require modification of usual psychopharmacological practices. For example, many terminally ill patients can no longer reliably take oral medications. Which of the following benzodiazepines can be administered rectally?

    A. Oxazepam.
    B. Midazolam.
    C. Alprazolam.
    D. Diazepam.
    E. Temazepam.

41.4   Terminally ill patients can present with a vexing combination of persistent anxiety, insomnia, and profound anorexia. Which of the following antidepressants is most appropriate for management of this constellation of symptoms?

    A. Mirtazapine.
    B. Bupropion.
    C. Citalopram.
    D. Fluoxetine.
    E. None of the above.

41.5 In regard to the use of psychostimulants in palliative care, which of the following statements is *true*?

    A. Psychostimulants can cause anorexia at therapeutic doses.
    B. Psychostimulants can cause insomnia at therapeutic doses.
    C. Psychostimulants should not be used in terminally ill patients with a substance abuse history.
    D. Psychostimulants reduce sedation associated with opioid use.
    E. Psychostimulants do not provide adjuvant analgesic affects.

41.6 Delirium in a terminally ill patient can be a very distressing experience for the patient and family members. In the Breitbart et al. (2002) study of delirium in the terminally ill,

    A. Twenty-five percent of patients recalled their delirium experience after recovery.
    B. More severe perceptual disturbances were associated with more recall of delirium symptoms.
    C. The most significant predictor of distress for patients was motor hyperactivity during delirium.
    D. Patients with hypoactive delirium were more distressed than hyperactive patients.
    E. Spouse distress was predicted by the patient's Karnofsky Performance Status.

41.7 Bereavement is an important aspect of palliative care, and an understanding of the terms used to describe various aspects of grief and mourning is helpful. Which of the following is defined as "a pathological outcome involving psychological, social, or physical morbidity"?

    A. Bereavement.
    B. Grief.
    C. Mourning.
    D. Disenfranchised grief.
    E. Complicated grief.

Chapter 1

Psychiatric Assessment and Consultation

Select the single best response for each question.

1.1 To function most effectively in a psychosomatic medicine clinical environment, the psychiatrist is advised to modify the style used to interview outpatients. Which of the following would *not* be a recommended interview style in the inpatient psychosomatic medicine environment?

A. Assume an active, open, and "spontaneous" interpersonal stance to establish rapport efficiently.
B. Do not allow long silences, as psychosomatic medicine patients may have limited stamina for the interview and essential data could be missed.
C. Immediately and in depth, seek to explore the experience and meaning of major trauma early in the therapeutic relationship.
D. Attempt to strike a pragmatic balance between a "biological" and a "psychodynamic" approach to clinical problems.
E. Elicit the patient's belief system about the presenting systemic illness.

The correct response is option C.

The process and content of the psychiatric interview must be adapted to the consultation setting. Deeply exploring traumatic events shortly after they occur may not be ideal; it is often sufficient to acknowledge the patient's past hardships and provide a perspective of what treatment after discharge can offer.

To establish rapport and to have a therapeutic impact, the psychiatrist should assume an engaging, more spontaneous stance (typically, after explaining the purpose of the visit and inquiring about the patient's physical complaints) and should deviate from the principles of anonymity, abstinence, and neutrality that help form the foundation for psychodynamic psychotherapy (see Perry and Viederman 1981). Long silences common in psychoanalytic psychotherapy are rarely appropriate in medical patients, who have not sought out psychiatric assessment and who lack the stamina for long interviews. Neither a rigidly biological approach (which can impede rapport) nor an exclusively psychoanalytic inquiry should be adopted. It is especially important to elicit the patient's beliefs about illness (what's wrong, what caused it, what treatment can do) so that emotional responses and behavior can be placed in perspective. Although the psychiatric consultant often works under pressure of time (e.g., conducting the evaluation between medical tests and procedures), an open-ended interview style should be used. **(p. 3)**

Perry S, Viederman M: Adaptation of residents to consultation-liaison psychiatry, I: working with the physically ill. Gen Hosp Psychiatry 3:141–147, 1981

1.2   The clinical examination in psychosomatic medicine differs from other clinical interviews by the needed focus on cognitive disorders and cognitive examination. Executive function, localized behaviorally to the frontal lobes, is tested by a series of useful bedside tests. Which of the following is *not* a test of executive function?

   A. Naming of visually recognized common objects.
   B. Listing as many animals as possible in 1 minute.
   C. Replicating three hand positions.
   D. The go/no-go task.
   E. Tests of abstraction.

The correct response is option A.

Visual recognition tasks and general-knowledge questions (e.g., "Who is the President?") draw upon declarative memory.

Executive function refers to the abilities that allow one to plan, initiate, organize, and monitor thought and behavior. These abilities, which localize broadly to the frontal lobes, are essential for normal social and professional performance but are difficult to test. Frontal lobe disorders often make themselves apparent in social interaction with a patient and are suspected when one observes disinhibition, impulsivity, disorganization, abulia, or amotivation. Tasks that can be used to gain some insight into frontal lobe function include verbal fluency, such as listing as many animals as possible in 1 minute; motor sequencing, such as asking the patient to replicate a sequence of three hand positions; the go/no-go task, which requires the patient to tap the desk once if the examiner taps once, but not to tap if the examiner taps twice; and tests of abstraction, including questions like "What do a tree and a fly have in common?" **(p. 6)**

1.3   Language disorders, or aphasias, are common in neurologically impaired patients and are associated with a high degree of comorbid psychiatric illness. A stroke patient presents with fluent speech that is largely sensible, and he appears to respond to examination instructions. He can name objects readily and accurately but shows a focal deficit in repetition; however, with rehearsal he can learn new material. This presentation is characteristic of which type of aphasia?

   A. Receptive.
   B. Expressive.
   C. Global.
   D. Anomic.
   E. Conduction.

The correct response is option E.

Language disorders result from lesions of the dominant hemisphere. In assessing language, one should first note characteristics of the patient's speech (e.g., nonfluency or paraphasic errors) and then assess comprehension.

Selective impairment of repetition characterizes conduction aphasia.

Receptive (Wernicke's or sensory) aphasia is characterized by fluent speech with both phonemic and semantic paraphasias (incorrect words that approximate the correct ones in meaning) and poor comprehension. The stream of incoherent speech and the lack of insight in patients with Wernicke's aphasia sometimes lead to misdiagnosis of a primary thought disorder and psychiatric referral; the clue to the diagnosis of a language disorder is the severity of the comprehension deficit.

Expressive (Broca's or motor) aphasia is characterized by effortful, nonfluent speech with use of phonemic paraphasias (incorrect words that approximate the correct ones in sound), reduced use of function words (e.g., prepositions and articles), and well-preserved comprehension.

Naming is impaired in both major varieties of aphasia, and anomia can be a clue to mild dysphasia. Reading and writing should also be assessed.

Global dysphasia combines features of Broca's and Wernicke's aphasias. **(p. 6)**

1.4   Advancements in neuroimaging have been part of the revolution in the clinical practice of psychosomatic medicine. The physician must be aware of the relative indications of various neuroimaging techniques for specific illnesses. Which of the following neurological lesions is better imaged by computed tomography (CT) than by magnetic resonance imaging (MRI)?

     A. Acute intracranial hemorrhage.
     B. Basal ganglia disease.
     C. Brain stem glioma.
     D. White matter disease.
     E. Tumor of the posterior fossa.

The correct response is option A.

Neuroimaging may aid in fleshing out the differential diagnosis of neuropsychiatric conditions, although it rarely establishes the diagnosis by itself (Dougherty and Rauch 2004). In most situations, MRI is preferred over CT.

CT is most useful in cases of suspected acute intracranial hemorrhage (having occurred within the previous 72 hours) or when MRI is contraindicated (in patients with metallic implants).

MRI provides greater resolution of subcortical structures (e.g., basal ganglia, amygdala, and other limbic structures) of particular interest to psychiatrists. It is also superior for detection of abnormalities of the brain stem and posterior fossa. Furthermore, MRI is better able to distinguish between gray matter and white matter lesions. **(p. 10)**

> Dougherty DD, Rauch SL: Neuroimaging in psychiatry, in Massachusetts General Hospital Psychiatry Update and Board Preparation, 2nd Edition. Edited by Stern TA, Herman JB. New York, McGraw-Hill, 2004, pp 227–232

1.5   Which of the following clinical scenarios would *not* routinely prompt early use of neuroimaging for evaluation?

     A. Acute onset of psychotic illness, without delirium, in a previously healthy patient.
     B. First presentation of apparent dementia.
     C. Pretreatment workup for electroconvulsive therapy (ECT) in a patient with psychotic depression.
     D. Mental status changes associated with lateralizing neurological signs.
     E. Delirium following documented overdose with anticholinergic medication with normal motor examination.

The correct response is option E.

Neuroimaging is not indicated in patients who have overdosed with anticholinergic medication.

Dougherty and Rauch (2004) suggest that the following conditions and situations merit consideration of neuroimaging: new-onset psychosis, new-onset dementia, delirium of unknown cause, prior to an initial course of ECT, and an acute mental status change with an abnormal neurological examination in a patient with either a history of head trauma or an age of 50 years or older. **(p. 10)**

> Dougherty DD, Rauch SL: Neuroimaging in psychiatry, in Massachusetts General Hospital Psychiatry Update and Board Preparation, 2nd Edition. Edited by Stern TA, Herman JB. New York, McGraw-Hill, 2004, pp 227–232

1.6   The Folstein Mini-Mental State Examination (MMSE) is a well-known instrument for rapid screening of cognitive impairment at the bedside. In assessment of temporoparietal and frontal lobe function, the MMSE may be usefully supplemented with the Mini-Cog, a convenient test that combines the Clock Drawing Test with which portion of the MMSE?

    A. Immediate memory (repeat three objects).
    B. Concentration (serial 100–7 or spell "world" backwards).
    C. Follow the three-step motor command.
    D. The five elements of place orientation.
    E. Three-minute recall of three objects.

The correct response is option E.

The Mini-Cog combines a portion of the MMSE (3-minute recall) with the Clock Drawing Test, as described by Critchley in 1953 (Scanlan and Borson 2001). In screening for dementia, the MMSE and the Mini-Cog have been shown to have similar sensitivity (76%–79%) and specificity rates (88%–89%) (Borson et al. 2003). However, the Mini-Cog is significantly shorter and enables screening temporoparietal and frontal cortical areas via the Clock Drawing Test, areas that are not fully assessed by the MMSE.

The MMSE is a 19-question test that provides an overview of a patient's cognitive function at a moment in time; it includes assessment of orientation, attention, and memory. It is of limited use without modification, however, in patients who are deaf or blind, are intubated, or do not speak English. The MMSE is also particularly insensitive in measuring cognitive decline in very intelligent patients, who may appear less impaired than they really are. **(pp. 13–14)**

> Borson S, Scanlan JM, Chen P, et al: The Mini-Cog as a screen for dementia: validation in a population-based sample. J Am Geriatr Soc 51:1451–1454, 2003
> Critchley M: The Parietal Lobes. New York, Hafner, 1953
> Scanlan J, Borson S: The Mini-Cog: receiver operating characteristics with expert and naive raters. Int J Geriatr Psychiatry 16:216–222, 200

1.7   The Patient Health Questionnaire (PHQ) is a self-administered questionnaire that can be useful in screening for psychiatric disorders in the primary care environment. This instrument reliably assesses all of the following psychiatric disorders *except*

    A. Cognitive disorders.
    B. Mood disorders.
    C. Anxiety disorders.
    D. Eating disorders.
    E. Somatoform disorders.

The correct response is option A.

The PHQ does not assess cognitive disorders.

The PHQ, an abbreviated form of the Primary Care Evaluation of Mental Disorders (PRIME-MD), consists of a three-page questionnaire that can be entirely self-administered by the patient (Spitzer et al. 1999). In addition to the assessment of mood, anxiety, eating, alcohol, and somatization disorders, the PHQ screens for posttraumatic stress disorder and common psychosocial stressors and also elicits a pregnancy history. The PHQ is valid and reliable and has improved the diagnosis of psychiatric conditions in primary care and other ambulatory medical settings (Spitzer et al. 1999); it may also have a role at the bedside. Subsets of the PHQ's items have been validated for specific screening purposes. **(p. 14)**

> Spitzer RL, Kroenke K, Williams JB: Validation and utility of a self-report version of PRIME-MD: the PHQ Primary Care Study. Primary Care Evaluation of Mental Disorders. Patient Health Questionnaire. JAMA 282:1737–1744, 1999

Chapter 2

Legal Issues

Select the single best response for each question.

2.1   What effect did the Health Insurance Portability and Accountability Act of 1996 (HIPAA) have upon confidentiality?

    A. It reinforced the concept of absolute confidentiality between physician and patient.
    B. It limited doctor–patient confidentiality if confidentiality is determined to be counter to public safety.
    C. It did not address the issue of confidentiality, but focused on other important issues.
    D. It recognized that the efficiency and effectiveness of the health care system need to be balanced against the safeguarding of protected health information.
    E. It reemphasized the concept of confidentiality as stated in the Hippocratic oath.

The correct response is option D.

Over time, the principle of strict or absolute confidentiality between one physician and one patient has eroded beyond the sharing of medical information with hospital personnel. The considerations of a complex society have increasingly led to an erosion of confidentiality as it was understood in the era of Hippocrates and subsequent centuries. Courts and legislatures have created limitations to doctor–patient confidentiality in circumstances where confidentiality is determined to be at odds with public safety or to be more harmful than beneficial for the patient. More recently, federal law has recognized efficiency and effectiveness of the health care system as a principle to be balanced with traditional management and safeguarding of protected health information under the Health Insurance Portability and Accountability Act of 1996 (HIPAA) (Brendel and Bryan 2004). **(p. 20)**

> Brendel RW, Bryan E: HIPAA for psychiatrists. Harv Rev Psychiatry 12:177–183, 2004
> Health Insurance Portability and Accountability Act of 1996, Public Law 104-191

2.2   Every U.S. jurisdiction identifies physicians as mandated reporters of suspected cases of *elder abuse and neglect*, which most states define as encompassing five categories of harm or risk of harm to an elderly person. Which of the following is *not* one of these categories?

    A. Refusal of medical care by an adult older than 65 years.
    B. Infliction of pain.
    C. Sexual assault.
    D. Financial exploitation.
    E. Infliction of emotional distress.

The correct response is option A.

While protecting patient information and confidentiality is the default rule, there are several situations in which physicians have an affirmative duty to disclose information to authorities. One such example is child and elder abuse and neglect reporting.

Beginning in the 1960s, legislation emerged out of the child protection model to protect vulnerable adults and by the mid-1970s, federal law was passed to establish adult protective services (Milosavljevic and Brendel 2008). Now, every U.S. jurisdiction identifies physicians as mandated reporters of suspected elder abuse and neglect. Akin to the jurisdictional variations in definitions of child abuse and neglect, the definition of elder abuse and neglect varies from state to state. That being said, most states use a standard incorporating five common elements: infliction of pain or injury, infliction of emotional or psychological harm, sexual assault, material or financial exploitation, and neglect (Kazim and Brendel 2004). **(p. 20)**

Kazim A, Brendel RW: Abuse and neglect, in Massachusetts General Hospital Psychiatry Update and Board Preparation, 2nd Edition. Edited by Stern TA, Herman JB. New York, McGraw-Hill, 2004, pp 539–544

Milosavljevic N, Brendel RW: Abuse and neglect, in Comprehensive Clinical Psychiatry. Edited by Stern TA, Rosenbaum JF, Fava M, et al. Philadelphia, PA, Mosby/Elsevier, 2008, pp 1133–1142

2.3   A 28-year-old man whom you have been treating confides that he intends to kill his ex-wife by shooting her next week, upon her return from a vacation. He has already revealed to you that the court has imposed a restraining order against him for previous assaults. He also has an unregistered handgun. In assessing whether you have a duty to warn the ex-wife of this patient, relevant considerations include all of the following *except*

   A. The patient has stated a specific threat.
   B. The patient has a past history of violence.
   C. The patient has identified the victim.
   D. The patient has a mental disorder.
   E. You have a basis for anticipatory violence if the wife is not warned.

The correct response is option D.

Whether or not a patient has a mental illness is not relevant when assessing the duty to warn third parties of potential physical harm.

In the more than three decades since the landmark California Supreme Court Decision of *Tarasoff v. Board of Regents* (1976), clinicians and lawmakers alike have debated the relative priority of patient confidentiality and public safety in defining the parameters of the duty, and whether the duty to warn or protect would apply in different jurisdictions.

Statutory methods by which the psychiatrist's duty to protect and potential liability may be circumscribed include requiring a specific threat to an identified or identifiable victim; a clinician's knowledge of the patient's having a past history of violence; and/or a reasonable basis to anticipate violence prior to invocation of the duty to protect. In addition to defining and/or limiting the circumstances in which the duty to protect arises, state laws may also specify what measures mental health clinicians may or must take in order to satisfactorily comply with their duty to protect. These measures often include notifying the police or another law enforcement agency, hospitalizing the patient, or warning the potential victim. **(p. 21)**

Tarasoff v Board of Regents of the University of California. 17 Cal.3d 425 (1976)

2.4   You are called by the surgical team to evaluate a patient's capacity to reject a surgical treatment for colon cancer that may prolong his life. In assessing this patient's decisional capacity, you elect to follow the four-pronged approach developed by Appelbaum and Grisso. Which of the following is *not* one of the four factors requiring consideration in this model?

   A. Rational manipulation of information.
   B. Absence of a serious mental disorder.
   C. Preference.
   D. Appreciation of the facts presented.
   E. Factual understanding of the procedure.

The correct response is option B.

A patient's decisional capacity depends on an understanding of the underlying illness, proposed interventions, prognosis, and consequences of treatment and nontreatment. The most established method of capacity determination for medical decision making is a practical four-pronged analysis developed by Appelbaum and Grisso (Appelbaum 2007; Appelbaum and Grisso 1988). Under this model, the four factors for consideration in determining decisional capacity are preference, factual understanding, appreciation of the facts presented (i.e., how they relate to the specific individual), and rational manipulation of information. All four elements must be met in order for the individual to demonstrate decisional capacity. In practice, a patient's decisional capacity is rarely questioned when the patient is in agreement with the proposed medical interventions. **(pp. 24–25)**

> Appelbaum PS: Clinical practice. Assessment of patients' competence to consent to treatment. N Engl J Med 357:1834–1840, 2007
>
> Appelbaum PS, Grisso T: Assessing patients' capacities to consent to treatment. N Engl J Med 319:1635–1638, 1988

2.5 An oncologist believes that a bone marrow transplant will benefit his patient with pancreatic cancer. In the course of the informed consent process, the physician summarizes the patient's diagnosis, outlines the expected benefits and risks of the procedure to the patient, and explains that the results of the treatment cannot be precisely predicted. Finally, he reviews the risks and benefits of alternative or no treatment. What important information did he forget to provide the patient?

    A. What he (the oncologist) would do if he were the patient.
    B. The cost of the treatment.
    C. The potential irreversibility of the treatment.
    D. An explanation of the procedure to the patient's wife.
    E. A discussion of recent journal articles published concerning the procedure.

The correct response is option C.

As a practical guide to sound clinical practice and risk management, the more information presented to the patient and the more extensive the communication about that information between the doctor and the patient, the better. There are six broad categories of information that, if presented to the patient, are generally accepted as meeting the standard of how much information needs to be presented, regardless of the particular jurisdictional standard (King and Moulton 2006):

- The diagnosis and the nature of the condition being treated
- The reasonably expected benefits from the proposed treatment
- The nature and likelihood of the risks involved
- The inability to precisely predict results of the treatment
- The potential irreversibility of the treatment
- The expected risks, benefits, and results of alternative, or no, treatment

There are limits to how much information physicians are required to share in the course of the informed consent process. Overall, the ideal of informed consent is a process incorporating a clear and frank discussion and exchange of information between doctor and patient (King and Moulton 2006). **(pp. 25–26)**

> King JS, Moulton BW: Rethinking informed consent: the case for shared medical decision-making. Am J Law Med 32:429–493, 2006

2.6   Advance directives are a legal means by which patients may make their treatment preferences known in case they later experience incapacity for decision making. Which of the following statements concerning advance directives is *true*?

     A. An advance directive may be prepared and executed by a patient even if he or she is incompetent.
     B. Once executed, an advance directive is considered active regardless of whether the patient is competent.
     C. Hospitals are encouraged, but not legally required, to ask patients whether they have an advance directive when they are admitted.
     D. Even if a patient regains capacity, the advance directive takes precedence when a medical decision needs to be made.
     E. If a patient does not have an advance directive, some states allow the use of a surrogate decision maker.

The correct response is option E.

In the absence of an advance directive, one of several pathways is generally followed. One legally recognized pathway available in some states is the use of a surrogate decision-making statute. In the absence of an advance directive, these laws give priorities to potential surrogate decision makers based on their relationship to the patient.

An advance directive is one common way of appointing a substitute decision maker. An advance directive is a document prepared and executed by an individual at a time when he or she is competent that either gives instructions to guide decisions or appoints a substitute decision maker, should the individual become incapacitated at some time in the future. Two types of advance directives are the health care proxy and the durable power of attorney for health care. Both are characterized by a "springing clause"—that is, once crafted, they remain inactive until such time as the patient, or principal, is incapacitated. At the time of incapacity and for the duration of the incapacity, the advance directive "springs" into effect. Should the patient regain capacity at a future time, the advance directive would again become inactive.

Since the passage of the federal Patient Self-Determination Act of 1990, hospitals have been legally required to inquire as to whether patients have an advance directive at the time the patient is admitted to the hospital and additionally required to provide information about advance directives. **(p. 27)**

     Patient Self-Determination Act of 1990, 42 USC 1395 cc(a); 60 C.F.R. 123 at 33294, 1995 (final rule)

Chapter 3

Ethical Issues

Select the single best response for each question.

3.1 Psychosomatic medicine psychiatrists who also serve as hospital ethics consultants are obliged to master two separate clinical roles, each requiring a different orientation and approach. In regard to these separate roles, which of the following statements is *false?*

A. Ethics consultants should avoid identifying unaddressed clinical problems, as doing so represents a violation of professional boundaries.
B. A psychiatric consultation follows the medical model of providing specific advice on diagnosis and treatment.
C. Health care professionals frequently expect ethics consultants to provide the same type of specific direction provided by medical specialty consultants.
D. The ethics community favors a more process-oriented type of consultation, as opposed to the traditional medical model.
E. A common result of an ethics consultation is the generation of a list of permissible options rather than a single "right answer."

The correct response is option A.

The ethics consultant who can identify unaddressed clinical concerns (e.g., is the patient depressed, anxious, or confused?) can help resolve an apparent ethical problem by bringing the prior clinical questions to the attention of the medical team or psychiatrist.

Psychiatric consultation follows the medical model of providing expert advice on diagnosis and therapy. Health care professionals often desire the same type of direction from an ethics consultant. However, within the bioethics community the traditional medical model is one of the least favored approaches to ethics consultation. Instead, most ethics committees and consultation services work to facilitate discussion and conflict resolution between the stakeholders in the case. The purpose of this process-oriented approach is to identify the range of ethically permissible options rather than to provide a single "right answer" or stipulate a specific course of action. **(p. 34)**

3.2 Ethics consultations benefit from an organizational framework to define the various domains of clinical ethics. Ethics discussions are organized around the major "principles of biomedical ethics" that may all be present in a particular case. Which of the following ethical principles covers the issue of informed consent?

A. Nonmaleficence.
B. Justice.
C. Respect for patient autonomy.
D. Beneficence.
E. Altruism.

The correct response is option C.

The most general moral considerations guiding ethical inquiry in medical contexts are the principles of biomedical ethics. The leading conception identifies four such principles (Beauchamp and Childress 2009):

1. *Respect for patient autonomy* requires that professionals recognize the right of competent adult individuals to make their own decisions about health care or research participation. This includes the obligation to obtain informed consent and the right of competent patients to refuse recommended diagnostic interventions or therapy, or to decline an invitation to enroll in research.
2. In the therapeutic context, *beneficence* directs professionals to promote the health and well-being of particular patients by offering and providing competent medical care; in research it directs investigators to produce valuable knowledge with the aim of improving medical care for future patients.
3. *Nonmaleficence* enjoins professionals to avoid harming patients or research subjects. Taken together, beneficence and nonmaleficence underlie the obligation of clinicians to assess the risk–benefit ratios of patient care and research interventions.
4. The principle of *justice* requires that medical care and research are performed in a way that is fair and equitable.

(p. 35)

Beauchamp TL, Childress JF: Principles of Biomedical Ethics, 6th Edition. New York, Oxford University Press, 2009

3.3 Psychiatrists are frequently consulted in ethically problematic cases regarding decision-making capacity (DMC). Whereas some clinical psychiatric syndromes are associated with fluctuating DMC, others characteristically involve stable DMC, and consulting clinicians must take this degree of clinical (hence capacity) stability into account in their assessments of DMC. In which of the following conditions is DMC more likely to be stable?

    A. Mania from steroids.
    B. Traumatic brain injury.
    C. Delirium.
    D. Depression.
    E. Dementia.

The correct response is option E.

Dementia involves stable or progressive cognitive impairment; thus, patients with dementia tend to have stable DMC. By contrast, patients with secondary mania, traumatic brain injury, delirium, or depression characteristically manifest fluctuating DMC. **(p. 36)**

3.4 Determination of decision-making capacity (DMC) requires the assessment of multiple domains of mental functioning. To date, the bulk of clinical research on DMC has focused on which of the following functional domains?

    A. Social functioning.
    B. Mood.
    C. Trust.
    D. Motivation.
    E. Cognitive function.

The correct response is option E.

Basic components of DMC include intellectual ability, memory, attention, concentration, conceptual organization, and aspects of "executive function," such as the ability to plan, solve problems, and make probability determinations. Most of the psychiatric literature on DMC has been focused on these cognitive functions and has employed psychometric approaches to the study of subjects with neuropsychiatric illnesses such as dementia, psychosis, major depression, and bipolar disorder (Chen et al. 2002).

In contrast, the contributions of mood, motivation, and other influences on risk assessment and decision making have received less attention but have clear implications for the process and quality of informed consent for both clinical procedures and research participation. The extent to which these factors—and less easily quantified concepts such as faith, intuition, trust, or ambivalence—affect the decision making process is not known. Although much work remains to be done to better understand the determinants of decision making, it is clear that focusing exclusively on measures of cognitive impairment is shortsighted. **(p. 36)**

Chen DT, Miller FG, Rosenstein DL: Enrolling decisionally impaired adults in clinical research. Med Care 40 (9 suppl):V20–V29, 2002

3.5   In recent years, the clinical and ethical appropriateness of the use of physical restraints in the medical setting has come under increasing scrutiny, leading to an evolution in medical and nursing practice regarding the use of restraints. In regard to the ethics of restraint use for an acutely agitated and confused medical patient, which of the following statements is *true*?

    A. Agitated and confused patients should never be restrained.
    B. Agitated and confused patients may be restrained only after a formal determination of decision-making capacity.
    C. Immediate safety concerns transcend ethics discussions and allow for restraint as the unequivocal standard of care in acute agitation and confusion.
    D. Restraints may be legally permissible but are always unethical.
    E. Refusal of care by an agitated and confused patient should be treated no differently from refusal of care by a competent and informed patient.

The correct response is option C.

In the case of an acutely agitated and confused patient, standard of care and legal precedent dictate immediate steps to ensure the patient's safety, even if this requires physical restraint. Compassionate care requires that the patient be treated with dignity and respect under such circumstances and that restraint should be continued only for as long as necessary. The critical distinction to be made at this juncture is between competent, informed refusal of care that warrants respect and refusal behavior due to compromised decision-making capacity.

Physical restraint of patients should be used only when no less restrictive method is available to protect them and staff from harm. The Centers for Medicare and Medicaid Services (U.S. Department of Health and Human Services 2006) and the Joint Commission (2009) require that hospitals have policies on physical restraint and seclusion. **(pp. 37–38)**

Joint Commission: Provision of care, treatment, and services, in Revised 2009 Accreditation Requirements as of March 26, 2009: Hospital Accreditation Program, Oakbrook Terrace, IL, Joint Commission Resources, 2009, pp 14–19

U.S. Department of Health and Human Services: Code of Federal Regulations, Title 42 (Public Health), Part 482 (Conditions of Participation for Hospitals), Section 13 (Patients' Rights), Standard e (Restraint for acute medical and surgical care). 71 FR 71426, Dec. 8, 2006. Available at: http://www.cms.gov/CFCsAndCoPs/downloads/finalpatientrightsrule.pdf. Accessed May 5, 2010.

3.6   Research on the use of advance directives and the behavior of substitute decision makers has found that

   A. Most patients welcome the opportunity to put into writing the kind of medical care they would like to receive if they were to become gravely ill and incompetent.
   B. Substitute decision makers tend to follow patients' stated preferences in their decisions.
   C. Substitute decision makers generally employ a *substituted judgment standard*, basing their decisions on what is in the best interests of the patient.
   D. Substitute decision makers do not base their decisions on what they would want for themselves.
   E. Only a minority of patients execute advance directives.

The correct response is option E.

Several studies found that only 15%–20% of patients fill out an advance directive for health care or research when given an opportunity to do so (Gross 1998; The SUPPORT Principal Investigators 1995; Wendler et al. 2002).

Regardless of the expressed wishes of patients, substitute decision makers tend to make decisions based on what they would want to happen to themselves or, alternatively, what they consider to be in the best interests of the patient rather than employing a substituted judgment standard (i.e., what the patient would have wanted) when making decisions for someone else (Li et al. 2007; Shalowitz et al. 2006). **(p. 38)**

   Gross MD: What do patients express as their preferences in advance directives? Arch Intern Med 158:363–365, 1998
   Li LL, Cheong KY, Yaw LK, et al: The accuracy of surrogate decisions in intensive care scenarios. Anaesth Intensive Care 35:46–51, 2007
   Shalowitz DI, Garrett-Mayer E, Wendler D: The accuracy of surrogate decision makers: a systematic review. Arch Intern Med 166:493–497, 2006
   The SUPPORT Principal Investigators: A controlled trial to improve care for seriously ill hospitalized patients: the Study to Understand Prognoses and Preferences for Outcomes and Risks of Treatments (SUPPORT). JAMA 274:1591–1598, 1995
   Wendler D, Martinez RA, Fairclough D, et al: Views of potential subjects toward proposed regulations for clinical research with adults unable to consent. Am J Psychiatry 159:585–591, 2002

3.7   A medically ill patient's mood symptoms may be of importance in a decision-making capacity (DMC) evaluation given the often "cognitive" presentation of mood disorders, especially in ill and geriatric patients. Depression in the medically ill is typically associated with all of the following *except*

   A. Reduced ability to tolerate discomfort.
   B. Difficulty maintaining hope.
   C. Poor adherence with medical care.
   D. Impaired DMC.
   E. Greater likelihood of considering physician-assisted suicide.

The correct response is option D.

Major depression in the medically ill usually does not render the patient incompetent. To be sure, the presence of depression may well influence the patient's ability to tolerate uncomfortable symptoms, maintain hope, or assess a treatment's risk–benefit ratio but will not necessarily render that patient unable to make medical decisions for him- or herself (Elliott 1997). Untreated depression has been linked to poor adherence with medical care, increased pain and disability, and a greater likelihood of considering euthanasia and physician-assisted suicide. Depression produces more subtle distortions of decision making than does delirium or psychosis, but refusal of even lifesaving treatment by a depressed patient cannot be assumed to constitute suicidality or lack of competence (Katz et al. 1995; Sullivan and Youngner 1994). Consequently, although a depressed patient should be strongly encouraged to accept treatment for depression, the decision to override a refusal of medical treatment should be based on whether the patient lacks DMC. **(p. 39)**

Elliott C: Caring about risks: are severely depressed patients competent to consent to research? Arch Gen Psychiatry 54:113–116, 1997

Katz M, Abbey S, Rydall A, et al: Psychiatric consultation for competency to refuse medical treatment: a retrospective study of patient characteristics and outcome. Psychosomatics 36:33–41, 1995

Sullivan MD, Youngner SJ: Depression, competence, and the right to refuse lifesaving medical treatment. Am J Psychiatry 151:971–978, 1994

3.8   Ethics methodology pertinent to the conduct of research with human participants takes pains to ensure that research design and consent procedures afford protection to participants considered to be "vulnerable to coercion or undue influence," including the "mentally disabled." Which of the following psychiatric illnesses is specifically included in the "mentally disabled" category?

A. Dementia.
B. Delirium.
C. Schizophrenia.
D. Mental retardation.
E. None of the above.

The correct response is option E.

The regulations governing federally funded human subjects research were written more than 20 years ago and mandated additional safeguards for research subjects considered "vulnerable to coercion or undue influence" (U.S. Department of Health and Human Services 1991). Included in this category of vulnerable subjects are the "mentally disabled." These regulations, known as the Common Rule, were clearly intended to prevent the exploitation of individuals for the sake of scientific progress. Unfortunately, the Common Rule does not include a definition of mental disability or of what would constitute the degree of mood, cognitive, or behavioral impairment that would render someone vulnerable in this respect. In practice, a psychiatric consultation often serves as an important additional safeguard by virtue of eliciting an expert opinion about a prospective research subject's decision-making capacity and ability to provide informed consent. **(p. 40)**

U.S. Department of Health and Human Services: Code of Federal Regulations, Title 45 (Public Welfare), Part 46 (Protection of Human Subjects). 56 FR 28012, 28022, June 18, 1991. Available at: http://www.hhs.gov/ohrp/human-subjects/guidance/45cfr46.htm. Accessed May 5, 2010.

C h a p t e r 4

Psychological Responses to Illness

Select the single best response for each question.

4.1 Which of the following is an example of stresses that a patient may experience when hospitalized?

    A. Lack of privacy.
    B. Bodily invasion.
    C. Pain.
    D. Separation from family.
    E. All of the above.

The correct response is option E.

All of the above are examples of stress experienced by hospitalized patients.

The lack of privacy in the hospital environment or clinic places significant stress on the patient (Kornfeld 1972). Bodily exposure evokes discomfort. Given only a thin gown to wear, patients may be subjected to repeated examinations by doctors, nurses, and medical students. Exposure of the most private aspects of life can occur (Perry and Viederman 1981).

Beyond simple exposure, the medical environment often involves experiences of bodily invasion that are very stressful for the patient (Gazzola and Muskin 2003). From the more invasive experiences of a colonoscopy, the placement of a nasogastric tube, or tracheal intubation, to ostensibly more benign procedures such as a fine-needle biopsy of a breast lump or a rectal examination, the fear and discomfort of such interventions are often not fully recognized by the physician for whom such procedures have become routine.

Pain should not be overlooked as a profound stressor that should be dealt with aggressively (Heiskell and Pasnau 1991). Even the most highly adapted patient with effective coping skills and strong social support can be taxed to the limit by extreme pain.

Separation from family or friends produces isolation, disconnection, and stress (Heiskell and Pasnau 1991; Strain and Grossman 1975). This can precipitate conscious or unconscious fears of abandonment. **(pp. 47–48)**

Gazzola L, Muskin PR: The impact of stress and the objectives of psychosocial interventions, in Psychosocial Treatment for Medical Conditions: Principles and Techniques. Edited by Schein LA, Bernard HS, Spitz HI, et al. New York, Brunner-Routledge, 2003, pp 373–406

Heiskell LE, Pasnau RO: Psychological reaction to hospitalization and illness in the emergency department. Emerg Med Clin North Am 9:207–218, 1991

Kornfeld DS: The hospital environment: its impact on the patient. Adv Psychosom Med 8:252–270, 1972

Perry S, Viederman M: Management of emotional reactions to acute medical illness. Med Clin North Am 65:3–14, 1981

Strain JJ, Grossman S: Psychological reactions to medical illness and hospitalization, in Psychological Care of the Medically Ill: A Primer in Liaison Psychiatry. New York, Appleton-Century-Crofts, 1975, pp 23–36

4.2   Attachment theory provides fruitful way of examining patients' interactions with the health care setting and their physicians. Among the four predominant attachment styles described by Bartholomew and Horowitz (1991), which attachment style is believed to derive from early experiences with unresponsive caregivers, leading individuals to excessively value self-reliance and to have difficulty trusting others?

        A. Fearful attachment style.
        B. Dismissing attachment style.
        C. Secure attachment style.
        D. Preoccupied attachment style.
        E. Histrionic attachment style.

The correct response is option B.

The dismissing attachment style is thought to derive from early experiences with consistently unresponsive caregivers. As an adaptation to such an environment, these individuals come to dismiss their need for others, value being "self-reliant" to an extreme, and have difficulty trusting others.

Hostile, rejecting, or abusive caregiving early in life is thought to originate the fearful attachment style, characterized by negative views of self and others and a desire for support but fear of rejection and difficulty trusting others. These individuals often alternate between help-seeking and help-rejecting behaviors and frequently demand care but are often nonadherent and miss appointments.

The individual with a secure attachment style is hypothesized to have experienced consistently responsive caregiving in early life and therefore has a positive expectation of others and comfort in depending on others for care.

Inconsistently responsive caregiving is proposed as the environmental antecedent to a preoccupied attachment style, characterized by increased effort on the part of the individual to elicit caregiving and a positive expectation of others, with a negative view of self. These individuals may be particularly vulnerable to consciously or unconsciously exaggerated illness behavior or high medical use (Ciechanowski et al. 2002). **(p. 49)**

> Bartholomew K, Horowitz LM: Attachment styles among young adults: a test of a four-category model. J Pers Soc Psychol 61:226–244, 1991
> Ciechanowski PS, Walker EA, Katon WJ, et al: Attachment theory: a model for health care utilization and somatization. Psychosom Med 64:660–667, 2002

4.3   Kahana and Bibring's (1964) seven personality types can provide a useful framework for understanding a patient's response to medical illness. Which of the following is *not* one of these seven personality types?

        A. Dependent.
        B. Paranoid.
        C. Antisocial.
        D. Obsessional.
        E. Schizoid.

The correct response is option C.

Although the most accurate and complete understanding of personality may be achieved through a dimensional model, the characterization of discrete personality types is useful in highlighting differences and providing vivid prototypical examples. Much of the literature on personality types has been contributions by psychodynamic psychiatry. Although this rich literature continues to be tremendously useful for psychiatrists working in the medical setting, it is often ignored unfortunately because of the current emphasis on biological and descriptive psychiatry. Kahana and Bibring's (1964) classic and still relevant paper "Personality Types in Medical Management," described seven personality types: 1) dependent, 2) obsessional, 3) histrionic, 4) masochistic, 5) paranoid, 6) narcissistic, and 7) schizoid. Kahana and Bibring's paper is so valuable because of the rich descriptions of these various personality types and the manner in which each type determines the individuals' subjective experiences of the meaning of illness. **(pp. 49–50)**

> Kahana RJ, Bibring G: Personality types in medical management, in Psychiatry and Medical Practice in a General Hospital. Edited by Zinberg NE. New York, International Universities Press, 1964, pp 108–123

4.4   The personality type of a hospitalized patient may elicit various countertransferance responses from the treating physician. A physician notices that she feels little connection with a patient and finds the patient difficult to engage. Which of the following personality types might elicit this countertransference response?

   A. Masochistic.
   B. Histrionic.
   C. Paranoid.
   D. Narcissistic.
   E. Schizoid.

The correct response is option E.

A doctor may feel little connection with and find it difficult to engage a schizoid patient.

The masochistic patient usually produces anger, hate, and frustration in the physician, who also may feel helpless. The histrionic patient may produce anxiety and impatience in the physician or elicit erotic responses. The paranoid patient causes the doctor to feel angry, attacked, or accused. The narcissistic patient frequently produces anger and the desire to counterattack in the doctor, who also may feel inferior. **(pp. 51–54; Table 4–1)**

4.5   Folkman et al. (1986) identified various categories of coping styles used by people faced with stressful situations. A patient who appears to expend considerable effort on harnessing his feelings and trying to keep his family members from knowing how ill he is might be exhibiting which of the following coping styles?

   A. Escape-avoidance.
   B. Distancing.
   C. Positive reappraisal.
   D. Self-controlling.
   E. Planful problem solving.

The correct response is option D.

Folkman et al. (1986) identified eight categories of coping styles in a factor analysis of the Ways of Coping Questionnaire–Revised: 1) confrontative coping (hostile or aggressive efforts to alter a situation), 2) distancing (attempts to detach oneself mentally from a situation), 3) self-controlling (attempts to regulate one's feelings or actions), 4) seeking social support (efforts to seek emotional support or information from others), 5) accepting responsibility (acknowledgment of a personal role in the problem), 6) using escape-avoidance (cognitive or behavioral efforts to escape or avoid the problem or situation), 7) planful problem solving (deliberate and carefully thought-out efforts to alter the situation), and 8) conducting positive reappraisal (efforts to reframe the situation in a positive light) (Penley et al. 2002). Research has shown that patients use multiple coping strategies in any given situation (Lazarus 1999). Individuals often prefer or habitually use certain strategies over others, but generally multiple strategies are used for a complex stressful situation such as a medical illness or hospitalization. **(pp. 54–55)**

> Folkman S, Lazarus RS, Dunkel-Schetter C, et al: The dynamics of a stressful encounter: cognitive appraisal, coping, and encounter outcomes. J Pers Soc Psychol 50:992–1003, 1986
> Lazarus RS: Stress and Emotion: A New Synthesis. New York, Springer, 1999
> Penley JA, Tomaka J, Wiebe JS: The association of coping to physical and psychological health outcomes: a meta-analytic review. J Behav Med 25:551–603, 2002

4.6   Vaillant (1993) proposed a hierarchy of defense mechanisms based on how much each defense distorts reality and how effectively it allows expression of the individual's wishes or needs without causing untoward external consequences. Patients with personality disorders, especially the Cluster B disorders, usually employ which of the following types of defenses?

      A. Neurotic defenses.
      B. Immature defenses.
      C. Psychotic defenses.
      D. Mature defenses.
      E. Adaptive defenses.

The correct response is option B.

Vaillant (1993) proposed a hierarchy of defense mechanisms ranked in four levels of adaptivity: psychotic, immature (or borderline), neurotic, and mature. This hierarchy is based on the degree to which each defense distorts reality and how effectively it enables the expression of wishes or needs without untoward external consequences. Patients often use many different defense mechanisms in different situations or under varying levels of stress. When a patient inflexibly and consistently uses lower-level defenses, this is often consistent with a personality disorder.

The *immature defenses* are characteristic of patients with personality disorders, especially the Cluster B personality disorders such as borderline personality disorder. Vaillant (1993) emphasized how many of these defenses are irritating to others and get under other people's skin.

In contrast to the immature defenses, the *neurotic defenses* do not typically irritate others and are more privately experienced—they are less interpersonal and often involve mental inhibitions. They distort reality less than do immature or psychotic defenses and may go unnoticed by the observer.

The *psychotic defenses* are characterized by the extreme degree to which they distort external reality. Patients in psychotic states usually employ these defenses; psychotherapy is generally ineffective in altering them, and antipsychotic medication may be indicated.

The *mature defenses* "integrate sources of conflict…and thus require no interpretation" (Vaillant 1993, p. 67). The use of mature defenses such as humor or altruism in the confrontation of a stressor such as medical illness often earns admiration from others and can be inspirational. **(p. 56)**

Vaillant GE: The Wisdom of the Ego. Cambridge, MA, Harvard University Press, 1993

4.7   An oncologist asks you to evaluate a patient with terminal cancer because he is concerned that her calm acceptance of treatment, courageous good humor, and lack of expressed fears indicate that she is "in denial." What type of defense mechanism might this patient be exhibiting?

      A. Suppression.
      B. Psychotic denial.
      C. Repression.
      D. Intermediate denial.
      E. Intellectualization.

The correct response is option A.

Psychiatrists are often called to see a patient "in denial" about a newly diagnosed illness and may be asked to assess the patient's capacity to consent to or refuse certain treatments. Denial can be adaptive, protecting the patient from being emotionally overwhelmed by an illness, or maladaptive, preventing or delaying diagnosis, treatment, and lifestyle changes. The severity of denial varies by the nature of what is denied, by the predominant defense mechanisms at work (e.g., suppression, repression, psychotic denial), and by the degree of accessibility to consciousness (Goldbeck 1997). Patients who use the mature defense of *suppression* in confronting an illness are not truly in denial. Rather, they have chosen to put aside their fears about illness and treatment until a later time. Their fears are not deeply unconscious but are easily accessible if patients choose to access them. These patients typically accept treatment, face their illnesses with courage, and do not let their emotions overtake them. Such "denial" is considered adaptive (Druss and Douglas 1988).

In contrast to suppression, the patient using *repression* as a defense is generally unaware of the internal experience (e.g., fear, thought, wish) being warded off. Repressed thoughts or feelings are not easily accessible to consciousness. Such a patient may feel very anxious without understanding why. For example, a 39-year-old man whose father died of a myocardial infarction at age 41 may become increasingly anxious as his 40th birthday approaches without being aware of the connection.

When it is more severe and pervasive, denial can result in patients flatly denying they are ill and not seeking medical care. If they are already in care, they decline treatment or are nonadherent. Repeated attempts by the medical team to educate them about their illness have no effect. Extreme denial may be severe enough to distort the perception of reality, sometimes described as *psychotic denial.* **(pp. 56–58)**

Druss RG, Douglas CJ: Adaptive responses to illness and disability: healthy denial. Gen Hosp Psychiatry 10:163–168, 1988

Goldbeck R: Denial in physical illness. J Psychosom Res 43:575–593, 1997

Chapter 5

Delirium

Select the single best response for each question.

5.1 In the diagnosis of delirium, it is phenomenologically important to distinguish delirium from similar neuropsychiatric disorders with which delirium can merge in clinical practice. A condition in which the patient has an intact level of arousal, a normal sleep–wake cycle, but a complete absence of apparent "awareness" both of the self and of the environment is considered to be

A. Hypoactive delirium.
B. Hyperactive delirium.
C. Coma.
D. Minimally conscious state.
E. Vegetative state.

The correct response is option E.

Delirium is an alteration of consciousness graded along a continuum between normal at one end and stupor and coma at the other end. Delirium must be distinguished from other brain states in which consciousness is lost or even more grossly impaired. *Vegetative state* includes arousal and intact sleep–wake cycle, but with complete absence of awareness of self or environment due to a disconnection between higher cortical regions and the brain stem/diencephalic areas.

Coma and *stupor* entail loss of consciousness and complete failure of arousal, without an intact sleep–wake cycle. Precise delineation between severe hypoactive delirium and stupor can be difficult.

Minimally conscious state is characterized by partial preservation of consciousness and an intact sleep–wake cycle, but intention is absent, and there is inconsistent ability to follow commands, visually track, verbalize (intelligibly), or gesture (Giacino et al. 2002). **(p. 71)**

> Giacino JT, Ashwal S, Childs N, et al: The minimally conscious state: definition and diagnostic criteria. Neurology 58:349–353, 2002

5.2 Delirium is associated with increased medical and surgical morbidity and greater medical resource consumption. In the review of delirium risk by Saravay and Strain (1994) which of the following patient groups had the *lowest* increase in hospital length of stay as a result of delirium?

A. General medical patients.
B. Elderly patients.
C. Stroke patients.
D. Cardiac surgery patients.
E. Hip fracture patients.

The correct response is option D.

The Academy of Psychosomatic Medicine (APM) Task Force on Mental Disorders in General Medical Practice (Saravay and Strain 1994) reviewed studies finding that comorbid delirium increased hospital length of stay

100% in general medical patients (Thomas et al. 1988), 114% in elderly patients (Schor et al. 1992), 67% in stroke patients (Cushman 1988), 300% in critical care patients (Kishi et al. 1995), 27% in cardiac surgery patients, and 200%–250% in hip surgery patients (Berggren et al. 1987). The APM task force noted that delirium contributed to increased length of stay via medical and behavioral mechanisms, including the following: decreased motivation to participate in treatment and rehabilitation, medication refusal, disruptive behavior, incontinence and urinary tract infection, falls and fractures, and decubiti. **(pp. 75–76)**

Berggren D, Gustafson Y, Eriksson B, et al: Postoperative confusion after anesthesia in elderly patients with femoral neck fractures. Anesth Analg 66:497–504, 1987

Cushman LA: Secondary neuropsychiatric implications of stroke: implications for acute care. Arch Phys Med Rehabil 69:877–879, 1988

Kishi Y, Iwasaki Y, Takezawa K, et al: Delirium in critical care unit patients admitted through an emergency room. Gen Hosp Psychiatry 17:371–379, 1995

Saravay SM, Strain JJ: Academy of Psychosomatic Medicine Task Force on Funding Implications of Consultation-Liaison Psychiatry Outcome Studies. Special series introduction: a review of outcome studies. Psychosomatics 35:227–232, 1994

Schor JD, Levkoff SE, Lipsitz LA, et al: Risk factors for delirium in hospitalized elderly. JAMA 267:827–831, 1992

Thomas RI, Cameron DJ, Fahs MC: A prospective study of delirium and prolonged hospital stay. Arch Gen Psychiatry 45:937–940, 1988

5.3   Dementia is a well established risk factor for delirium. Which of the following dementia subtypes is considered to have a particularly high risk for the development of delirium?

    A. Alzheimer's disease of early onset.
    B. Alzheimer's disease of late onset.
    C. Dementia due to head trauma.
    D. Dementia due to hypothyroidism.
    E. Dementia due to Parkinson's disease.

The correct response is option B.

Up to two-thirds of the cases of delirium occur superimposed on preexisting cognitive impairment (Wahlund and Bjorlin 1999) which has been reported to increase risk ninefold, making it the strongest risk factor for prevalent delirium (Korevaar et al. 2005). The absence of dementia can be considered an important predictor of recovery (Cole et al. 2007). Delirium is 2.0–3.5 times more common in patients with dementia compared with control subjects without dementia (Erkinjuntti et al. 1986; Jitapunkul et al. 1992). Delirium risk appears to be greater in Alzheimer's disease of late onset and dementia of vascular origin as compared with other dementias, with this increased risk perhaps reflecting the relatively widespread neuronal disturbance associated with these conditions (Robertsson et al. 1998). **(p. 81)**

Cole M, McCusker J, Ciampi A, et al: An exploratory study of diagnostic criteria for delirium in older medical inpatients. J Neuropsychiatry Clin Neurosci 19:151–156, 2007

Erkinjuntti T, Wikström J, Parlo J, et al: Dementia among medical inpatients: evaluation of 2000 consecutive admissions. Arch Intern Med 146:1923–1926, 1986

Jitapunkul S, Pillay I, Ebrahim S: Delirium in newly admitted elderly patients: a prospective study. Q J Med 83:307–314, 1992

Korevaar JC, van Munster BC, de Rooij SE: Risk factors for delirium in acutely admitted elderly patients: a prospective cohort study. BMC Geriatr 5:6, 2005

Robertsson B, Blennow K, Gottfries CG, et al: Delirium in dementia. Int J Geriatr Psychiatry 13:49–56, 1998

Wahlund L, Bjorlin GA: Delirium in clinical practice: experiences from a specialized delirium ward. Dement Geriatr Cogn Disord 10:389–392, 1999

5.4 A clinically useful model for understanding and modifying delirium risk was described by Inouye and Charpentier (1996). This predictive model addresses both predisposing and precipitating factors in the development of delirium. According to this model, which of the following items is considered to be a *precipitating* factor?

  A. More than three medications added.
  B. Cognitive impairment before the development of delirium.
  C. Severe systemic illness.
  D. Dehydration.
  E. Visual impairment.

The correct response is option A.

Inouye and Charpentier (1996) developed a predictive model for delirium risk that included four predisposing factors (cognitive impairment, severe illness, visual impairment, dehydration) and five precipitating factors (more than three medications added, catheterization, use of restraints, malnutrition, and any iatrogenic event). These factors predicted a 17-fold variation in the relative risk of developing delirium. **(p. 81)**

> Inouye SK, Charpentier PA: Precipitating factors for delirium in hospitalized elderly persons: predictive model and interrelationships with baseline vulnerability. JAMA 275:852–857, 1996

5.5 While not routinely used in the majority of delirium cases, the electroencephalogram (EEG) is typically abnormal in delirium. Furthermore, the type of delirium may be associated with specific EEG findings. Which EEG pattern is suggestive of delirium tremens due to alcohol withdrawal?

  A. Bilateral diffuse slowing.
  B. Frontocentral spikes and polyspikes.
  C. Left or bilateral slowing or delta bursts.
  D. Generalized epileptiform activity.
  E. Low-voltage fast activity.

The correct response is option E.

Although generalized slowing is the typical EEG pattern for both hypoactive and hyperactive presentations of delirium and for most etiologies, delirium tremens is characterized by low-voltage fast activity (Kennard et al. 1945) that is superimposed on slow waves. **(p. 92)**

> Kennard MA, Bueding E, Wortis WB: Some biochemical and electroencephalographic changes in delirium tremens. Q J Stud Alcohol 6:4–14, 1945

5.6 The distinction between delirium and dementia is an important clinical decision, often made more complex by the high rates of comorbidity and the overlapping symptom profiles of these disorders of cognition. Which dementia type, characterized by fluctuations in symptoms, visual hallucinations, attention deficits, altered levels of consciousness, and delusions, can be particularly challenging to distinguish from delirium?

  A. Vascular dementia.
  B. Dementia due to Parkinson's disease.
  C. Dementia due to multiple sclerosis.
  D. Alzheimer's disease.
  E. Lewy body dementia.

The correct response is option E.

The most difficult differential diagnosis for delirium is dementia—the other cause of generalized cognitive impairment. Particularly challenging can be diagnosing dementia with Lewy bodies because it may mimic delirium with fluctuation of symptom severity, visual hallucinations, attentional impairment, alteration of consciousness, and delusions (Robinson 2002). Despite this substantial overlap, delirium and dementia can be reliably distinguished by a combination of careful history taking for symptom onset, examination of the patient, and selected clinical tests. Abrupt onset and fluctuating course are highly characteristic of delirium. In addition, level of consciousness and attention are markedly disturbed in delirium but remain relatively intact in uncomplicated dementia. **(p. 97)**

Robinson MJ: Probable Lewy body dementia presenting as delirium. Psychosomatics 43:84–86, 2002

5.7   Management of delirium routinely includes the use of antipsychotic medications. A serious side effect of many of these medications (particularly intravenous haloperidol) is prolonged QTc interval and torsade des pointes. Risk factors for antipsychotic-induced torsade des pointes include all of the following *except*

   A. Male gender.
   B. Heart disease.
   C. Hypokalemia.
   D. Higher antipsychotic doses.
   E. History of long QT syndrome.

The correct response is option A.

Cases of prolonged QTc interval and torsade de pointes (multifocal ventricular tachycardia) have been increasingly recognized and attributed to intravenously administered haloperidol, even in young patients, and therefore patients need to be monitored (Hatta et al. 2001; Kriwisky et al. 1990; Metzger and Friedman 1993; O'Brien et al. 1999; Perrault et al. 2000). Risk factors include female sex, heart disease, hypokalemia, higher doses of the offending agent, concomitant use of a QT-prolonging drug, and a history of long QT syndrome (Justo et al. 2005). **(p. 101)**

Hatta K, Takahashi T, Nakamura H, et al: The association between intravenous haloperidol and prolonged QT interval. J Clin Psychopharmacol 21:257–261, 2001

Justo D, Prokhorov V, Heller K, et al: Torsade de pointes induced by psychotropic drugs and the prevalence of its risk factors. Acta Psychiatr Scand 111:171–176, 2005

Kriwisky M, Perry GY, Tarchitsky D, et al: Haloperidol-induced torsades de pointes. Chest 98:482–484, 1990

Metzger E, Friedman R: Prolongation of the corrected QT and torsades de pointes cardiac arrhythmia associated with intravenous haloperidol in the medically ill. J Clin Psychopharmacol 13:128–132, 1993

O'Brien JM, Rockwood RP, Suh KI: Haloperidol-induced torsade de pointes. Ann Pharmacother 33:1046–1050, 1999

Perrault LP, Denault AY, Carrier M, et al: Torsades de pointes secondary to intravenous haloperidol after coronary artery bypass graft surgery. Can J Anaesth 47:251–254, 2000

Chapter 6

Dementia

Select the single best response for each question.

6.1 Which of the following statements regarding the epidemiology of dementia in the United States is *false?*

    A. The estimated prevalence rate for all dementias in the U.S. population older than 65 years is 19.8%.

    B. The incidence of dementia of the Alzheimer's type (DAT) is 56.1 per 1,000 person-years in the population older than 90 years.

    C. In one large-scale study, approximately 9.1% of patients 55 years and older who were admitted to a teaching hospital medical service had dementia.

    D. The prevalence of minor cognitive impairment in individuals 65 years or older ranges between 3% and 19%.

    E. Approximately one-third of patients referred to memory clinics have minor cognitive impairment.

The correct response is option A.

The adjusted prevalence estimate for all dementias in the U.S. population after age 65 years is 9.6% and for DAT is 6.5% (Breitner et al. 1999).

Incidence estimates of dementia show that DAT rates rise from 2.8 per 1,000 person-years (age group: 65–69 years) to 56.1 per 1,000 person-years (age group: older than 90 years) (Kukull et al. 2002).

Dementia is commonly found in general hospitals. A large-scale study documented that 9.1% of patients aged 55 years and older admitted to a teaching hospital medical service had dementia, but the prevalence was 31.2% in patients ages 85 years and older (Erkinjuntti et al. 1986).

The prevalence of minor cognitive impairment ranges between 3% and 19% in population studies in individuals age 65 years or older (Gauthier et al. 2006). It may account for more than one-third of the patients referred to memory clinics (Wahlund et al. 2003). **(p. 117)**

Breitner JC, Wyse BW, Anthony JC, et al: APOE-epsilon4 count predicts age when prevalence of AD increases, then declines: the Cache County Study. Neurology 53:321–331, 1999

Erkinjuntti T, Wikstrom J, Palo J, et al: Dementia among medical inpatients: evaluation of 2000 consecutive admissions. Arch Intern Med 146:1923–1926, 1986

Gauthier S, Reisberg B, Zaudig M, et al: Mild cognitive impairment. International Psychogeriatric Association Expert Conference on mild cognitive impairment. Lancet 367:1262-1270, 2006

Kukull WA, Higdon R, Bowen JD, et al: Dementia and Alzheimer disease incidence: a prospective cohort study. Arch Neurol 59:1737–1746, 2002

Wahlund LO, Pihlstrand E, Jonhagen ME: Mild cognitive impairment: experience from a memory clinic. Acta Neurol Scand Suppl 179:21–24, 2003

6.2 Which of the following is a confirmed protective factor for dementia of the Alzheimer's type (DAT)?

    A. Low cholesterol level.

    B. Aspirin use.

    C. Diet high in vitamin E and antioxidants.

    D. Apolipoprotein $\varepsilon2$ allele.

    E. Moderate alcohol consumption.

The correct response is option D.

The apolipoprotein ε2 allele is a confirmed protective factor for DAT. Low cholesterol levels, diets high in vitamin E and antioxidants, and moderate alcohol consumption are presumed protective, while aspirin has no protective effect. **(p. 119 [Table 6–4])**

6.3   A number of clinical characteristics differentiate cortical and subcortical dementia syndromes. Which of the following is indicative of subcortical dementia as opposed to cortical dementia?

   A. Aphasia.
   B. Agnosia.
   C. Apathy.
   D. Alexia.
   E. Apraxia.

The correct response is option C.

Apathy is a clinical characteristic of subcortical dementia. Other early characteristics are extrapyramidal signs, abnormal gait, psychomotor retardation, and the presence of affective syndromes. **(p. 122; Table 6–6)**

6.4   A 70-year-old male patient presents with parkinsonian features, fluctuating cognitive performance, hallucinations, and delusions. He also has a history of frequent falls and transient, unexplained episodes of loss of consciousness. Which of the following is the most likely diagnosis?

   A. Frontotemporal dementia.
   B. Parkinson's disease.
   C. Wilson's disease.
   D. Normal-pressure hydrocephalus.
   E. Dementia with Lewy bodies.

The correct response is option E.

Psychotic syndromes and confusional states are common in patients with dementia with Lewy bodies (DLB) and may be the presenting symptomatology. Other characteristics include relative preponderance of visuospatial and frontal lobe signs and clear day-to-day fluctuations in symptoms and cognitive performance. Parkinsonian features, together with fluctuation in cognitive performance, hallucinations, and delusions are core features for the diagnosis (McKeith et al. 2005). Patients who have DLB have frequent falls and/or transient, unexplained episodes of loss of consciousness. They have a characteristic vulnerability to neuroleptics, which frequently exacerbate extrapyramidal dysfunction.

The most characteristic features that distinguish frontotemporal dementia (FTD) from dementia of the Alzheimer's type (DAT) are personality changes and neuropsychiatric symptoms, which may be quite marked and precede the cognitive decline by several years. Psychiatric symptoms include marked irritability; poor judgment; defective control of impulses, including violent impulses in some cases; disinhibition; and a general disregard for the conventional rules of social conduct. Restlessness and hyperorality also have been reported. Social withdrawal or overt depression may be the first symptom in some patients.

A typical subcortical, progressive dementia syndrome may occur in patients with Parkinson's disease, and recent studies suggest it may eventually affect most patients (Aarsland et al. 2003). Classic parkinsonian signs in a patient with dementia point to the diagnosis. Apathy is particularly prominent and may advance to an akinetic mute state.

Subcortical dementia with characteristic extrapyramidal signs also may be seen in Wilson's disease. This combination of symptoms, together with onset during adolescence or early adulthood, should suggest the diagnosis. Cognitive deficits are usually mild, and psychosis is infrequent. However, depressive syndromes, irritability, disinhibition, personality changes, and poor impulse control are common, with the severity paralleling the severity of the neurological signs (Shanmugiah et al. 2008).

Normal-pressure hydrocephalus can present as a very characteristic neuropsychiatric syndrome, a triad of clinical symptoms combining motoric and psychopathological features (Folstein and McHugh 1983; McHugh 1966): 1) an early gait disturbance, resembling the stiff steps of spastic paraparesis; 2) subcortical dementia with particularly severe apathetic features; and 3) urinary incontinence that may not appear until late in the course. **(pp. 123–125)**

Aarsland D, Andersen K, Larsen JP, et al: Prevalence and characteristics of dementia in Parkinson disease: an 8-year prospective study. Arch Neurol 60:387–392, 2003

Folstein MF, McHugh PR: The neuropsychiatry of some specific brain disorders, in Handbook of Psychiatry 2, Mental Disorders and Somatic Illness. Edited by Lader MH. London, Cambridge University Press, 1983, pp 107–118

McHugh PR: Hydrocephalic dementia. Bull N Y Acad Med 42:907–917, 1966

McKeith IG, Dickson DW, Lowe J, et al: Diagnosis and management of dementia with Lewy bodies: third report of the DLB Consortium. Neurology 65:1863–1872, 2005

Shanmugiah A, Sinha S, Taly AB, et al. Psychiatric manifestations in Wilson's disease: a cross-sectional analysis. J Neuropsychiatry Clin Neurosci 20:81–85, 2008

6.5   Clinical characteristics suggestive of vascular dementia include all of the following *except*

   A. Gradual onset with a slow decline.
   B. Emotional lability.
   C. Uneven cognitive deterioration.
   D. Focal neurological signs and symptoms.
   E. Relative preservation of insight and judgment.

The correct response is option A.

The onset of vascular dementia is abrupt, not gradual. Other characteristics include uneven cognitive deterioration, relative preservation of insight and judgment, emotional incontinence and lability, history of strokes, history of cardiovascular risk factors, and focal neurological signs and symptoms. **(p. 125; Table 6–10)**

Chapter 7

Aggression and Violence

Select the single best response for each question.

7.1 The association of violence and psychiatric disorders has been the subject of various studies. However, not all psychiatric disorders confer the same risk of violence. In the study by Swanson et al. (1990), which of the following psychiatric disorders was associated with the *lowest* risk of violence?

   A. Anxiety disorders.
   B. Substance abuse.
   C. Substance dependence.
   D. Mood disorders.
   E. Schizophrenia.

The correct response is option A.

Violence is common among individuals with psychiatric disorders. A 1990 community-based study found that 55.5% of the respondents who reported violent behavior in the previous year had a psychiatric diagnosis, compared with 19.6% of the nonviolent respondents (Swanson et al. 1990). In that study, 8.9%–21.1% of the men and 3.3%–21.7% of the women who had a psychiatric diagnosis reported violent behavior, in contrast to 2.7% of the men and 1.1% of the women who did not have such diagnosis. The association was lowest for anxiety disorders and highest for substance use disorders, major affective disorders, and schizophrenia. **(p. 154)**

> Swanson JW, Holzer CE 3rd, Ganju VK, et al: Violence and psychiatric disorder in the community: evidence from the Epidemiologic Catchment Area surveys. Hosp Community Psychiatry 41:761–770, 1990

7.2 Aggressive behavior can be viewed as the product of an interaction between a *host* with a baseline propensity for aggression and specific provocations (*agents*) in particular contexts (*circumstances*). Within this framework, which of the following would be a *circumstance* associated with violence, rather than an *agent*?

   A. Threats by others.
   B. Misperceptions.
   C. Conflicts.
   D. Physical discomfort.
   E. Hospitalization for serious illness.

The correct response is option E.

The *host–agent–context* framework describes the setting and sequence of events leading to an episode of aggressive behavior, while simultaneously placing these events in the context of the specific circumstances and the individual's psychological assets and liabilities.

From a pathogenetic perspective, aggression is a heterogeneous behavior associated with genetic, familial, and social determinants. These include unfavorable prenatal, perinatal, and rearing experiences (such as childhood experience of neglect or abuse); genetic determinants; poor education; and negative cultural and peer influences (Volavka 1999). These factors, and others acquired, such as Axis I conditions, brain injury syndromes, and personality disorders, can be viewed as coalescing in the individual to yield a *host* with a baseline propensity for aggression that interacts with specific provocations (*agents*) and occurs in environments or *circumstances* to produce aggressive behaviors. Examples of *agents* include threats by others, misperceptions, conflicts, or physical discomfort. *Circumstances* are *contexts*, such as intense (or distant) interpersonal relationships, personal losses, or hospitalization for serious illness, that are captured in a narrative that reveals a vulnerable patient's maladaptive interactions with his or her environment.

This framework allows for enhanced understanding of any patient and his or her observed aggressive behavior. In some cases, an aggressive episode is the latest in a pattern of recurring impulsive, predatory, or pathological acts, which may (or may not) be associated with identifiable triggers, in an individual with cognitive or emotional vulnerabilities. In other cases, the act may be an easily discerned complication of the patient's primary condition or a not-so-surprising reaction to distressing circumstances. **(pp. 156–157)**

Volavka J: The neurobiology of violence: an update. J Neuropsychiatry Clin Neurosci 11:307–314, 1999

7.3 The prefrontal cortex is functionally implicated in the control of aggression and the maintenance of self-control and prosocial behavior. Patients with which of the following types of dementia characteristically exhibit disinhibited behavior, including impulsivity and aggressive outbursts?

    A. Parkinson's dementia.
    B. Vascular dementia.
    C. Lewy body dementia.
    D. Alzheimer's dementia.
    E. Frontotemporal dementia.

The correct response is option E.

The role of the prefrontal cortex in maintaining self-control and prosocial behavior has been recognized for more than a century and a half, ever since the classic case of Phineas Gage (Harlow 1848, 1868), who underwent a dramatic personality change (manifesting as a coarse manner, jocularity, impulsivity, and aggressive outbursts) after sustaining orbitofrontal cortical injury from a projectile. Patients who suffer frontotemporal dementia, a neurodegenerative condition characterized by focal degeneration of the frontal and temporal cortices, frequently manifest a similar phenotype. **(p. 157)**

Harlow JM: Passage of an iron rod through the head. Boston Med Surg J 39:389–393, 1848
Harlow JM: Recovery from the passage of an iron rod through the head. Publications of the Massachusetts Medical Society 2:327–347, 1868

7.4 Violence associated with personality disorders is best understood as being consistent with the patient's habitual range of behaviors. Which of the following personality disorders is most frequently associated with habitual aggression?

    A. Narcissistic personality disorder.
    B. Borderline personality disorder.
    C. Antisocial personality disorder.
    D. Schizoid personality disorder.
    E. Paranoid personality disorder.

The correct response is option C.

Violence associated with personality disorders is usually embedded in the individual's behavioral repertoire. Antisocial personality is most likely associated with habitual aggression. Antisocial individuals usually are thrill-seeking, have low frustration tolerance, and have high rates of substance abuse, criminal behavior, and violence. **(p. 161)**

7.5 Various substances of abuse are associated with violent behavior, with the effects usually mediated by the psychoactive properties of the particular substance. Which of the following substances is the *least* associated with violent behavior?

A. LSD.
B. Alcohol.
C. Cocaine.
D. Amphetamine.
E. Phencyclidine.

The correct response is option A.

Individuals who have taken lysergic acid diethylamide (LSD), ecstasy, or other hallucinogens are the least likely to engage in violent behavior.

Alcohol is the psychoactive substance most often associated with violence. Alcohol-related violence may result from a severely intoxicated state that produces gross impairment of self-restraint and judgment and/or a blackout. Pathological intoxication, which occurs in vulnerable individuals following the ingestion of only modest amounts of alcohol, may be associated with disorganized behavior, emotional lability, and violent outbursts. In severe cases, pathological intoxication may be accompanied by a delirium with hyperarousal, hallucinations, delusions, and terror, followed by amnesia for the event after recovery. Alcohol withdrawal also can be accompanied by irritability and low frustration tolerance, which predispose to directed aggression, or by seizures that are followed by aggression during a postictal state. Patients who develop delirium tremens may show poorly coordinated, resistive, or preemptive violence in response to hyperarousal, hallucinations, and terror.

Intoxication with other substances also can result in violence. Cocaine and amphetamine abuse is common and can produce impulsive, disinhibited intoxicated states during which violence may occur. Patients undergoing opioid, sedative, or cocaine withdrawal may experience anxious tension and irritability, during which interpersonal conflict or frustration may result in violent behavior. Although phencyclidine is not commonly abused, phencyclidine intoxication can manifest with severe impulsively directed violence. **(p. 162)**

7.6 A phenomenon that may link seizure disorder with violent behavior is postictal psychosis, which although usually transient may become persistent. Which of the following statements regarding postictal psychosis is *false*?

A. Symptoms of postictal psychosis may include mania or depression with mood-congruent psychosis.
B. Patients with postictal psychosis may manifest a formal thought disorder.
C. Patients with postictal psychosis may experience hallucinations.
D. Delusions in postictal psychosis are commonly of a paranoid nature.
E. Violence is less likely in postictal psychosis than in interictal psychosis or postictal confusion.

The correct response is option E.

Violence is more likely to occur in individuals with postictal psychosis, compared with those with interictal psychosis or postictal confusion (Kanemoto et al. 1999).

Postictal psychosis usually manifests as grandiose affective psychoses (mania or depression with mood-congruent psychotic phenomena) or with thought disorder, hallucinations, and paranoid ideational psychoses reminiscent of schizophrenia. Although usually transient (of no longer than several hours' duration), these states may last up to several weeks. Postictal psychosis has a tendency to recur and may become chronic. Violence in the context of postictal psychosis may be motivated by paranoid delusions and hallucinations, in which case it manifests as well-directed violence. Most episodes of postictal psychosis resolve spontaneously or following treatment with low doses of an antipsychotic, and improved control of the epilepsy then becomes the focus of treatment. However, some patients require chronic maintenance treatment with antipsychotics. **(p. 163)**

Kanemoto K, Kawasaki J, Mori E: Violence and epilepsy: a close relation between violence and postictal psychosis. Epilepsia 40:107–109, 1999

7.7   Dementia in elderly patients is unfortunately associated with aggressive behavior, which can complicate clinical management and may require changes in the care model and living arrangements. Which of the following aggressive behaviors is *less* common in elderly people with dementia?

   A. Throwing objects.
   B. Pushing and shoving.
   C. Kicking.
   D. Scratching.
   E. Goal-directed destruction of property.

The correct response is option E.

It is unusual for elderly persons with dementia to have well-coordinated and goal-directed physical aggression, but such violence does occur and can be serious, especially when committed by younger patients with dementia.

   In elders with dementia, aggression generally manifests as relatively simple behaviors such as throwing objects, pushing, shoving, kicking, pinching, biting, and scratching; destruction of property is uncommon (Cohen-Mansfield and Billig 1986). Impulsive, intrusive, aggressive sexual behaviors may be manifest, and intimacy-seeking sexual behaviors may also be complicated by reactive aggression when the patient is thwarted (de Medeiros et al. 2008). **(p. 164)**

Cohen-Mansfield J, Billig N: Agitated behaviors in the elderly, I: a conceptual review. J Am Geriatr Soc 34:711–721, 1986

de Medeiros K, Rosenberg PB, Baker AS, et al: Improper sexual behaviors in elders with dementia living in residential care. Dement Geriatr Cogn Disord 26:370–377, 2008

7.8   The psychosomatic medicine consultant is often called upon to offer psychopharmacological interventions for patients with a history of violent behavior. In the Citrome et al. (2001) randomized study comparing the anti-aggressive effects of various antipsychotics, which of the following agents was found to be most effective?

   A. Clozapine.
   B. Olanzapine.
   C. Risperidone.
   D. Haloperidol.
   E. Aripiprazole.

The correct response is option A.

In a randomized comparative study, clozapine was the most efficacious agent (independent of effectiveness in relieving psychosis); olanzapine, risperidone, and haloperidol were equal in effectiveness (Citrome et al. 2001). Although these results would seem to recommend clozapine as a first choice for treating aggression in psychotic patients, in practice, the drug is typically reserved for severe or treatment-resistant cases because of its adverse-effect profile. **(p. 169)**

Citrome L, Volavka J, Czobor P, et al: Effects of clozapine, olanzapine, risperidone, and haloperidol on hostility among patients with schizophrenia. Psychiatr Serv 52:1510–1514, 2001

Chapter 8

Depression

Select the single best response for each question.

8.1 It has been hypothesized that the prevalence of major depressive disorder (MDD) in medical settings increases progressively with the severity of the medical disease. What is the prevalence of MDD in patients hospitalized on an inpatient medical unit?

    A. 2%–4%.
    B. 6%–14%.
    C. 15%–20%.
    D. 21%–25%.
    E. 26%–31%.

The correct response is option B.

The prevalence of MDD in medical inpatient settings ranges from 6% to 14%.

Depressive disorders are extremely common in the general population, with up to 17% of adults in the United States having had at least one episode of major depressive disorder (MDD) during their lifetime (Kessler et al. 2003), and 2%–4% suffering from a current MDD (Burvill 1995). Medical illness has been consistently shown to be a risk factor for depression.

Presumably based on differences in medical disease severity, the prevalence of MDD has been found to increase progressively from community samples (2%–4%), to primary care settings (5%–10%), to medical inpatient settings (6%–14%) (Burvill 1995). Similarly, the risk of a depressive episode in patients in primary care (Barkow et al. 2002) and in the community (Wilhelm et al. 1999) rises with the number of comorbid medical diseases. **(p. 176)**

> Barkow K, Maier W, Ustun TB, et al: Risk factors for new depressive episodes in primary health care: an international prospective 12-month follow-up study. Psychol Med 32:595–607, 2002
> Burvill PW: Recent progress in the epidemiology of major depression. Epidemiol Rev 17:21–31, 1995
> Kessler RC, Berglund P, Demler O, et al: The epidemiology of major depressive disorder: results from the National Comorbidity Survey Replication (NCS-R). JAMA 289:3095–3105, 2003
> Wilhelm K, Parker G, Dewhurst-Savellis J, et al: Psychological predictors of single and recurrent major depressive episodes. J Affect Disord 54:139–147, 1999

8.2 Various approaches have been proposed to diminish the confounding effect of medical symptoms in the diagnosis of major depressive disorder (MDD). In one approach, symptoms that are more likely to be confused with medical illness, such as loss of energy, weight loss, and impaired concentration, are replaced by symptoms more likely to be affective in origin, such as irritability, tearfulness, social withdrawal, and feeling punished. What is this approach called?

    A. Exclusive.
    B. Etiological.
    C. Dimensional.
    D. Substitutive.
    E. Categorical.

The correct response is option D.

Various approaches have been proposed to diminish the confounding effect of medical symptoms in the diagnosis of MDD. In the "substitutive" approach (Endicott 1984), symptoms that are more likely to be affective in origin—such as irritability, tearfulness, social withdrawal, and feeling punished—are substituted for symptoms that are most likely to be confounded with the effects of medical illness, such as loss of energy, weight loss, and impaired concentration. This substitution eliminates the need to distinguish symptoms of medical illness from those of depression but may underestimate depression prevalence by excluding some somatic symptoms that are core manifestations of more severe forms of depression. Furthermore, the criteria to determine which symptoms should be substituted are not clearly established, and this approach has not been widely adopted.

DSM-IV-TR (American Psychiatric Association 2000) suggests a combined "exclusive" and "etiological" approach, which specifies exclusion of symptoms that are judged by the clinician to be etiologically related to a general medical condition or that are not more frequent in depressed than nondepressed patients (Bukberg et al. 1984). This approach is intended to avoid attributing symptoms of physical illness to a depressive syndrome, although the wording in DSM-IV-TR leaves unclear whether the exclusion applies only to the physiological consequences of the medical condition or also extends to psychological reactions to the condition (Koenig et al. 1997). In practice, the exclusive approach is usually applied only to the somatic symptoms of depression, although this does not take into account that depressed medical patients report significantly more physical symptoms than matched nondepressed medical patients (Simon and Von Korff 2006). In any case, the criteria for determining which symptoms are due to a medical illness and which are due to other factors unrelated to the medical illness are unclear. **(p. 178)**

American Psychiatric Association: Diagnostic and Statistical Manual of Mental Disorders, 4th Edition, Text Revision. Washington, DC, American Psychiatric Association, 2000

Bukberg J, Penman D, Holland JC: Depression in hospitalized cancer patients. Psychosom Med 46:199–212, 1984

Endicott J: Measurement of depression in patients with cancer. Cancer 53:2243–2249, 1984

Koenig HG, George LK, Peterson BL, et al: Depression in medically ill hospitalized older adults: prevalence, characteristics, and course of symptoms according to six diagnostic schemes. Am J Psychiatry 154:1376–1383, 1997

Simon GE, Von Korff M: Medical co-morbidity and validity of DSM-IV depression criteria. Psychol Med 36:27–36, 2006

8.3   Various rating scales have been developed to measure depressive symptoms in medically ill patients. One widely used self-report screening instrument was originally developed as a measure of symptom severity in psychiatric patients but has been used and found to be accurate in numerous studies of depression in the medically ill. What is the name of this instrument?

   A. Hospital Anxiety and Depression Scale (HADS).
   B. Patient Health Questionnaire Depression Module (PHQ-9).
   C. Center for Epidemiologic Studies Depression Scale (CES-D).
   D. Primary Care Evaluation of Mental Disorders (PRIME-MD).
   E. Beck Depression Inventory–II (BDI-II).

The correct response is option E.

The BDI-II is the most widely accepted measure of depressive distress. Originally developed as a measure of symptom severity in psychiatric patients, this 21-item self-report scale has been used in numerous studies of depression in the medically ill. Several studies evaluating the accuracy of the BDI-II as a screening instrument in medically ill samples found it to be an accurate self-report measure of depressive symptoms (Berard et al. 1998; Craven et al. 1987). The cutoff most commonly recommended in the medically ill is 15–16 (Berard et al. 1998).

The HADS is a 14-item self-report scale specifically designed for use in the medically ill, with separate 7-item subscales for anxiety and depression. The depression subscale emphasizes anhedonia and does not include somatic items. The HADS is highly acceptable to patients and has been extensively used in the medically ill (Herrmann 1997).

The CES-D Scale is a 20-item self-report measure of depressive symptoms, in which only 4 of the 20 items are somatic. Originally designed as a measure of depressive distress in nonpsychiatric community samples, it has also been extensively used in medically ill samples with evidence of good psychometric properties. A cutoff score of 17 was originally recommended to identify subjects with clinically significant depression (Radloff 1977), but the low positive predictive value of the CES-D suggests that it might be a better measure of general distress than of depression.

The PHQ-9 is the nine-item depression module of the PHQ, which is a self-administered version of the PRIME-MD, a freely available diagnostic instrument for common mental disorders specifically designed for use in primary care settings. When assessed against an independent structured interview performed by mental health professionals, a PHQ-9 score of 10 or greater had a sensitivity of 88% and a specificity of 88% for the diagnosis of major depressive disorder. PHQ-9 scores of 5, 10, 15, and 20 represented mild, moderate, moderately severe, and severe depression, respectively (Spitzer et al. 1999). **(pp. 180–182)**

Berard RM, Boermeester F, Viljoen G: Depressive disorders in an out-patient oncology setting: prevalence, assessment, and management. Psychooncology 7:112–120, 1998

Craven JL, Rodin GM, Johnson L, et al: The diagnosis of major depression in renal dialysis patients. Psychosom Med 49:482–492, 1987

Herrmann C: International experiences with the Hospital Anxiety and Depression Scale—a review of validation data and clinical results. J Psychosom Res 42:17–41, 1997

Radloff L: The CES-D Scale: a self-report depression scale for research in the general population. Appl Psychol Meas 1:385–401, 1977

Spitzer RL, Kroenke K, Williams JB: Validation and utility of a self-report version of PRIME-MD: the PHQ primary care study. Primary Care Evaluation of Mental Disorders. Patient Health Questionnaire. JAMA 282:1737–1744, 1999

8.4   The association of depression with specific medical diseases is of concern because of its impact on the treatment, course, and outcome of these conditions. Which of the following statements concerning depression and its treatment in patients with serious and chronic medical illnesses is *false*?

   A. Antidepressants and psychotherapeutic treatment of depression in cancer patients improve survival.
   B. The majority of trials of antidepressants and psychotherapeutic interventions have failed to demonstrate beneficial effects on cardiac outcomes.
   C. Depression in individuals with diabetes mellitus has been associated with poorer adherence to diabetic dietary and medication regimens.
   D. Depressive disorders in patients with Parkinson's disease are associated with increased impairment of cognitive function and lower perceived quality of life.
   E. Depressive symptoms in older adults have been associated with an increased risk for the development of mild cognitive impairment.

The correct response is option A.

Evidence that treatment of depression in cancer improves medical outcomes is limited. In a randomized controlled trial of a 6-month course of fluoxetine versus placebo in early-stage breast cancer patients undergoing adjuvant therapy, Navari et al. (2008) reported that fluoxetine reduced depressive symptoms, improved quality of life, and increased the percentage of patients who successfully completed adjuvant treatment. Studies have yet to be published on recurrence or survival rates associated with treatment of major depressive disorder. Although the question of whether psychotherapy can improve survival in cancer has been a hotly debated one

(Kraemer et al. 2009), the preponderance of the evidence demonstrates that the psychosocial interventions that are effective in reducing depressive symptoms do not confer a survival benefit in cancer (Kissane 2009).

Randomized trials of antidepressant treatment, such as the Sertraline AntiDepressant Heart Attack Randomized Trial (SADHART; Glassman et al. 2002), and the Myocardial INfarction and Depression—Intervention Trial (MIND-IT; van den Brink et al. 2002) failed to demonstrate a reduction in risk for cardiac events. Similarly, no beneficial effects on cardiac outcomes were found in studies of psychotherapeutic interventions such as the Montreal Heart Attack Readjustment Trial (MHART; Frasure-Smith 1995) and the Enhancing Recovery in Coronary Heart Disease Patients (ENRICHD; Berkman et al. 2003) trials. More recently, the first study to demonstrate a reduction in major adverse cardiac events (4% vs. 13%) in patients with acute coronary syndrome who were treated for depression was reported (Davidson et al. 2010). Unique aspects of this study were a flexible treatment model (in which patients could choose problem-solving therapy and/or antidepressants) and selection for persistent (>3 months) depression. A better understanding of the temporal and mechanistic relationships between depression and CAD will be crucial for the design of future trials in order to clarify potential medical effects of antidepressant treatment (Dickens et al. 2007).

Depression in individuals with diabetes mellitus is an important risk factor because it is associated with poorer adherence to the diabetic dietary and medication regimen and with poorer quality of life (Van Tilburg et al. 2001). Depression has also been associated with an increased risk of diabetes-related medical complications, including sexual dysfunction, retinopathy, nephropathy, heart disease, and stroke (de Groot et al. 2001), and with increased mortality (Milano and Singer 2007).

Depressive disorders in patients with Parkinson's disease have been associated with increased impairment of fine motor performance, decrements in cognitive function, and reduced perceived quality of life (McDonald et al. 2003).

In older adults, depressive symptoms have been associated with an increased risk for the development of mild cognitive impairment (Barnes et al. 2006). **(pp. 182–186)**

Barnes DE, Alexopoulos GS, Lopez OL, et al: Depressive symptoms, vascular disease, and mild cognitive impairment: findings from the Cardiovascular Health Study. Arch Gen Psychiatry 63:273–279, 2006

Berkman LF, Blumenthal J, Burg M, et al: Effects of treating depression and low perceived social support on clinical events after myocardial infarction: the Enhancing Recovery in Coronary Heart Disease Patients (ENRICHD) Randomized Trial. JAMA 289:3106–3116, 2003

Davidson KW, Rieckmann N, Clemow L, et al: Enhanced depression care for patients with acute coronary syndrome and persistent depressive symptoms: coronary psychosocial evaluation studies randomized controlled trial. Arch Intern Med 170:600–608, 2010

de Groot M, Anderson R, Freedland KE, et al: Association of depression and diabetes complications: a meta-analysis. Psychosom Med 63:619–630, 2001

Dickens C, McGowan L, Percival C, et al: Depression is a risk factor for mortality after myocardial infarction: fact or artifact? J Am Coll Cardiol 49:1834–1840, 2007

Frasure-Smith N: The Montreal Heart Attack Readjustment Trial (MHART). J Cardiopulm Rehabil 15:103–106, 1995

Glassman AH, O'Connor CM, Califf RM, et al: Sertraline treatment of major depression in patients with acute MI or unstable angina. JAMA 288:701–709, 2002

Kissane D: Beyond the psychotherapy and survival debate: the challenge of social disparity, depression and treatment adherence in psychosocial cancer care. Psychooncology 18:1–5, 2009

Kraemer HC, Kuchler T, Spiegel D: Use and misuse of the consolidated standards of reporting trials (CONSORT) guidelines to assess research findings: comment on Coyne, Stefanek, and Palmer (2007). Psychol Bull 135:173–178; discussion 179–182, 2009

McDonald WM, Richard IH, DeLong MR: Prevalence, etiology, and treatment of depression in Parkinson's disease. Biol Psychiatry 54:363–375, 2003

Milano AF, Singer RB: Mortality in comorbidity (II)—excess death rates derived from a follow-up study on 10,025 subjects divided into 4 groups with or without depression and diabetes mellitus. J Insur Med 39:160–166, 2007

Navari RM, Brenner MC, Wilson MN: Treatment of depressive symptoms in patients with early stage breast cancer undergoing adjuvant therapy. Breast Cancer Res Treat 112:197–201, 2008

van den Brink RH, van Melle JP, Honig A, et al: Treatment of depression after myocardial infarction and the effects on cardiac prognosis and quality of life: rationale and outline of the Myocardial INfarction and Depression—Intervention Trial (MIND-IT). Am Heart J 144:219–225, 2002

Van Tilburg MA, McCaskill CC, Lane JD, et al: Depressed mood is a factor in glycemic control in type 1 diabetes. Psychosom Med 63:551–555, 2001

8.5   Which of the following medications or medication classes have been shown in randomized controlled trials to be effective in treating depression in patients with medical illnesses such as cardiac disease, stroke, and cancer?

   A. Venlafaxine.
   B. Mirtazapine.
   C. Selective serotonin reuptake inhibitors (SSRIs).
   D. Bupropion.
   E. Duloxetine.

The correct response is option C.

SSRIs are generally regarded as first-line treatment in the management of depression in the medically ill because of their tolerability and relative safety. Randomized controlled trials have shown various SSRIs to be effective and safe in patients with cardiac disease (Glassman et al. 2002), stroke (Wiart et al. 2000), cancer (Pezzella et al. 2001), HIV infection (Rabkin et al. 1999), Alzheimer's disease (Lyketsos et al. 2000), multiple sclerosis (Mohr et al. 2001), and diabetes (Lustman et al. 2000).

Novel antidepressants such as venlafaxine, duloxetine, bupropion, and mirtazapine have become increasingly popular as alternatives to SSRIs in the medically ill, although there is little empirical evidence supporting their specific advantages in this population. **(pp. 186–187)**

Glassman AH, O'Connor CM, Califf RM, et al: Sertraline treatment of major depression in patients with acute MI or unstable angina. JAMA 288:701–709, 2002

Lustman PJ, Freedland KE, Griffith LS, et al: Fluoxetine for depression in diabetes: a randomized double-blind placebo-controlled trial. Diabetes Care 23:618–623, 2000

Lyketsos CG, Sheppard JM, Steele CD, et al: Randomized, placebo-controlled, double-blind clinical trial of sertraline in the treatment of depression complicating Alzheimer's disease: initial results from the Depression in Alzheimer's Disease study. Am J Psychiatry 157:1686–1689, 2000

Mohr DC, Goodkin DE, Islar J, et al: Treatment of depression is associated with suppression of nonspecific and antigen-specific T(H)1 responses in multiple sclerosis. Arch Neurol 58:1081–1086, 2001

Pezzella G, Moslinger-Gehmayr R, Contu A: Treatment of depression in patients with breast cancer: a comparison between paroxetine and amitriptyline. Breast Cancer Res Treat 70:1–10, 2001

Rabkin JG, Wagner GJ, Rabkin R: Fluoxetine treatment for depression in patients with HIV and AIDS: a randomized, placebo-controlled trial. Am J Psychiatry 156:101–107, 1999

Wiart L, Petit H, Joseph PA, et al: Fluoxetine in early poststroke depression: a double-blind placebo-controlled study. Stroke 31:1829–1832, 2000

Chapter 9

Suicidality

Select the single best response for each question.

9.1 Mann's (1998) diathesis–stress model of suicidal behavior is a useful clinical construct, wherein diathesis represents more long-standing components, while stress relates to more momentary circumstances. Suicidality is felt to result when an acute stress is "superimposed" on a suicide diathesis. Which of the following components would be considered a *stress* rather than a *diathesis* component of suicidal behavior?

    A. Genetic predisposition.
    B. Early life experiences.
    C. Chronic substance abuse.
    D. Family and social dynamics.
    E. Chronic illness.

The correct response is option D.

Noting that two groups of patients, each with the same severity of depressive illness, attempt suicide at different rates, Mann (1998), in his diathesis–stress model of suicidal behavior, proposed suicide diathesis components, including genetic predisposition, early life experience, chronic illness, chronic substance abuse, and certain dietary factors.

Extreme stress alone, which Mann defined as acute psychiatric illness, intoxication, medical illness, or family and social stresses, is not typically enough to invoke suicidal behavior. A suicidal individual already has the predisposition, or diathesis, on which the stress is superimposed, resulting in the suicide attempt. **(pp. 199–200)**

    Mann J: The neurobiology of suicide. Nat Med 4:25–30, 1998

9.2 Serotonin hypofunction has been correlated with suicidal behavior and has been proposed as a biological marker for suicide risk. Factors associated with lower serotonergic activity and greater suicide risk include all of the following *except*

    A. History of childhood abuse.
    B. Family history of depression.
    C. Substance abuse.
    D. High serum cholesterol.
    E. Traumatic brain injury.

The correct response is option D.

The search for possible biological markers for suicide has focused on the midbrain dorsal and median raphe nuclei, with their serotonergic inputs to the ventral prefrontal cortex. Responsible for dampening aggressive or impulsive behavior, the ventral prefrontal cortex exerts its inhibitory effects on suicidal behavior less effectively when serotonergic hypofunction occurs (Kamali et al. 2001). A history of child abuse, a familial depression history, substance abuse, head injury, genetic variants, and low cholesterol levels are all associated with both lower serotonergic activity and greater suicide risk (Mann 1998). **(p. 200)**

Kamali M, Oquendo M, Mann J: Understanding the neurobiology of suicidal behavior. Depress Anxiety 14:164–176, 2001

Mann J: The neurobiology of suicide. Nat Med 4:25–30, 1998

9.3   Kishi and Kathol (2002) described four "pragmatic reasons" for suicidal acts. Which of the following is *not* one of these four reasons?

   A. Despair at losing cognitive function in early dementia.
   B. Psychosis.
   C. Depression.
   D. Poor impulse control.
   E. Philosophical reasons.

The correct response is option A.

Kishi and Kathol (2002) identified four "pragmatic reasons" for suicidality: 1) psychosis, 2) depression, 3) poor impulse control, and 4) philosophical reasons. **(p. 201)**

Kishi Y, Kathol RG: Assessment of patients who attempt suicide. Prim Care Companion J Clin Psychiatry 4:132–136, 2002

9.4   An understanding of the epidemiology of suicide can be useful in clinical decision making. Which of the following statements regarding suicide rates is *true*?

   A. The known suicide rate today is at least 1.5 times the rate in 1900.
   B. Between 1990 and 2001, the suicide rate increased in every age category.
   C. The current suicide rate in the United States is approximately 20 per 100,000 population.
   D. Suicide is the third leading cause of death in 15- to 24-year-olds in the United States.
   E. Nonwhite Americans have twice the rate of suicide of white Americans.

The correct response is option D.

In 15- to 24-year-olds, suicide ranks behind only accidents and homicide as a leading cause of death (McIntosh 2009). The suicide rate among men is 3.8 times higher than among women.

   The known suicide rate today is nearly identical to what it was in 1900 (Monk 1987), but the epidemiology of suicide has been shifting over the past few decades. Between 1990 and 2001, suicide rates decreased in every age category, with the overall annual rate in the United States declining from 12.4 to 10.8 per 100,000. Over the most recent 5 years for which statistics are available, however, the rate has ticked up in several age groups, as has the overall rate to 11.1 per 100,000. Nonwhite Americans killed themselves in 2006 at less than half the rate of white Americans (McIntosh 2009). **(p. 201)**

McIntosh J: U.S.A. Suicide: Suicide Data, 2006. Washington, DC, American Association of Suicidology, 2009

Monk M: Epidemiology of suicide. Epidemiol Rev 9:51–69, 1987

9.5   Findings from the Misono et al. (2008) study of suicide risk in cancer patients included all of the following *except*

   A. The standardized mortality ratio of suicide in cancer patients was 1.9 relative to the general population.
   B. The highest suicide rate reported was for cancers of the larynx (5.75).
   C. Older white male cancer patients were at especially high risk for suicide.
   D. Suicide risk was highest in the first 5 years after diagnosis of cancer.
   E. Cancer patients continued to have an elevated suicide risk 15 years after their diagnosis.

The correct response is option B.

In the Misono et al. (2008) study, the highest rate of suicide was reported for lung and bronchial (standardized mortality ratio [SMR] = 5.74), stomach (SMR = 4.68), oral–pharyngeal (SMR = 3.66), and laryngeal cancer (SMR = 2.83).

Recent populations studies replicate what has been known for decades: cancer patients have an elevated suicide risk relative to the general population. In a U.S. cohort of nearly 3.6 million individuals diagnosed with cancer between 1973 and 2002, the SMR for suicide was 1.9 relative to the general population.

As in the general population, aged white men with cancer were at particularly high risk. The first 5-year period after diagnosis was the time of highest risk, although elevated risk persisted after 15 years (Misono et al. 2008). **(p. 207)**

Misono S, Weiss NS, Fann JR, et al: Incidence of suicide in persons with cancer. J Clin Oncol 26:4731–4738, 2008

9.6   In a recent survey by Ganzini et al. (2009) of patients' motivations for seeking physician-assisted death (PAD), the reason most commonly cited was

   A. Desire to control timing of death and to avoid loss of independence.
   B. Concerns about future unbearable pain.
   C. Worry about compromised quality of life.
   D. Limited social support.
   E. Current physical and mental symptoms.

The correct response is option A.

Recent work by Ganzini et al. (2009) contradicts the notion that present physical discomfort or interpersonal issues drive patients' interest in PAD. In this survey of 56 Oregonians who had expressed interest in physician-assisted suicide at end of life, the most important motivations were desire to control the timing and location of death and desire to avoid loss of independence. Worries about future pain, compromised quality of life, and dependence on others for care came next. Least important were limited supports or current physical or mental symptoms. The overall portrait of a typical PAD requester was of a rugged individualist determined to be in charge of his or her destiny, even unto the moment of death. **(p. 212)**

Ganzini L, Goy E, Dobscha S: Oregonians' reasons for requesting physician aid in dying. Arch Intern Med 169:489–492, 2009

Chapter 10

Psychosis, Mania, and Catatonia

Select the single best response for each question.

10.1 Hallucinations are a hallmark of a psychotic disorder due to a medical condition. A visually impaired patient who remains aware of the abnormal nature of his hallucinations, and as a result is hesitant to divulge information about them, is likely experiencing which of the following?

   A. Hypnopompic hallucinations.
   B. Peduncular hallucinosis.
   C. Pseudohallucinations.
   D. Functional hallucinations.
   E. Hypnagogic hallucinations.

The correct response is option C.

Hallucinations can occur in any sensory modality. If patients retain their insight into the abnormal nature of their hallucinations, the term *pseudohallucinations* is sometimes used (Berrios and Dening 1996). A good example of hallucinations that occur in patients who remain insightful (and as a consequence hesitant to divulge information about the experience unless specifically asked for fear of being labeled as insane) is the Charles Bonnet syndrome (Menon 2005), in which generally pleasant, complex visual hallucinations occur in visually impaired individuals who are cognitively intact.

Another example of complex visual hallucinations is *peduncular hallucinosis*, in which vivid, scenic images can emerge after focal damage to the thalamus or mesencephalic structures (Benke 2006; Mocellin et al. 2006). Some hallucinations occur only under very specific conditions. For example, auditory hallucinations heard only when the air conditioner is running are called *functional hallucinations*. *Hypnagogic* or *hypnopompic hallucinations* occur only in the transition to sleep or awakening, respectively. **(p. 220)**

> Benke T: Peduncular hallucinosis: a syndrome of impaired reality monitoring. J Neurol 253:1561–1571, 2006
> Berrios GE, Dening TR: Pseudohallucinations: a conceptual history. Psychol Med 26:753–763, 1996
> Menon GJ: Complex visual hallucinations in the visually impaired: a structured history-taking approach. Arch Ophthalmol 123:349–355, 2005
> Mocellin R, Walterfang M, Velakoulis D: Neuropsychiatry of complex visual hallucinations. Aust N Z J Psychiatry 40:742–751, 2006

10.2 Delusions are often classified by their content and style. A syndrome in which the patient believes that a family member or close friend has been replaced by an exact double is called

   A. Othello syndrome.
   B. Ganser syndrome.
   C. Charles Bonnet syndrome.
   D. Capgras' delusion.
   E. Cotard's syndrome.

The correct response is option D.

The presence of a belief in duplicates and replacements is typical for a group of delusions known as delusional misidentification syndromes (Weinstein 1994). For example, in the Capgras' delusion, a patient believes that a family member or close friend has been replaced by an exact double.

Some delusional syndromes are best known by their eponyms such as the delusions of infidelity (Othello syndrome) or delusions of nihilism (Cotard's syndrome) (Freudenreich 2007). As with hallucinations, however, the type of delusion lacks diagnostic specificity. For example, although the morbid jealousy in the Othello syndrome is traditionally associated with male alcoholic patients, it can occur as both a primary psychiatric disorder and a manifestation of organic etiology (Yusim et al. 2008). **(p. 220)**

Freudenreich O: Psychotic Disorders: A Practical Guide. Baltimore, MD, Lippincott Williams & Wilkins, 2007
Weinstein EA: The classification of delusional misidentification syndromes. Psychopathology 27:130–135, 1994
Yusim A, Anbarasan D, Bernstein C, et al: Normal pressure hydrocephalus presenting as Othello syndrome: case presentation and review of the literature. Am J Psychiatry 165:1119–1125, 2008

10.3 A form of catatonia characterized by fever, autonomic dysfunction with tachycardia and elevated blood pressure, rigidity, mutism, and stupor is called

    A. Catatonic withdrawal.
    B. Neuroleptic malignant syndrome (NMS).
    C. Catatonic excitement.
    D. Lethal catatonia.
    E. Malignant catatonia.

The correct response is option B.

NMS is a form of malignant catatonia characterized by fever, autonomic dysfunction with tachycardia and elevated blood pressure, rigidity, mutism, and stupor. NMS usually develops over the course of a few days (Caroff 1980; Mann and Caroff 1990). It commonly begins with rigidity and mental status changes, followed by signs of a hypermetabolic state. Hyperthermia, which can climb to higher than 42°C, is reported in 98% of the cases. The patient with NMS may be alert, delirious, stuporous, or comatose.

Catatonic withdrawal, with posturing, rigidity, mutism, and repetitive actions, is the most commonly recognized form of *catatonia*, occasionally referred to as the "Kahlbaum syndrome" (Fink and Taylor 2009). Patients with severe catatonia will be stuporous and may even present with low Glasgow Coma Scale scores. However, patients also can present with hyperactivity, hyperproductive pressured speech, and restless, agitated behavior accompanied by catatonic features (bizarre stereotypies, mannerisms, grimacings, echo phenomena, perseverations) and an acute confusional state.

Catatonic excitement has at times been called "delirious mania" or "Bell's mania" (Bell 1849; Fink 1999).

In 1934, Stauder described a syndrome of "lethal catatonia." It was marked by the acute onset of a manic delirium, high fever, and catatonic stupor and a mortality rate of greater than 50%. Because not all cases are lethal, Philbrick and Rummans (1994) suggested the term *malignant catatonia* to describe critically ill cases marked by autonomic instability or hyperthermia, in contrast to cases of "simple, nonmalignant catatonia." **(pp. 230–231)**

Bell L: On a form of disease resembling some advanced stages of mania and fever. Am J Insanity 6:97–127, 1849
Caroff S: The neuroleptic malignant syndrome. J Clin Psychiatry 41:79–83, 1980
Fink M: Delirious mania. Bipolar Disord 1:54–60, 1999
Fink M, Taylor MA: The catatonia syndrome: forgotten but not gone. Arch Gen Psychiatry 66:1173–1177, 2009
Mann S, Caroff SN: Lethal catatonia and the neuroleptic malignant syndrome, in Psychiatry: A World Perspective. Edited by Stefanis C, Soldatos C, Rambazilas A. Amsterdam, The Netherlands, Elsevier Science, 1990, pp 287–292
Philbrick K, Rummans T: Malignant catatonia. J Neuropsychiatry Clin Neurosci 6:1–13, 1994
Stauder K: Die tödliche Katatonie. Arch Psychiatry Nervenkr 102:614–634, 1934

10.4 The modified Bush-Francis Catatonia Rating Scale (BFCRS) is commonly used to evaluate the signs and symptoms of catatonia. According to symptom definitions provided in this instrument, motor activity that is perseverative, non-goal-directed, and not inherently abnormal, such as playing with fingers, is called

    A. Stereotypy.
    B. Mannerisms.
    C. Negativism.
    D. *Mitgehen.*
    E. Excitement.

The correct response is option A.

As defined in the modified BFCRS (Bush et al. 1996; Fricchione et al. 2004), *stereotypy* is a perseverative, non-goal-directed, not inherently abnormal motor activity (e.g., playing with fingers, or repetitively touching, patting, or rubbing oneself). *Mannerisms* are bizarre, inherently abnormal movements (e.g., hopping or walking on tiptoe, saluting those passing by, or exaggerating caricatures of mundane movements). *Negativism* is a seemingly motiveless resistance to instructions or attempts to move or examine the patient; patient does the exact opposite of the instruction. *Mitgehen* is an exaggerated arm raising in response to light pressure of finger, despite instructions to the contrary; like an "Anglepoise lamp." *Excitement* is severe hyperactivity, and constant motor unrest, which is manifestly purposeless (not to be attributed to akathisia or goal-directed agitation). **(p. 231; Table 10–5)**

> Bush G, Fink M, Petrides G, et al: Catatonia, I: rating scale and standardized examination. Acta Psychiatr Scand 93:129–136, 1996
>
> Fricchione GL, Huffman JC, Stern TA, et al: Catatonia, neuroleptic malignant syndrome, and serotonin syndrome, in Massachusetts General Hospital Handbook of General Hospital Psychiatry, 5th Edition. Edited by Stern TA, Fricchione GL, Cassem NH, et al. Philadelphia, PA, Mosby/Elsevier, 2004, pp 513–530

10.5 Which of the following medications has been found to be most effective in the treatment of catatonia?

    A. Selective serotonin reuptake inhibitors.
    B. Beta-blockers.
    C. Second-generation antipsychotics.
    D. Mood stabilizers.
    E. Benzodiazepines.

The correct response is option E.

Catatonia, when properly treated, typically resolves completely, but an underlying psychosis will often remain. Benzodiazepines and electroconvulsive therapy (ECT) are the most frequently recommended treatments. Bush et al. (1996) in an open trial with 13 acutely catatonic patients reported that 2 mg of intravenous lorazepam reduced catatonia scores on the Bush-Francis Catatonia Rating Scale (BFCRS) by 60% within 10 minutes. Although no published randomized controlled trials for acute catatonia are available, many case series and prospective open trials over the past 20 years with parenteral or oral benzodiazepines (such as lorazepam) showed a response rate of 60%–80% within hours or days (Rosebush and Mazurek 2004). Given the consistent benefit with low risk in these studies along with extensive clinical experience, a benzodiazepine given parenterally has been advocated as appropriate initial treatment for catatonia (Bush et al. 1996; Rosebush and Mazurek 2004). Arguments favoring benzodiazepines include familiarity in contemporary psychiatric practice, a favorable therapeutic index, and the availability of flumazenil, a specific antagonist for benzodiazepines. It is of interest that flumazenil reversed the benefit of lorazepam in a case of catatonia (Wetzel et al. 1987). Initial dosages of 2–6 mg/day of lorazepam by any route of administration are recommended, but some patients may require higher doses. **(p. 235)**

Bush G, Fink M, Petrides G, et al: Catatonia, II: treatment with lorazepam and electroconvulsive therapy. Acta Psychiatr Scand 93:137–143, 1996

Rosebush P, Mazurek M: Pharmacotherapy, in Catatonia: From Psychopathology to Neurobiology. Edited by Caroff SN, Mann SC, Francis A, et al. Washington, DC, American Psychiatric Publishing, 2004, pp 141–150

Wetzel H, Heuser I, Benkert O: Stupor and affective state: alleviation of psychomotor disturbances by lorazepam and recurrence of symptoms after Ro 15-1788. J Nerv Ment Dis 175:240–242, 1987

Chapter 11

Anxiety Disorders

Select the single best response for each question.

11.1   Anxiety symptoms are common in medical patients; for this reason, it is a good clinical practice to use validated screening instruments to assist in the identification of anxiety disorder cases. The Generalized Anxiety Disorder–7 (GAD-7) scale is an effective screen for all of the following anxiety disorders *except*

    A. Generalized anxiety disorder (GAD).
    B. Panic disorder.
    C. Posttraumatic stress disorder (PTSD).
    D. Obsessive-compulsive disorder (OCD).
    E. Social phobia.

The correct response is option D.

A 7-item anxiety screen, the Generalized Anxiety Disorder (GAD)-7 scale, has been reported to be an effective screen for GAD, panic, PTSD, and social phobia (Kroenke et al. 2007), but not for OCD. **(p. 241)**

> Kroenke K, Spitzer RL, Williams JB, et al: Anxiety disorders in primary care: prevalence, impairment, comorbidity, and detection. Ann Intern Med 146:317–325, 2007

11.2   Posttraumatic stress disorder (PTSD) has a higher prevalence in medical/surgical settings than in the general population. Findings from studies of PTSD in medical settings have included all of the following *except*

    A. PTSD has been reported in 20%–45% of burn patients.
    B. Approximately one-third of motor vehicle accident victims reported PTSD symptoms.
    C. Patients with stimulant intoxication reported higher PTSD symptom levels.
    D. Female trauma patients had more PTSD symptoms than male patients.
    E. In patients with implanted cardioverter defibrillators, PTSD was associated with greater morbidity but not greater mortality.

The correct response is option E.

In one recent study of patients with an implanted cardioverter defibrillator, high levels of PTSD symptoms were associated with increased mortality over an average of 5 years of follow-up (Ladwig et al. 2008).

It is not surprising that PTSD symptoms are common among individuals who experience acute physical traumas. For example, burn victims have been reported to have PTSD at rates ranging from 20% to 45% (Difede et al. 2002; McKibben et al. 2008; Yu and Dimsdale 1999). In one study, 30%–40% of survivors of a motor vehicle crash or an assault reported PTSD symptoms for months after the trauma. Higher symptom levels were associated with female gender, stimulant intoxication, and greater prior trauma (Zatzick et al. 2002). **(p. 243)**

> Difede J, Ptacek JT, Roberts J, et al: Acute stress disorder after burn injury: a predictor of posttraumatic stress disorder? Psychosom Med 64:826–834, 2002

Ladwig KH, Baumert J, Marten-Mittag B, et al: Posttraumatic stress symptoms and predicted mortality in patients with implantable cardioverter-defibrillators: results from the prospective living with an implanted cardioverter-defibrillator study. Arch Gen Psychiatry 65:1324–1330, 2008

McKibben JB, Bresnick MG, Wiechman Askay SA, et al: Acute stress disorder and posttraumatic stress disorder: a prospective study of prevalence, course, and predictors in a sample with major burn injuries. J Burn Care Res 29:22–35, 2008

Yu BH, Dimsdale JE: Posttraumatic stress disorder in patients with burn injuries. J Burn Care Rehabil 20:426–433, 1999

Zatzick DF, Kang SM, Muller HG, et al: Predicting posttraumatic distress in hospitalized trauma survivors with acute injuries. Am J Psychiatry 159:941–946, 2002

11.3 Given the often life-threatening nature of the illness, it is not surprising that posttraumatic stress disorder (PTSD) has been reported in patients being treated for cancer. In this context, which of the following variables is *not* associated with a greater risk of PTSD?

    A. Past psychological trauma.
    B. Severity of the cancer.
    C. Prior psychiatric illness.
    D. Lower levels of social support.
    E. Other recent psychosocial stressors.

The correct response is option B.

Severity of cancer is not a strong predictor of the development of PTSD.

The likelihood of developing PTSD symptoms after cancer treatment has been shown to be increased among individuals with past trauma, prior psychiatric diagnoses, lower levels of social support, and recent life stressors (Green et al. 2000; Jacobsen et al. 2002). **(p. 243)**

Green BL, Krupnick JL, Rowland JH, et al: Trauma history as a predictor of psychologic symptoms in women with breast cancer. J Clin Oncol 18:1084–1093, 2000

Jacobsen PB, Sadler IJ, Booth-Jones M, et al: Predictors of posttraumatic stress disorder symptomatology following bone marrow transplantation for cancer. J Consult Clin Psychol 70:235–240, 2002

11.4 One of the prototypical models in psychosomatic medicine is the relationship between thyroid disease and many psychiatric disorders, notably anxiety disorders. In regard to this relationship, which of the following statements is *false?*

    A. Anxiety due to hyperthyroidism is accompanied by persistent tachycardia.
    B. Anxiety due to hyperthyroidism is associated with cold, "clammy" palms.
    C. Complaints of fatigue are associated with a desire to be active.
    D. Hyperthyroidism is associated with cognitive impairment as well as anxiety.
    E. Anxiety treatment should be instituted while hyperthyroidism is treated medically.

The correct response is option B.

Anxiety symptoms commonly occur among individuals with thyroid disease. Patients with subclinical and clinical hyperthyroidism have been shown to have elevated anxiety levels (Gulseren et al. 2006; Sait Gönen et al. 2004). Hyperthyroidism may be difficult to distinguish from a primary anxiety disorder.

Signs that may be suggestive of thyrotoxicosis include persistent tachycardia, palms that are warm and dry (not cold and clammy), and fatigue accompanied by the desire to be active (Colon and Popkin 2002). Some individuals with hyperthyroidism also may have cognitive impairment. Improvement in anxiety usually parallels successful treatment of the hyperthyroidism. Therefore, specific antianxiety treatment may not be necessary.

Nonetheless, antianxiety treatment should be considered during normalization of thyroid hormone levels, particularly for individuals with moderate to severe symptoms. Beta-blockers, which are used routinely for acute treatment of hyperthyroidism, will relieve peripheral manifestations of anxiety. **(pp. 246–249)**

Colon EA, Popkin MK: Anxiety and panic, in The American Psychiatric Publishing Textbook of Consultation-Liaison Psychiatry, 2nd Edition. Edited by Wise MG, Rundell JR. Washington, DC, American Psychiatric Publishing, 2002, pp 393–415

Gulseren S, Gulseren L, Hekimsoy Z, et al: Depression, anxiety, health-related quality of life, and disability in patients with overt and subclinical thyroid dysfunction. Arch Med Res 37:133–139, 2006

Sait Gönen M, Kisakol G, Savas Cilli A, et al: Assessment of anxiety in subclinical thyroid disorders. Endocr J 51:311–315, 2004

11.5 Yalom (1980) has written on the phenomenon of death anxiety in the context of life-threatening and/or terminal illness. Which of the following statements regarding the management of death anxiety is *false?*

   A. Open, frank discussions about death should be avoided, as they increase anxiety and distress.
   B. Maintenance of hope is important in managing death anxiety.
   C. Therapy goals for death anxiety may target accomplishment of specific short-term goals rather than attainment of full recovery.
   D. Helping patients find meaning despite their suffering is an important therapy goal.
   E. Placing emphasis on the importance of patients to their families may decrease anxiety.

The correct response is option A.

Patients confronting life-threatening or terminal illnesses such as cancer may experience death anxiety (Yalom 1980). Open discussions with patients about death help to reduce anxiety and distress (Spiegel et al. 1981), and psychological interventions alone can help patients manage their death anxiety (Payne and Massie 2000).

Maintaining hope is an important aspect of minimizing anxiety, although goals can change from full recovery to having more time to accomplish specific short-term goals. Helping patients find meaning and value in their lives, despite their illness and suffering, helps to relieve emotional distress (Frankl 1987). For example, anxiety can be reduced when patients see that they are still important to their families or that they still have unfinished business to address. **(p. 250)**

Frankl V: Man's Search for Meaning. London, Hoddard-Stoughton, 1987

Payne D, Massie MJ: Anxiety in palliative care, in Handbook of Psychiatry in Palliative Medicine. Edited by Chochinov HM, Breitbart W. New York, Oxford University Press, 2000, pp 63–74

Spiegel D, Bloom J, Yalom I: Group support for patients with metastatic cancer. Arch Gen Psychiatry 38:527–533, 1981

Yalom I: Death and Dying. New York, Basic Books, 1980

11.6 The pharmacological management of anxiety is an important intervention in psychosomatic medicine. However, pharmacological agents delivered in the context of systemic illness need to be chosen carefully. Which benzodiazepine has the advantages of oral, intravenous, or intramuscular administration; a conjugation metabolism; and no active metabolite?

   A. Alprazolam.
   B. Oxazepam.
   C. Lorazepam.
   D. Temazepam.
   E. Midazolam.

The correct response is option C.

Because lorazepam can be given orally, intravenously, or intramuscularly and does not have an active metabolite, it is often a preferred medication in hospitalized patients. Lorazepam can be given in an intravenous bolus or drip, but as doses increase to provide sedation and treat delirium tremens, respiratory status must be watched closely. Lorazepam and oxazepam are metabolized through conjugation, and temazepam is metabolized almost exclusively through conjugation (Trevor and Way 2007). As a result, those benzodiazepines may be less problematic in patients with liver disease than are the other benzodiazepines, which are oxidatively metabolized (Crone et al. 2006).

Alprazolam works rapidly and is eliminated quickly, but as a result there may be rebound anxiety and withdrawal symptoms.

Midazolam, a benzodiazepine with a very short half-life that can only be given intravenously or intramuscularly, is used for short-term procedures such as bone marrow biopsies, endoscopies, and magnetic resonance imaging scans in claustrophobic patients. **(p. 251)**

Crone CC, Gabriel GM, DiMartini A: An overview of psychiatric issues in liver disease for the consultation-liaison psychiatrist. Psychosomatics 47:188–205, 2006

Trevor AJ, Way WL: Sedative-hypnotic drugs, in Basic and Clinical Pharmacology, 10th Edition. Edited by Katzung BG. New York, McGraw-Hill, 2007, pp 347–362

Chapter 12

Somatization and Somatoform Disorders

Select the single best response for each question.

12.1 Etiological factors posited to contribute to the development of somatization and somatoform disorders include all of the following *except*

    A. Childhood exposure to parental chronic illness.
    B. Negative affectivity.
    C. Alexithymia.
    D. Sexual or physical abuse.
    E. Anger or hostility.

The correct response is option E.

Although repressed anger or aggression was thought by classical psychodynamic theorists to be important, Kellner et al. (1985) found no evidence that anger or hostility plays a specific etiological role in somatization and hypochondriasis.

The cognitive appraisals patients make of somatic symptoms often have some of their roots in early family experiences. Childhood exposure to parental chronic illness or abnormal illness behavior appears to increase the risk of somatization in later life (Bass and Murphy 1995; Craig et al. 1993; Gilleland et al. 2009).

Negative affectivity, a construct based on negative mood, poor self-concept, and pessimism, is also considered an important contributor to somatization (De Gucht et al. 2004) and was found to be a prospective predictor of somatization among victims of acute trauma (Elklit and Christiansen 2009).

Alexithymia refers to impairment in the ability to verbalize affect and elaborate fantasies that results from deficits in the cognitive processing and regulation of emotions (Taylor 2000). It has been implicated as a mechanism of some forms of somatization.

Sexual and physical abuse, in both childhood and adulthood, have been linked with somatization, medically unexplained symptoms, and somatoform disorders in numerous studies since the late 1980s. The mechanisms by which physical and sexual trauma is associated with somatization are poorly understood. **(pp. 266–267)**

Bass C, Murphy M: Somatoform and personality disorders; syndromal comorbidity and overlapping developmental pathways. J Psychosom Res 39:403–427, 1995

Craig TK, Boardman AP, Mills K, et al: The South London somatisation study, I: longitudinal course and the influence of early life experiences. Br J Psychiatry 163:579–588, 1993

De Gucht V, Fischler B, Heiser W: Personality and affect as determinants of medically unexplained symptoms in primary care: a follow-up study. J Psychosom Res 56(3):279–285, 2004

Elklit A, Christiansen DM: Predictive factors for somatization in a trauma sample. Clin Pract Epidemiol Ment Health 5:1, 2009

Gilleland J, Suveg C, Jacob ML, et al: Understanding the medically unexplained: emotional and familial influences on children's somatic functioning. Child Care Health Dev 35:383–390, 2009

Kellner R, Slocumb J, Wiggins RG, et al: Hostility, somatic symptoms and hypochondriacal fears and beliefs. J Nerv Ment Dis 173:554–560, 1985

Taylor GJ: Recent developments in alexithymia theory and research. Can J Psychiatry 45:134–142, 2000

12.2   Which of the following statements concerning the epidemiology of somatization disorder is *true?*

   A. The disorder usually develops when patients are in their 40s.
   B. There is no cultural variability in the presentation of somatization disorder.
   C. The prevalence of somatization disorder is higher in medical settings.
   D. The disorder is more common in men than in women.
   E. Patients with somatization disorder are excellent historians who provide detailed and precise descriptions of their medical history.

The correct response is option C.

The lifetime prevalence of somatization disorder has varied widely across studies, ranging from 0.2% to 2.0% among women and less than 0.2% in men (American Psychiatric Association 2000), reflecting variations in research methodology and study samples. Because patients with somatization disorder actively seek medical help, the prevalence in medical settings is higher than in the general population.

Somatization disorder is based on the earlier diagnosis of Briquet's syndrome, which required 25 of 59 physical symptoms, an illness onset before age 30 years, and a pattern of recurrent physical complaints, and was shown to have validity, reliability, and internal consistency (Feighner et al. 1972).

There is cultural variability in the presentation of somatization disorder. Symptoms used in DSM-IV-TR are those that have been found to be most diagnostic in the United States (American Psychiatric Association 2000). The disorder is uncommon in American men (Golding et al. 1991), although in an American sample, women and men with somatization disorder had similar clinical characteristics, including comorbid psychopathology (Golding et al. 1991).

Patients with somatization disorder are often difficult historians who provide dramatic and colorful but vague descriptions of their medical history (Cassem and Barsky 1991) and may present as odd or anxious (Rost et al. 1992). There is often more to be learned in a review of their medical records. **(pp. 269–270)**

American Psychiatric Association: Diagnostic and Statistical Manual of Mental Disorders, 4th Edition, Text Revision. Washington, DC, American Psychiatric Association, 2000

Cassem NH, Barsky AJ: Functional somatic symptoms and somatoform disorders, in Massachusetts General Hospital Handbook of General Hospital Psychiatry, 3rd Edition. Edited by Cassem NH. St. Louis, MO, Mosby Year Book, 1991, pp 131–157

Feighner JP, Robins E, Guze SB, et al: Diagnostic criteria for use in psychiatric research. Arch Gen Psychiatry 26:57–63, 1972

Golding JM, Smith GR Jr, Kashner TM: Does somatization disorder occur in men? Clinical characteristics of women and men with multiple unexplained somatic symptoms. Arch Gen Psychiatry 48:231–235, 1991

Rost KM, Akins RN, Brown FW, et al: The comorbidity of DSM-III-R personality disorders in somatization disorder. Gen Hosp Psychiatry 14:322–326, 1992

12.3   Which of the following statements regarding the epidemiology of conversion disorder is *true?*

   A. The prevalence is higher in men than in women.
   B. Conversion symptoms usually begin slowly and innocuously.
   C. The disorder has been reported to occur in 1%–4.5% of hospitalized neurological and medical patients.
   D. Symptoms, if unilateral, usually occur on the right side of the body.
   E. The disorder is typically diagnosed when patients are in their 30s.

The correct response is option C.

The reported prevalence of conversion disorder has varied and is likely influenced by several factors. Toone's 1990 review noted rates of 0.3% in the general population, 1%–3% in medical outpatients, and 1%–4.5% in hospitalized neurological and medical patients.

Much higher prevalence rates have been described in developing countries (Murphy 1990) and in isolated rural American settings (Ford 1983). Women outnumber men with the disorder in a ratio varying from 2:1 to 10:1 (Murphy 1990).

Conversion symptoms typically begin abruptly and dramatically. Common conversion symptoms include motor symptoms (e.g., paralysis, disturbances in coordination or balance, localized weakness, akinesia, dyskinesia, aphonia, urinary retention, and dysphagia), sensory symptoms (e.g., blindness, double vision, anesthesia, paresthesia, deafness), and seizures or convulsions that may have voluntary motor or sensory components.

Unilateral symptoms may be more likely to occur on the left side of the body, as may be true for other somatoform disorders, although the neurophysiological basis for this finding is unclear (Toone 1990) and not all data support it (Roelofs et al. 2000; Stone et al. 2002).

Onset is typically in adolescence or early adulthood, but cases have been described in children as well as in older adults. **(pp. 272–273)**

Ford CV: The Somatizing Disorders: Illness as a Way of Life. New York, Elsevier, 1983

Murphy MR: Classification of the somatoform disorders, in Somatization: Physical Symptoms and Psychological Illness. Edited by Bass C. Boston, MA, Blackwell Scientific, 1990, pp 10–39

Roelofs K, Naring GW, Moene FC, et al: The question of symptom lateralization in conversion disorder. J Psychosom Res 49:21–25, 2000

Stone J, Sharpe M, Carson A, et al: Are functional motor and sensory symptoms really more frequent on the left? A systematic review. J Neurol Neurosurg Psychiatry 73:578–581, 2002

Toone BK: Disorders of hysterical conversion, in Somatization: Physical Symptoms and Psychological Illness. Edited by Bass C. Boston, MA, Blackwell Scientific, 1990, pp 207–234

12.4   Which of the following statements regarding the epidemiology of hypochondriasis is *false?*

    A. Patients have a high rate of psychiatric comorbidity.
    B. Primary hypochondriasis is an acute condition that responds readily to treatment.
    C. High medical utilization is common.
    D. Patients often have compromised occupational functioning.
    E. Interpersonal relationships are usually impaired.

The correct response is option B.

The clinical course and prognosis of hypochondriasis are poorly understood. There appear to be multiple pathways to the diagnosis. Primary hypochondriasis appears to be a chronic condition, and therefore some have argued that it might be better classified as a personality style or trait (Barsky and Klerman 1983; Fallon and Feinstein 2001; Mayou et al. 2003; Tyrer et al. 1990). In DSM-IV-TR, the course is described as "usually chronic, with waxing and waning symptoms, but complete recovery sometimes occurs" (American Psychiatric Association 2000, p. 506).

Patients with hypochondriasis have a high rate of psychiatric comorbidity, with the most common comorbid diagnoses being generalized anxiety disorder, dysthymia, major depressive disorder, somatization disorder, and panic disorder (Barsky et al. 1992). Personality disorders, as assessed by questionnaire, were three times more likely to be diagnosed in hypochondriacal patients compared with a control group (Barsky et al. 1992).

High medical utilization is common, and the potential exists for iatrogenic damage from repeated investigations. Involvement with complementary health care practices is common.

Occupational functioning is often compromised, with increased time taken off from work and decreased performance when the individual is at work because of the preoccupation with disease.

Interpersonal relationships typically deteriorate because of the preoccupation with disease. **(p. 275)**

American Psychiatric Association: Diagnostic and Statistical Manual of Mental Disorders, 4th Edition, Text Revision. Washington, DC, American Psychiatric Association, 2000

Barsky AJ, Klerman GL: Overview: hypochondriasis, bodily complaints, and somatic styles. Am J Psychiatry 140:273–283, 1983

Barsky AJ, Wyshak G, Klerman GL: Psychiatric comorbidity in DSM-III-R hypochondriasis. Arch Gen Psychiatry 49:101–108, 1992

Fallon BA, Feinstein S: Hypochondriasis, in Somatoform and Factitious Disorders (Review of Psychiatry Series, Vol 20, No 3; Oldham JM and Riba MB, series editors). Edited by Phillips KA. Washington, DC, American Psychiatric Press, 2001, pp 27–66

Mayou R, Levenson J, Sharpe M: Somatoform disorders in DSM-V. Psychosomatics 44:449–451, 2003

Tyrer P, Fowler-Dixon R, Ferguson B, et al: A plea for the diagnosis of hypochondriacal personality disorder. J Psychosom Res 34:637–642, 1990

12.5 The psychiatric disorder most frequently comorbid with body dysmorphic disorder (BDD) is

A. Major depressive disorder.
B. Social phobia.
C. Obsessive-compulsive disorder.
D. Substance use disorder.
E. Panic disorder.

The correct response is option A.

BDD has substantial comorbidity. Major depressive disorder is the most common comorbid disorder, with a current comorbidity rate of about 60% and a lifetime rate of more than 80% (Phillips and Diaz 1997).

Other disorders with lifetime rates of more than 30% include social phobia, substance use disorders, and obsessive-compulsive disorder. Some case series have lower rates of comorbidity (Veale et al. 1996). Social phobia usually begins before the onset of BDD, whereas depression and substance use disorders typically develop after the onset of BDD (Gunstad and Phillips 2003). Personality disorder is common (Phillips 2001), with the most common diagnosis being avoidant personality disorder (Veale et al. 1996). **(p. 276)**

Gunstad J, Phillips KA: Axis I comorbidity in body dysmorphic disorder. Compr Psychiatry 44:270–276, 2003

Phillips KA: Body dysmorphic disorder, in Somatoform and Factitious Disorders (Review of Psychiatry Series, Vol 20, No 3; Oldham JM and Riba MB, series editors). Edited by Phillips KA. Washington, DC, American Psychiatric Press, 2001, pp 67–94

Phillips KA, Diaz SF: Gender differences in body dysmorphic disorder. J Nerv Ment Dis 185:570–577, 1997

Veale D, Boocock A, Gournay K, et al: Body dysmorphic disorder. A survey of fifty cases. Br J Psychiatry 169:196–201, 1996

12.6 Which of the following has been found to be most effective in treating somatoform disorders?

A. Interpersonal psychotherapy.
B. Motivational therapy.
C. Brief psychodynamic psychotherapy.
D. Hypnosis.
E. Cognitive-behavioral therapy.

The correct response is option E.

A systematic review of 34 randomized controlled trials of treatments for somatoform disorders, almost all published in 1995–2007, concluded that cognitive-behavioral therapy (CBT) is "the best established treatment for a variety of somatoform disorders" (Kroenke 2007). CBT was effective in 11 of 13 studies and antidepressants were effective in 4 of 5 studies. For the treatment of somatization disorder, 3 of 4 studies found that a psychiatric consultation letter to the primary care physician was effective in improving the patient's functional status, though none found this intervention to reduce the patient's psychological distress. **(p. 277)**

Kroenke K: Efficacy of treatment for somatoform disorders: a review of randomized controlled trials. Psychosom Med 69:881–888, 2007

Chapter 13

Deception Syndromes
Factitious Disorders and Malingering

Select the single best response for each question.

13.1 Factitious disorder, the conscious, surreptitious fraudulent production of symptoms or signs for the purpose of assuming the sick role and to obtain medical care, is commonly classified as either common factitious disorder or Munchausen syndrome. These subtypes can be quite different in terms of clinical appearance and contributory risk factors. Characteristic features of common factitious disorder include all of the following *except*

    A. Female gender.
    B. Unmarried status.
    C. Age in the 30s.
    D. Employment (current or past) in a health care occupation.
    E. Use of alias identity and frequent travel to seek medical care.

The correct response is option E.

Risk factors for factitious disorder vary according to the subtype of the clinical syndrome. The most common subtype is common factitious disorder (or nonperegrinating factitious disorder), in which the person does not use aliases or travel from hospital to hospital. In this syndrome, female gender, unmarried status, age in the 30s, prior work or experience in the health care professions (e.g., nursing), and Cluster B personality disorders with borderline features are frequently found. **(p. 292)**

13.2 Munchausen syndrome patients may present in classic ways to the health care system, and their behavior while in patient status may help the physician to make the diagnosis. Characteristic features of Munchausen syndrome include all of the following *except*

    A. Travel among many hospitals.
    B. Use of alias identity and possible multiple medical records.
    C. Frequent emergency department presentation.
    D. Presentation with dramatic symptoms of multiple apparently serious disease states.
    E. Refusal to undergo diagnostic studies for presenting symptoms.

The correct response is option E.

The Munchausen patient is usually willing to undergo multiple diagnostic studies.
    Classic Munchausen syndrome consists of three essential components: the simulation or self-induction of disease, pseudologia fantastica, and travel from hospital to hospital, often using aliases to disguise identity. These patients frequently present in the emergency department with dramatic symptoms such as hemoptysis, acute chest pain suggesting a myocardial infarction, or coma from self-induced hypoglycemia. Among the most common presentations are chest pain, endocrine disorders such as hyperthyroidism or Cushing's syndrome, coagulopathies, infections, and neurological symptoms. In addition, the patient may call attention to himself or herself by providing false information such as claiming to be a former professional football player, a recipient of the

Medal of Honor, or perhaps the president of a foreign university. Despite such reputed prominence, these patients and their physicians rarely receive telephone calls from concerned family members or friends. **(p. 293)**

13.3 Ganser's syndrome, a rarely encountered condition that has similarities to and some overlap with factitious disorder, should be considered in the differential diagnosis of cases of apparent factitious disorder. Which of the following characteristics is quite specific to this syndrome?

  A. Amnesia.
  B. Disorientation.
  C. Visual hallucinations.
  D. Approximate answers to questions.
  E. Olfactory hallucinations.

The correct response is option D.

Ganser's syndrome is closely related to factitious disorder, with predominantly psychological symptoms (Wirtz et al. 2008). This syndrome is characterized by the provision of approximate answers (*Vorbeireden*) to questions (e.g., the examiner asks, "What is the color of snow?" and the patient answers, "Green").

Complaints of amnesia, disorientation, and perceptual disturbance are generally present as well. This syndrome was originally described by the nineteenth-century German psychiatrist Sigbert Ganser (1965) as a form of malingering seen in prisoners, but it also has been described in other settings, including general hospital units (Dalfen and Anthony 2000; Weiner and Braiman 1955). **(p. 294)**

Dalfen AK, Anthony F: Head injury, dissociation and the Ganser syndrome. Brain Inj 14:1101–1105, 2000
Ganser SJM: A peculiar hysterical state (translated by Schorer CE). Br J Criminol 5:120–126, 1965
Weiner H, Braiman A: The Ganser syndrome. Am J Psychiatry 111:767–773, 1955
Wirtz G, Baas U, Hofer H, et al: Psychopathology of Ganser's syndrome: literature review and case report [in German]. Nervenarzt 79:543–557, 2008

13.4 Which is the most common psychiatric comorbidity in factitious disorder?

  A. Schizophrenia.
  B. Major depression.
  C. Cluster A personality disorder.
  D. Cluster B personality disorder.
  E. Cluster C personality disorder.

The correct response is option D.

The large majority of patients with factitious disorder have an underlying severe personality disorder, usually of the Cluster B type. Factitious behavior can be seen as a form of acting out, similar to other acting-out behaviors seen in Cluster B personality disorders. Axis I comorbidity, including major depression and schizophrenia, has been described, but is not common. **(p. 295)**

13.5 Munchausen syndrome by proxy is a recently appreciated and very disruptive problem seen primarily in child psychosomatic medicine practice. In the review by Sheridan (2003), findings included all of the following *except*

  A. Victims were primarily female.
  B. Most victims were age 4 years or younger.
  C. Most cases involved active production of symptoms rather than mere misrepresentation of them.
  D. The most commonly produced symptom was apnea.
  E. There was an extremely high rate of death in victim's siblings.

The correct response is option A.

The typical presentation of Munchausen syndrome by proxy is that of a child admitted to a hospital with symptoms such as seizures, bleeding, diarrhea, or respiratory difficulties (including apnea). Sheridan (2003) reviewed and summarized published data from 451 cases of Munchausen syndrome by proxy. Her findings indicated no gender bias of the child victims, who were usually age 4 years or younger. In most of the situations, the perpetrator actively produced symptoms by smothering or poisoning the child, although some instances involved exaggeration or lying about symptoms. The most frequently noted symptoms of the child victims were, in order, apnea, anorexia, feeding problems, diarrhea, seizures, and cyanosis. The mortality rate for identified children victims was 6.0%, but 25% of known siblings were known to be dead. **(p. 297)**

Sheridan MS: The deceit continues: an updated literature review of Munchausen syndrome by proxy. Child Abuse Negl 27:431–451, 2003

13.6   Psychometric testing can be a very helpful adjunct in the diagnosis of malingering. Which of the following assessment instruments, by virtue of its forced-choice format and statistical norming, is a useful test for patients who distort symptoms?

   A. Rorschach.
   B. Minnesota Multiphasic Personality Inventory–2 (MMPI-2).
   C. Beck Depression Inventory (BDI).
   D. Hamilton Rating Scale for Depression (HAM-D).
   E. Hopkins Symptom Checklist–90.

The correct response is option B.

Psychological testing is often helpful in identifying malingering patients. The MMPI-2 is a useful test for patients who distort their presentations (Arbisi and Butcher 2004; McCaffrey and Bellamy-Campbell 1989; Wetzler and Marlowe 1990). This test and others have diagnostic value in assessing those who exaggerate physical and psychological symptoms (Cliffe 1992; Rawling 1992; Walters et al. 2008).

Screening instruments with face validity such as the BDI and the Hopkins Symptom Checklist–90 are easily distorted by patients who embellish their symptoms (Lees-Haley 1989a, 1989b), and these instruments have very limited value in the determination of malingering. Forced-choice psychological tests may be valuable in detecting malingering. If a person makes more errors than would be expected by chance, a statistical probability can be determined as to whether the person actually knew the correct answers. **(p. 300)**

Arbisi PA, Butcher JN: Psychometric perspectives on detection of malingering of pain: use of the Minnesota Multiphasic Personality Inventory–2. Clin J Pain 20:383–391, 2004

Cliffe MJ: Symptom-validity testing of feigned sensory or memory deficits: a further elaboration for subjects who understand the rationale. Br J Clin Psychol 31:207–209, 1992

Lees-Haley PR: Malingering emotional distress on the SCL-90R: toxic exposure and cancerphobia. Psychol Rep 65:1203–1208, 1989a

Lees-Haley PR: Malingering traumatic mental disorder on the Beck Depression Inventory: cancerphobia and toxic exposure. Psychol Rep 65:623–626, 1989b

McCaffrey RJ, Bellamy-Campbell R: Psychometric detection of fabricated symptoms of combat-related post-traumatic stress disorder: a systematic replication. J Clin Psychol 45:76–79, 1989

Rawling PJ: The Simulation Index: a reliability study. Brain Inj 6:381–383, 1992

Walters GD, Rogers R, Berry DTR, et al: Malingering as a categorical or dimensional construct: the latent structure of feigned psychopathology as measured by the SIRS and MMPI-2. Psychol Assess 20:238–247, 2008

Wetzler S, Marlowe D: "Faking bad" on the MMPI, MMPI-2, and Millon-II. Psychol Rep 67:1117–1118, 1990

Chapter 14

Eating Disorders

Select the single best response for each question.

14.1 Which of the following statements concerning the diagnosis of anorexia nervosa is *false?*

    A. Patients must manifest a weight markedly (≥15%) lower than expected for gender and height.
    B. Amenorrhea is no longer a requirement for postmenarchal women.
    C. The diagnosis requires an overconcern with weight and shape.
    D. Many patients with anorexia nervosa are compulsive exercisers.
    E. Patients with anorexia nervosa are often rigid and perfectionistic.

The correct response is option B.

Amenorrhea is a requirement for postmenarchal women.

    To receive a diagnosis of anorexia nervosa, patients must manifest weight loss, or the absence of expected weight gain, leading to a state of significant undernourishment, as reflected by a weight markedly (i.e., at least 15%) lower than expected for gender and height. In addition to severely restricting their intake of food, many individuals with anorexia nervosa are also compulsive exercisers. Patients with anorexia nervosa are often rigid and perfectionistic, not only in their adherence to restrictive eating and compulsive exercise practices but also in other areas of life. The diagnosis requires an overconcern with weight and shape, which may or may not take the form of an actual misperception of body fatness but must reflect an overinvestment in thinness as a central feature of one's self-worth. **(p. 306)**

14.2 Which of the following points should clinicians keep in mind when evaluating a patient for bulimia nervosa?

    A. Progression from anorexia nervosa to bulimia nervosa is quite rare.
    B. Individuals who simultaneously meet criteria for anorexia nervosa and bulimia nervosa are diagnosed as having anorexia nervosa, binge-eating/purging type.
    C. The diagnosis of bulimia nervosa cannot be made in overweight or obese individuals.
    D. Most individuals who present for treatment of bulimia nervosa are more than 15% below their expected weight.
    E. In more than half of cases, normal-weight individuals with bulimia nervosa progress to anorexia nervosa.

The correct response is option B.

Under the current diagnostic system, individuals who simultaneously meet criteria for anorexia nervosa and bulimia nervosa are diagnosed as having anorexia nervosa, binge-eating/purging type.

    Bulimia nervosa, first described as a variant of anorexia nervosa (Russell 1979) and later applied to individuals of normal weight, comprises regular, uncontrolled consumption of objectively large amounts of food (binge eating), regular use of unhealthy compensatory methods intended to undo the effects of eating, and preoccupation with weight and/or shape as a central component of self-worth.

    Although most individuals who present for treatment for bulimia nervosa are of normal weight, the diagnosis can also be made in overweight or obese individuals.

The progression from anorexia nervosa to bulimia nervosa is quite common, occurring in about one-half of patients with restricting anorexia nervosa (Bulik et al. 1997). Normal-weight patients with bulimia nervosa progress to anorexia nervosa somewhat less frequently. **(p. 306)**

Bulik CM, Sullivan PF, Fear J, et al: Predictors of the development of bulimia nervosa in women with anorexia nervosa. J Nerv Ment Dis 185:704–707, 1997

Russell GFM: Bulimia nervosa: an ominous variant of anorexia nervosa. Psychol Med 9:429–448, 1979

14.3   A parent brings her 10-year-old daughter to your office and states that her daughter will eat only a small number of foods. The child's growth and development are normal. What is the most likely diagnosis?

   A.   Food phobia.
   B.   Food avoidance emotional disorder.
   C.   Functional dysphagia.
   D.   Pervasive refusal syndrome.
   E.   Selective eating disorder.

The correct response is option E.

As is the case for adult eating disorders, the classification of child and adolescent eating disturbances is the subject of active debate (Bravender et al. 2007). Disordered eating patterns occurring before puberty include food avoidance emotional disorder, selective eating, pervasive refusal syndrome, food phobias, functional dysphagia, and full-syndrome anorexia nervosa (Lask and Bryant-Waugh 1997; Nicholls and Bryant-Waugh 2009; Rosen 2003).

Selective eating is diagnosed in children who eat only a small number of foods but whose growth and development are generally normal.

Food avoidance emotional disorder is similar to, but less severe than, anorexia nervosa and carries a better prognosis.

Children with *functional dysphagia* avoid food due to a fear of swallowing, choking, or vomiting for which no organic etiology can be identified.

Pervasive refusal syndrome is a severe disorder in which refusal to eat is accompanied by refusal to function in other spheres (e.g., walking, talking, self-care) and is probably not best viewed as an eating disorder.

Specific *food phobias* are often reflective of more pervasive anxiety disorders, and obsessional fears related to food may be particularly common in boys presenting with childhood anorexia nervosa. **(pp. 308–309)**

Bravender T, Bryant-Waugh R, Herzog D, et al: Classification of child and adolescent eating disturbances. Workgroup for Classification of Eating Disorders in Children and Adolescents (WCEDCA). Int J Eat Disord 40 (suppl):S117–S122, 2007

Lask B, Bryant-Waugh R: Prepubertal eating disorders, in Handbook of Treatment for Eating Disorders, 2nd Edition. Edited by Garner DM, Garfinkel PE. New York, Guilford, 1997, pp 476–483

Nichols D, Bryant-Waugh R: Eating disorders of infancy and childhood: definition, symptomatology, epidemiology, and comorbidity. Child Adolesc Psychiatric Clin N Am 18:17–30, 2009

Rosen DS: Eating disorders in children and young adolescents: etiology, classification, clinical features, and treatment. Adolesc Med 14:49–59, 2003

14.4   Which of the following statements concerning the course and outcome of anorexia nervosa is *false*?

   A.   Mortality rates are as high as 5% per decade of illness.
   B.   Among surviving patients, fewer than half recover fully.
   C.   Approximately one-fifth of patients remain chronically ill.
   D.   Patients treated as adolescents have a worse outcome.
   E.   The risk of suicide is pronounced.

The correct response is option D.

The outcome of patients treated for anorexia nervosa as adolescents appears to be more favorable (Strober et al. 1997), underscoring the importance of early intervention or, ideally, prevention.

Studies of the long-term course of anorexia nervosa suggest that there is no typical outcome. Rather, the illness tends to require long-term treatment, with some patients achieving full recovery, others experiencing a longer course of partially remitted or unremitted illness, and some dying as a direct or indirect result of the illness (Pike 1998), with risk of suicide particularly pronounced (Berkman et al. 2007). Mortality rates are as high as 5% per decade of illness in the longest follow-up studies (Nielsen 2001); of surviving patients, fewer than half recover fully, one-quarter to one-third recover partially, and one-fifth remain chronically ill (Steinhausen 2002, 2009). These figures are cross-nationally consistent (Lee et al. 2003). **(p. 310)**

> Berkman ND, Lohr KN, Bulik CM: Outcomes of eating disorders: a systematic review of the literature. Int J Eat Disord 40:293–309, 2007
>
> Lee S, Chan YYL, Hsu LKG: The intermediate term outcome of Chinese patients with anorexia nervosa in Hong Kong. Am J Psychiatry 160:967–972, 2003
>
> Nielsen S: Epidemiology and mortality of eating disorders. Psychiatr Clin North Am 24:201–214, 2001
>
> Pike KM: Long-term course of anorexia nervosa: response, relapse, remission, and recovery. Clin Psychol Rev 18:447–475, 1998
>
> Steinhausen HC: The outcome of anorexia nervosa in the 20th century. Am J Psychiatry 159:1284–1293, 2002
>
> Steinhausen HC: Outcome of eating disorders. Child Adolesc Psychiatric Clin N Am 18:225–242, 2009
>
> Strober M, Freeman R, Morrell W: The long-term course of severe anorexia nervosa in adolescents: survival analysis of recovery, relapse, and outcome predictors over 10–15 years in a prospective study. Int J Eat Disord 22:339–360, 1997

14.5   The most serious complication of weight restoration in patients with anorexia nervosa is

    A. Refeeding syndrome.
    B. Hypercholesterolemia.
    C. Hypercortisolism.
    D. Low white blood cell count.
    E. Abnormal thyroid hormone status.

The correct response is option A.

One of the most serious complications of weight restoration is the refeeding syndrome, characterized by marked fluid and electrolyte abnormalities, including low serum phosphate levels. The combination of depletion of total body phosphate stores during catabolic starvation and increased cellular influx of phosphate during anabolic refeeding leads to severe extracellular hypophosphatemia. This well-recognized complication of refeeding, particularly in individuals with very low body weight, can lead to cardiac arrhythmias, delirium, and even sudden death (Solomon and Kirby 1990). Other potential symptoms of the refeeding syndrome include abnormal sodium and fluid balance; alterations in the metabolism of glucose, protein, and fat; thiamine deficiency; hypokalemia; and hypomagnesemia (Mehanna et al. 2008). This syndrome has most often been noted in refeeding with total parenteral nutrition but can be seen with oral and nasogastric refeeding regimens as well (American Psychiatric Association 2006).

Cholesterol levels in anorexia nervosa are usually normal or high despite low cholesterol intake. These levels do not result from the de novo synthesis of cholesterol. Rather, abnormal thyroid hormone status, low serum estrogen levels, hypercortisolism, and impaired clearance of cholesterol explain or contribute to hypercholesterolemia in this setting. Weight restoration is typically accompanied by reduction in cholesterol level and apolipoprotein B (Feillet et al. 2000), and no effort should be made to further reduce dietary fat or cholesterol (Rock and Curran-Celentano 1996). Other laboratory abnormalities that characterize starvation and early recovery such as low white blood cell count or elevated liver transaminases typically normalize with weight recovery. **(p. 322)**

American Psychiatric Association: Practice guideline for the treatment of patients with eating disorders (revision). American Psychiatric Association Work Group on Eating Disorders. Am J Psychiatry 163 (suppl):1–54, 2006

Feillet F, Feillet-Coudray C, Bard JM, et al: Plasma cholesterol and endogenous cholesterol synthesis during refeeding in anorexia nervosa. Clin Chim Acta 294:45–56, 2000

Mehanna JM, Moledina J, Travis J: Refeeding syndrome: what it is and how to treat it. BMJ 336:1495–1498, 2008

Rock CL, Curran-Celentano JC: Nutritional management of eating disorders. Psychiatr Clin North Am 19:701–713, 1996

Solomon SM, Kirby DF: The refeeding syndrome: a review. JPEN J Parenter Enteral Nutr 14:90–97, 1990

C h a p t e r   1 5

Sleep Disorders

Select the single best response for each question.

15.1   Patients with disrupted sleep usually spend most of the night

  A. In stage N1 with much rapid eye movement (REM) sleep.
  B. In stage N2 with much REM sleep.
  C. In stage N3 with little REM sleep.
  D. In stages N1 and N2 with little REM sleep.
  E. In stage N3 with much REM sleep.

The correct response is option D.

Patients with disrupted sleep often spend most of the night in stages N1 and N2 and have little slow-wave or REM sleep. **(p. 336)**

15.2   The multiple sleep latency test (MSLT) is a useful tool for evaluating patients with excessive daytime sleepiness. Which of the following statements regarding the MSLT is *false?*

  A. The MSLT needs to be completed before an overnight sleep study.
  B. Patients need 6 hours of sleep before the MSLT.
  C. The leads attached to the patient are the electroencephalographic, electromyographic, and electro-oculographic leads.
  D. The test measures initial sleep latency and initial rapid eye movement (REM) latency.
  E. Patients must stay awake between the examined naps.

The correct response is option A.

The MSLT is used to identify disorders of excessive daytime sleepiness, including narcolepsy (Krahn et al. 2001). Patients must first undergo an overnight sleep study for exclusion of other sleep disorders caused by disrupted nocturnal sleep.

If the patient has had, at minimum, 6 hours of sleep to preclude sleep deprivation, then a valid MSLT can be conducted the next day. Patients are asked to take four or five scheduled naps wearing a simplified set of leads including only electroencephalographic, electromyographic, and electro-oculographic leads. The test is used to measure initial sleep latency and initial REM latency, if present, for each nap. Patients are asked to stay awake between naps, to refrain from stimulants such as caffeine and prescribed medications, and to undergo drug screening for occult sedative use. **(p. 340)**

> Krahn L, Black J, Silber M: Narcolepsy: new understanding of irresistible sleep. Mayo Clinic Proc 76:185–194, 2001

15.3   Which of the following statements regarding narcolepsy is *false?*

     A. Patients have excessive daytime sleepiness.
     B. Patients have episodic, sudden "sleep attacks."
     C. The majority of patients experience cataplexy.
     D. During cataplexy, consciousness is lost.
     E. Patients commonly experience sleep paralysis.

The correct response is option D.

There is no loss of consciousness during cataplexy.

Narcolepsy is characterized by chronic excessive daytime sleepiness with episodic sleep attacks. Approximately 65%–75% of patients with narcolepsy have cataplexy, which is a condition in which an emotional trigger, most commonly laughter, provokes abrupt muscle atonia without loss of consciousness. Other associated symptoms of narcolepsy include sleep paralysis (isolated loss of muscle tone associated with rapid eye movement in normal sleep) and hypnagogic and hypnopompic hallucinations (vivid dreaming occurring at the time of sleep onset and awakening that can be difficult to distinguish from reality). **(p. 341)**

15.4   Which of the following treatments for narcolepsy was initially approved by the U.S. Food and Drug Administration (FDA) for cataplexy and later approved for all narcolepsy symptoms?

     A. Methylphenidate.
     B. Dextroamphetamine.
     C. Modafinil.
     D. Sodium oxybate.
     E. Armodafinil.

The correct response is option D.

Sodium oxybate (also known as gamma-hydroxybutyrate), approved by the FDA in 2002, is a medication indicated for the treatment of narcolepsy. This novel hypnotic was approved initially for the treatment of cataplexy and subsequently permitted for all narcoleptic symptoms. An endogenous substance, sodium oxybate increases slow-wave sleep and also improves sleep continuity (Lammers et al. 1993). Although somewhat counterintuitive, clinical trials in narcolepsy have demonstrated that sodium oxybate decreases excessive daytime sleepiness by increasing sleep (Black and Houghton 2006).

Pharmacological treatment options for narcolepsy include methylphenidate or amphetamines, which target excessive daytime sleepiness (Mitler and Hayduk 2002). Extended-release preparations of methylphenidate and amphetamines have the advantage of continuous drug delivery, which reduces the daytime variability in alertness that may occur with the immediate-release forms, which are taken twice or three times a day. Modafinil is a unique wake-promoting medication that was approved by the FDA in 1999. Because it lacks sympathomimetic activity, it is not considered a psychostimulant.

Recently, armodafinil, the longer-acting R-enantiomer of modafinil, was shown to reduce excessive daytime sleepiness in narcolepsy and to be more suitable than modafinil for administration once a day (Keam and Walker 2007). **(p. 342)**

Black J, Houghton W: Sodium oxybate improves excessive daytime sleepiness in narcolepsy. Sleep 29:939–946, 2006
Keam S, Walker MC: Therapies for narcolepsy with or without cataplexy: evidence-based review. Curr Opin Neurol 20:699–703, 2007
Lammers GJ, Arends J, Declerck AC, et al: Gamma-hydroxybutyrate and narcolepsy: a double blind placebo-controlled study. Sleep 16:216–220, 1993
Mitler M, Hayduk R: Benefits and risks of pharmacotherapy for narcolepsy. Drug Saf 25:790–809, 2002

15.5 Which of the following is *not* a characteristic feature of Kleine-Levin syndrome?

    A. Male patient.
    B. Young patient.
    C. Periods of profound anorexia.
    D. Periodic hypersomnia.
    E. Approximately 50% risk of concurrent depressed mood.

The correct response is option C.

Anorexia is not a characteristic of patients with Kleine-Levin syndrome.

Kleine-Levin syndrome, also known as recurrent hypersomnia, is an important part of the differential diagnosis of idiopathic hypersomnia. Patients with recurrent hypersomnia are generally male adolescents who engage in binge eating and have periodic hypersomnia that lasts several weeks (Minvielle 2000). The typical pattern is recurrent episodes each lasting approximately a week, spanning 8 years. Depressed mood has been reported in 48% of affected patients (Arnulf et al. 2005). In the absence of any randomized controlled trials in Kleine-Levin syndrome, psychostimulants and lithium have been reported to prevent relapses (Oliveira et al. 2009). **(p. 243)**

    Arnulf I, Zeitzer JM, File J, et al: Kleine-Levin syndrome: a systematic review of 186 cases in the literature. Brain 128:2763–2776, 2009
    Minvielle S: Klein-Levin syndrome: a neurological disease with psychiatric symptoms [in French]. Encephale 26:71–74, 2000
    Oliveira MM, Conti C, Saconato H, et al: Pharmacological treatment for Kleine-Levin syndrome. Cochrane Database Syst Rev (2):CD006685, 2009

15.6 Which neurotransmitter abnormality is associated with restless legs syndrome?

    A. Increased dopamine levels.
    B. Increased serotonin levels.
    C. Decreased gamma-aminobutyric acid levels.
    D. Decreased dopamine levels.
    E. Decreased serotonin levels.

The correct response is option D.

Restless legs syndrome is believed to be a condition associated with decreased dopamine levels. Treatment with dopamine antagonists aggravates the symptoms, and this syndrome occurs with increased frequency in Parkinson's disease. Positron emission tomographic studies of restless legs syndrome have shown decreased dopaminergic functioning in the caudate and putamen regions of the brain (Ruottinen et al. 2000). Treatment with dopaminergic agonists, even low doses, leads to marked improvement. **(p. 348)**

    Ruottinen HM, Partinen M, Hublin C, et al: An FDOPA PET study in patients with periodic limb movement disorder and restless legs syndrome. Neurology 54:502–504, 2000

Chapter 16

Sexual Dysfunction

Select the single best response for each question.

16.1 In a retrospective analysis of 32,616 healthy male participants from a 1986 study, erectile dysfunction was found to be associated with a fourfold increase in the risk of developing which disease?

    A. Stroke.
    B. Prostate cancer.
    C. Renal failure.
    D. Parkinson's disease.
    E. Diabetes.

The correct response is option D.

Sexual dysfunction can be a harbinger of otherwise asymptomatic systemic disease. Among 32,616 healthy male participants reporting erectile dysfunction (ED) in a U.S. study in 1986, a fourfold higher risk of developing Parkinson's disease was found over the next 16 years of follow-up, suggesting that erectile difficulties can precede the onset of the classic motor features of parkinsonism by a substantial margin (Gao et al. 2007). **(p. 361)**

> Gao X, Chen H, Schwarzschild MA, et al: Erectile function and risk of Parkinson's disease. Am J Epidemiol 166:1446–1450, 2007

16.2 Sexual dysfunction can occur in individuals following a myocardial infarction (MI), in part because patients are concerned about the risks of resuming sexual activity. In regard to this issue, which of the following statements is *false?*

    A. Energy requirements for sexual intercourse and orgasm are estimated to be similar to climbing a flight of stairs.
    B. The risk of a recurrent MI after sex in a 50-year-old patient is two chances in a thousand per hour.
    C. Exercise will increase tolerance for sexual activity.
    D. The risk of further cardiac damage from sexual activity is low and short-lasting.
    E. Threatening symptoms of a recurrent MI are unlikely to occur during sexual activity if no cardiac symptoms arise during exercise testing to 6 metabolic equivalents (METs).

The correct response is option B.

The risk of recurrent MI, during the period of 2 hours after sex, in a patient with a previous MI at age 50, has been calculated to increase from 10 chances to 20 chances in a million per hour (Muller et al. 1996).

Most patients report reduced frequency of sexual activity after MI, and 10%–54% do not resume it at all (Drory et al. 2000). However, it is important to advise that risk of further cardiac damage is low and short-lasting. Energy requirements for sexual stimulation, intercourse, and orgasm are estimated to be 3–4 METs—similar to climbing a flight of stairs.

The patient can be advised that threatening symptoms are unlikely to occur if no cardiac symptoms arise during exercise testing to 6 METs. Prescribing exercise will increase tolerance for sexual activity. **(p. 365)**

Drory Y, Karvetz S, Weingarten M: First acute myocardial infarction: comparison of sexual activity of women and men after first acute myocardial infarction. Am J Cardiol 85:1283–1287, 2000

Muller JE, Mittleman MA, Maclure M, et al: Triggering myocardial infarction by sexual activity. Low absolute risk and prevention by regular physical exertion. Determinants of Myocardial Infarction Onset Study Investigators. JAMA 275:1405–1409, 1996

16.3   Sexual dysfunction after traumatic brain injury is common. Which of the following is the single most sensitive predictor of sexual functioning after traumatic brain injury?

   A. Location of brain injury.
   B. Presence of posttraumatic stress disorder.
   C. Duration of coma.
   D. Presence of psychosis.
   E. Presence of depression.

The correct response is option E.

Depression is the most sensitive single predictor of sexual functioning after mechanical injury to the brain (Hibbard et al. 2000).

Whether from trauma or from stroke, brain injury is frequently associated with sexual problems, the prevalence of which can be difficult to estimate when the patient has extensive bodily injuries other than to the brain or when the patient who has had a stroke has comorbid impairment of genital blood supply because of vascular disease. Depression affecting sexuality is common in both vascular injury and traumatic injury to the brain. Published prevalence levels of depression in the chronic phase following moderate and severe brain injuries are as high as 50% (Kelly et al. 2006).

There is no clear relationship between the focality of brain injury or the duration of coma and the degree of sexual impairment (Sandel et al. 1996). Prevalence figures range from 36% to 54% for more severe head injuries compared with 15% for healthy control subjects (Ponsford 2003). **(p. 369)**

Hibbard MR, Gordon WA, Flanagan S, et al: Sexual dysfunction after traumatic brain injury. NeuroRehabilitation 15:107–120, 2000

Kelly DF, McArthur DL, Levin H, et al: Neurobehavioral and quality of life changes associated with growth hormone insufficiency after complicated mild, moderate, or severe traumatic brain injury. J Neurotrauma 223:928–942, 2006

Ponsford J: Sexual changes associated with traumatic brain injury. Neuropsychol Rehabil 13:275–289, 2003

Sandel ME, Williams KS, Dellapietra L, et al: Sexual functioning following traumatic brain injury. Brain Inj 10:719–728, 1996

16.4   Dopamine agonists, especially when combined with L-dopa, have been reported to produce

   A. Compulsive gambling.
   B. Anorgasmia in women.
   C. Depression.
   D. Erectile dysfunction in men.
   E. Lack of sexual desire.

The correct response is option A.

Aberrant sexual behavior has been reported in patients with Parkinson's disease. The term *hedonistic homeostatic dysregulation* has been coined to signify exhibitionism and excessive use of phone-sex lines, prostitution services, and sex shops. Eventually, there can be a vicious cycle of dysregulation of brain reward systems, resulting in compulsive use of dopamine agonist medications promoting other behavior disorders, such as pathological gambling, obsessive shopping, and aggression (Giovannoni et al. 2000). It is currently thought that administration of dopamine agonists, especially if combined with L-dopa, may cause these disorders through excessive stimulation of D_2 receptors and particularly the D_3 subclass (Klos et al. 2005). Of 300 patients with Parkinson's disease taking dopamine agonists including ropinirole and pramipexole, 25 had sexual compulsions and 28 had comorbid or separate compulsive gambling, of whom 17 met criteria for pathological gambling. These concerns were more common in men than in women (Singh et al. 2007). **(p. 370)**

Giovannoni G, O'Sullivan JD, Turner K, et al: Hedonistic homeostatic dysregulation in patients with Parkinson's disease on dopamine replacement therapies. J Neurol Neurosurg Psychiatry 68:423–428, 2000

Klos KJ, Bower JH, Josephs KA, et al: Pathological hypersexuality predominantly linked to adjuvant dopamine agonist therapy in Parkinson's disease and multiple system atrophy. Parkinsonism Relat Disord 11:381–386, 2005

Singh A, Kandimala G, Dewey RB, et al: Risk factors for pathologic gambling and other compulsions among Parkinson's disease patients taking dopamine agonists. J Clin Neurosci 14:1178–1181, 2007

16.5   The most common sexual dysfunction in women with end-stage renal disease is

    A. Dyspareunia.
    B. Vaginal dryness.
    C. Low sexual desire.
    D. Lack of orgasm.
    E. Reduced vaginal sensation.

The correct response is option C.

Low sexual desire is present in up to 100% of women with end-stage renal disease and those undergoing hemodialysis and is as high as 80% posttransplantation (Basson et al. 2010). Multiple factors are involved including anemia, negative outcomes to sexual interactions, estrogen deficiency with vaginal atrophy, high prolactin, depression, chronic pain, and psychosexual and interpersonal issues. In addition, 40% of women with end-stage renal disease are totally amenorrheic, and fewer than 10% have regular menstrual periods. Premature menopause is common. **(p. 373)**

Basson R, Rees P, Wang R, et al: Sexual function in chronic illness. J Sex Med 7(1 Pt 2):374–388, 2010

Chapter 17

Substance-Related Disorders

Select the single best response for each question.

17.1 The benzodiazepine antagonist flumazenil is an emergency treatment for acute benzodiazepine intoxication. Which of the following statements concerning flumazenil's clinical use is *false?*

  A. Nausea and vomiting are common side effects of flumazenil.
  B. Flumazenil may not completely reverse benzodiazepine-associated respiratory depression.
  C. Flumazenil carries some risk of seizure provocation in benzodiazepine-dependent patients.
  D. In mixed overdoses with tricyclic antidepressants (TCAs), flumazenil may precipitate arrhythmias.
  E. Flumazenil should be routinely administered in all comatose patients when it is not known what drugs were ingested.

The correct response is option E.

Flumazenil, a benzodiazepine antagonist, is available for the treatment of acute benzodiazepine intoxication. Flumazenil should not routinely be administered to comatose patients when the identity of ingested drug(s) is not certain.

Nausea and vomiting are its most common side effects. It may not completely reverse respiratory depression and may provoke withdrawal seizures in patients with benzodiazepine dependence. In a mixed overdose with TCAs, flumazenil can precipitate arrhythmias that had been suppressed by the sedative (Weinbroum et al. 1997). Flumazenil appears safe in patients with stable ischemic heart disease (Croughwell et al. 1990). Flumazenil should be withheld in patients with a history of or current seizures and in patients who have overdosed on drugs that lower the seizure threshold. Repeat doses should be administered slowly in patients who are physically dependent on benzodiazepines. Flumazenil is short-acting and sedation may recur after an initial awakening. This can be treated by repeating doses at 20-minute intervals, as needed. **(p. 384)**

> Croughwell ND, Reves JG, Will CJ, et al: Safety of rapid administration of flumazenil in patients with ischaemic heart disease. Acta Anaesthesiol Scand Suppl 92:55–58, 1990
> Weinbroum AA, Flaishon R, Sorkine P, et al: A risk-benefit assessment of flumazenil in the management of benzodiazepine overdose. Drug Saf 17:181–196, 1997

17.2 Opioid intoxication is a common emergency presentation that may prompt a psychosomatic medicine evaluation. Common physical signs of opioid intoxication include all of the following *except*

  A. Dilated pupils.
  B. Decreased respiration.
  C. Decreased level of consciousness.
  D. Miotic pupils.
  E. Absent bowel sounds.

The correct response is option A.

Acute opioid intoxication is characterized by decreased level of consciousness, substantially decreased respiration, miotic pupils, and absent bowel sounds. **(p. 389)**

17.3   Hepatitis C virus (HCV) infection is a common cause of liver failure, leading to the need for transplantation. Because many patients with HCV-induced liver disease are on methadone maintenance or buprenorphine treatment, challenging clinical decisions can ensue. Which of the following statements regarding treatment for opioid dependence and comorbid HCV is *false*?

A. The rate of HCV among methadone maintenance patients is 70%.
B. Methadone maintenance should be continued while evaluation for liver transplantation is under way.
C. Methadone maintenance should be discontinued after liver transplantation.
D. Methadone maintenance is associated with better outcomes (in terms of relapse to heroin use postoperatively) compared with tapering and discontinuing.
E. Opioid-dependent patients on buprenorphine should continue taking the drug throughout the transplant evaluation process.

The correct response is option C.

The standard of care for patients with severe liver disease on methadone maintenance is to continue methadone during evaluation, transplant surgery, and thereafter, rather than attempting to taper the patient off methadone (Lucey and Weinrieb 2009).

Chronic infection with HCV can lead to cirrhosis and the need for liver transplant, and the rate of HCV infection among methadone maintenance patients is 70% (Weaver et al. 2005). Accurate data about drug and alcohol use among patients with liver disease or liver transplant candidates are difficult to obtain because patients believe that divulging this information will harm their chances of receiving further care, especially access to a liver transplant (Weinrieb et al. 2000). Continuation of methadone maintenance has superior outcomes in terms of relapse to heroin use when compared with tapering off methadone (Ball and Ross 1991). Therefore, it is inappropriate to require patients who are stable on methadone (or buprenorphine) to discontinue this treatment prior to any surgical procedure or other intervention. **(p. 390)**

Ball J, Ross A: The Effectiveness of Methadone Maintenance Treatment. New York, Springer-Verlag, 1991
Lucey MR, Weinrieb RM: Alcohol and substance abuse. Semin Liver Dis 29:66–73, 2009
Weaver MF, Cropsey KL, Fox S: HCV prevalence in methadone maintenance: self-report versus serum test. Am J Health Behav 29:387–394, 2005
Weinrieb RM, Van Horn DH, McLellan AT, et al: Interpreting the significance of drinking by alcohol-dependent liver transplant patients: fostering candor is the key to recovery. Liver Transpl 6:769–776, 2000

17.4   Drug interactions may be problematic with the clinical use of methadone, due to hepatic metabolism pathways. Which of the following medications has been shown to lower serum methadone levels, producing opioid withdrawal?

A. Risperidone.
B. Diazepam.
C. Fluoxetine.
D. Erythromycin.
E. None of the above.

The correct response is option A.

Many different medications affect methadone metabolism, primarily because it is metabolized by cytochrome P450 (CYP) 3A4. Risperidone, rifampicin, and many antiretrovirals can lower serum methadone levels, resulting in opioid withdrawal symptoms. These interactions usually do not have life-threatening consequences for patients, other than acute discomfort and risk of relapse to opioid abuse (Ferrari et al. 2004).

Diazepam, fluoxetine, and erythromycin can elevate methadone serum levels and increase the risk of opioid intoxication. Methadone use can prolong the QTc interval. (p. 391)

Ferrari A, Coccia CP, Bertolini A, et al: Methadone—metabolism, pharmacokinetics and interactions. Pharmacol Res 50:551–559, 2004

17.5   Which of the following statements regarding buprenorphine is *true?*

   A. It is a full opioid agonist at the mu receptor.
   B. It is known to commonly increase the QTc interval.
   C. It is marketed in a combination product with naltrexone.
   D. Buprenorphine does not elevate hepatic transaminases in patients with hepatitis C virus (HCV).
   E. It has fewer drug interactions than methadone.

The correct response is option E.

Buprenorphine has fewer drug interactions than methadone, so it is safer when used for patients with medical comorbidities such as HIV on antiretroviral medications. However, buprenorphine may cause elevation of liver transaminases in patients with chronic HCV infection (Petry et al. 2000), which has a very high prevalence among patients who have injected opioids and are receiving maintenance treatment, so monitoring of liver enzymes may be necessary. Buprenorphine toxicity has been linked to use of benzodiazepines (Tracqui et al. 1998).

Buprenorphine, a partial opioid agonist, reduces illicit opioid use with long-term therapy (Kakko et al. 2003). Buprenorphine is taken sublingually. It is available alone or in a combination preparation with naloxone, an opioid antagonist that has poor oral absorption. Buprenorphine has a lower potential for causing respiratory depression than does methadone, and the typical treatment dose (16–32 mg) can be tolerated by opioid-naive users. It does not appear to prolong the QTc interval (Wedam et al. 2007), unlike methadone. (p. 391)

Kakko J, Svanborg KD, Kreek MJ, et al: 1-year retention and social function after buprenorphine-assisted relapse prevention treatment for heroin dependence in Sweden: a randomised, placebo-controlled trial. Lancet 361:662–668, 2003

Petry NM, Bickel WK, Piasecki D, et al: Elevated liver enzyme levels in opioid-dependent patients with hepatitis treated with buprenorphine. Am J Addict 9:265–269, 2000

Tracqui A, Kintz P, Ludes B: Buprenorphine-related deaths among drug addicts in France: a report on 20 fatalities. J Anal Toxicol 22:430–434, 1998

Wedam EF, Bigelow GE, Johnson RE, et al: QT-interval effects of methadone, levomethadyl, and buprenorphine in a randomized trial. Arch Intern Med 167:2469–2475, 2007

17.6   Eye movements, a subtle neurological sign, can be useful in diagnosis of certain drug-related states based on physical examination. Which of the following drugs is associated with a classic vertical nystagmus?

   A. Marijuana.
   B. Cocaine.
   C. Phencyclidine.
   D. Methamphetamine.
   E. Heroin.

The correct response is option C.

Intoxication with phencyclidine (PCP, angel dust) causes a characteristic vertical nystagmus (it can also cause horizontal or rotatory nystagmus), which helps to identify it as the cause when a patient presents with intoxication by an unknown drug (Weaver and Schnoll 2007). In general, acute physiological complications of hallucinogen intoxication rarely require medical treatment. However, malignant hyperthermia and seizures may occur with hallucinogen intoxication. Warning signs for hallucinogen hyperthermia are agitation, dry skin, and increased muscle tension. **(p. 395)**

Weaver MF, Schnoll SH: Phencyclidine and ketamine, in Treatments of Psychiatric Disorders, 4th Edition. Edited by Gabbard GO. Washington, DC, American Psychiatric Publishing, 2007, pp 271–280

Chapter 18

Heart Disease

Select the single best response for each question.

18.1   The most common psychiatric disorder found in patients with coronary artery disease (CAD) is

    A. Generalized anxiety disorder.
    B. Posttraumatic stress disorder.
    C. Major depression.
    D. Panic disorder.
    E. Acute stress disorder.

The correct response is option C.

Depression appears to be the most common psychiatric disorder in CAD patients (Barth et al. 2004; Glassman and Shapiro 1998; Rugulies 2002; van Melle et al. 2004; Wulsin and Singal 2003). Numerous surveys of patients with established coronary disease, acute myocardial infarction (MI), and unstable angina consistently indicate a point prevalence of depression in the range of 15%–20% (Barth et al. 2004; Shapiro et al. 1997; van Melle et al. 2004).

Many studies indicate the widespread failure to diagnose and treat depression in CAD patients (Frasure-Smith et al. 1993; Luutonen et al. 2002). In a Finnish study (Luutonen et al. 2002) of 85 consecutive post-MI patients with 18-month follow-up, the prevalence of Beck Depression Inventory (BDI) scores of 10 or greater was 21% in the hospital, 30% at 6 months, and 33.9% at 18 months. Only 6 patients received mental health treatment; 2 received benzodiazepines; none received adequate antidepressant therapy. **(p. 408)**

Barth J, Schumacher M, Herrmann-Lingen C: Depression as a risk factor for mortality in patients with coronary heart disease: a meta-analysis. Psychosom Med 66:802–813, 2004

Frasure-Smith N, Lesperance F, Talajic M: Depression following myocardial infarction. Impact on 6-month survival. JAMA 270:1819–1825, 1993

Glassman AH, Shapiro PA: Depression and the course of coronary artery disease. Am J Psychiatry 155:4–11, 1998

Luutonen S, Holm H, Salminen JK, et al: Inadequate treatment of depression after myocardial infarction. Acta Psychiatr Scand 106:434–439, 2002

Rugulies R: Depression as a predictor for coronary heart disease: a review and meta-analysis. Am J Prev Med 23:51–61, 2002

Shapiro PA, Lidagoster L, Glassman AH: Depression and heart disease. Psychiatr Ann 27:347–352, 1997

van Melle JP, de Jonge P, Spijkerman TA, et al: Prognostic association of depression following myocardial infarction with mortality and cardiovascular events: a meta-analysis. Psychosom Med 66:814–822, 2004

Wulsin LR, Singal BM: Do depressive symptoms increase the risk for the onset of coronary disease? A systematic quantitative review. Psychosom Med 65:201–210, 2003

18.2 The proposed association of mitral valve prolapse and panic disorder has been supported by which of the following findings?

    A. Panic occurs at higher-than-expected rates in patients with electrocardiogram (ECG) mitral valve prolapse.

    B. Mitral valve prolapse rarely occurs in populations with other psychiatric disorders.

    C. A systemic review conducted in 2008 found substantial evidence of the association.

    D. Genetic studies have established a possible link between panic disorder and mitral valve prolapse and other medical conditions.

    E. A high percentage (60%–70%) of patients with panic disorder have ECG findings of prolapse.

The correct response is option D.

An association of mitral valve prolapse with panic was proposed in the past on the basis of symptoms associated with prolapse (fluttering or palpitation experiences) in patients with panic disorder and echocardiographic findings of prolapse (Carney et al. 1990; Gorman et al. 1988). Depending on the echocardiographic criteria employed, 5%–20% or more of patients with panic disorder have mitral valve prolapse (Dager et al. 1986; Liberthson et al. 1986; Margraf et al. 1988). Individuals with mitral valve prolapse may be asymptomatic or may experience occasional palpitations or "fluttering" sensations in the precordium, and it has been proposed that these sensations give rise to catastrophic cognitions that stimulate panic attacks in predisposed individuals (Barlow 1988). The link has been questioned, however, because panic does not occur at higher-than-expected rates in patients with echocardiographic mitral valve prolapse, and because mitral valve prolapse occurs in many other psychiatric disorder populations. A systematic review found the evidence of association inconclusive at best (Filho et al. 2008). A possible link, in at least some cases, comes from genetic studies in panic disorder that have identified a syndrome of joint hyperlaxity, bladder and renal abnormalities, mitral valve prolapse, and panic attacks that is linked to chromosome 13 (Hamilton et al. 2003; Martin-Santos et al. 1998). **(p. 409)**

Barlow DH: Anxiety and Its Disorders. New York, Guilford, 1988

Carney RM, Freedland KE, Ludbrook PA, et al: Major depression, panic disorder, and mitral valve prolapse in patients who complain of chest pain. Am J Med 89:757–760, 1990

Dager SR, Comess KA, Dunner DL: Differentiation of anxious patients by two-dimensional echocardiographic evaluation of the mitral valve. Am J Psychiatry 143:533–535, 1986

Filho AS, Maciel BC, Martín-Santos R, et al: Does the association between mitral valve prolapse and panic disorder really exist? Prim Care Companion J Clin Psychiatry 10:38–47, 2008

Gorman JM, Goetz RR, Fyer M, et al: The mitral valve prolapse–panic disorder connection. Psychosom Med 50:114–122, 1988

Hamilton SP, Fyer AJ, Durner M, et al: Further genetic evidence for a panic disorder syndrome mapping to chromosome 13q. Proc Natl Acad Sci U S A 100:2550–2555, 2003

Liberthson R, Sheehan DV, King ME, et al: The prevalence of mitral valve prolapse in patients with panic disorders. Am J Psychiatry 143:511–515, 1986

Margraf J, Ehlers A, Roth WT: Mitral valve prolapse and panic disorder: a review of their relationship. Psychosom Med 50:93–113, 1988

Martin-Santos R, Bulbena A, Porta M, et al: Association between joint hypermobility syndrome and panic disorder. Am J Psychiatry 155:1578–1583, 1998

18.3 Risk factors for experiencing delirium after open-heart surgery include all of the following *except*

    A. Cerebrovascular disease.

    B. Use of dexmedetomidine for postoperative sedation.

    C. Metabolic abnormalities.

    D. Older age.

    E. Prolonged postoperative sedation.

The correct response is option B.

Predictors of delirium after open-heart surgery include older age, cerebrovascular disease, prolonged sedation, metabolic derangement, and narcotic use (Giltay et al. 2006; Kazmierski et al. 2008; Norkiene et al. 2007). Off-pump coronary bypass surgery has been studied as a means of reducing delirium and neuropsychological impairment after surgery (Diegeler et al. 2000). Avoidance of the heart-lung bypass machine reduces the production of inflammatory cytokines and reduces emboli to the brain; these factors appear to correlate with, at best, modestly improved neuropsychological outcome (Lee et al. 2003; Van Dijk et al. 2002, 2007). Delirium after heart surgery is commonly related to the duration of postoperative sedation with narcotics and benzodiazepines. Substitution of dexmedetomidine for fentanyl, midazolam, or lorazepam sedation reduces the incidence of delirium (Maldonado et al. 2009; Pandharipande et al. 2007). **(p. 411)**

Diegeler A, Hirsch R, Schneider F, et al: Neuromonitoring and neurocognitive outcome in off-pump versus conventional coronary bypass operation. Ann Thorac Surg 69:1162–1166, 2000

Giltay EJ, Huijskes RVHP, Kho KH, et al: Psychotic symptoms in patients undergoing coronary artery bypass grafting and heart valve operation. Eur J Cardio-Thorac Surg 30:140–147, 2006

Kazmierski J, Kowman M, Banach M, et al: Clinical utility and use of DSM-IV and ICD-10 criteria and the Memorial Delirium Assessment Scale in establishing a diagnosis of delirium after cardiac surgery. Psychosomatics 49:73–76, 2008

Lee JD, Lee SJ, Tsushima WT, et al: Benefits of off-pump bypass on neurologic and clinical morbidity: a prospective randomized trial. Ann Thorac Surg 76:18–25, 2003

Maldonado JR, Wysong A, van der Starre PJ, et al: Dexmedetomidine and the reduction of postoperative delirium after cardiac surgery. Psychosomatics 50:206–217, 2009

Norkiene I, Ringaitiene D, Misiuriene I, et al: Incidence and precipitating factors of delirium after coronary artery bypass grafting. Scand Cardiovasc J 41:180–185, 2007

Pandharipande PP, Pun BT, Herr DL, et al: Effect of sedation with dexmedetomidine vs lorazepam on acute brain dysfunction in mechanically ventilated patients: the MENDS randomized controlled trial. JAMA 298:2644–2653, 2007

Van Dijk D, Jansen EWL, Hijman R, et al: Cognitive outcome after off-pump and on-pump coronary artery bypass graft surgery: a randomized trial. JAMA 287:1405–1412, 2002

van Dijk D, Spoor M, Hijman R, et al: Cognitive and cardiac outcomes 5 years after off-pump vs on-pump coronary artery bypass graft surgery. JAMA 297:701–708, 2007

18.4   The cardiologist on the inpatient medical unit asks you to evaluate a post–myocardial infarction patient who is experiencing visual hallucinations manifesting as yellow rings around objects. You review the cardiac medications the patient is receiving and immediately identify an agent capable of producing the side effects that the patient is experiencing. The medication responsible is likely

   A. Amiodarone.
   B. An angiotensin-converting enzyme inhibitor.
   C. A beta-blocker.
   D. An angiotensin II receptor blocker.
   E. Digoxin.

The correct response is option E.

Side effects of digoxin include visual hallucinations, delirium, and depression (see Table 18–1). **(p. 411)**

Table 18–1. Selected psychiatric side effects of cardiac drugs

Drug/class	Effects
Digoxin	Visual hallucinations (classically, yellow rings around objects), delirium, depression
Beta-blockers	Fatigue, sexual dysfunction
Alpha-blockers	Depression, sexual dysfunction
Lidocaine	Agitation, delirium, psychosis
Carvedilol	Fatigue, insomnia
Methyldopa	Depression, confusion, insomnia
Reserpine	Depression
Clonidine	Depression
ACE inhibitors	Mood elevation or depression (rare)
Pressors (dobutamine, milrinone, dopamine)	Psychiatric effects (rare)
Angiotensin II receptor blockers	Psychiatric effects (rare)
Amiodarone	Mood disorders secondary to thyroid effects
Diuretics	Hypokalemia, hyponatremia resulting in anorexia, weakness, apathy

Note. ACE = angiotensin-converting enzyme.

18.5   The combination of tendency to experience negative affects and to inhibit expression of negative emotions in social interactions has been termed

   A. Type A personality.
   B. Type B personality.
   C. Type C personality.
   D. Type D personality.
   E. Type E personality.

The correct response is option D.

The combination of tendency to experience negative affects and to inhibit expression of negative emotions in social interactions has been coined Type D (for "distressed") personality (Denollet 2005; Pelle et al. 2009). This construct, explored almost exclusively in European studies, has been repeatedly associated with increased coronary disease risk (Denollet et al. 1995, 1996, 2006). **(p. 416)**

> Denollet J: DS14: standard assessment of negative affectivity, social inhibition, and Type D personality. Psychosom Med 67:89–97, 2005
>
> Denollet J, Sys S, Brutsaert DL: Personality and mortality after myocardial infarction. Psychosom Med 57:582–591, 1995
>
> Denollet J, Sys SU, Stroobant N, et al: Personality as independent predictor of long-term mortality in patients with coronary heart disease. Lancet 347:417–421, 1996
>
> Denollet J, Pedersen SS, Vrints CJ, et al: Usefulness of type D personality in predicting five-year cardiac events above and beyond concurrent symptoms of stress in patients with coronary heart disease. Am J Cardiol 97:970–973, 2006
>
> Pelle AJ, Denollet J, Zwisler AD, et al: Overlap and distinctiveness of psychological risk factors in patients with ischemic heart disease and chronic heart failure: are we there yet? J Affect Disord 113:150–156, 2009

18.6   Following cardiac bypass surgery, a patient is placed on a thiazide diuretic, an angiotensin-converting enzyme (ACE) inhibitor, and warfarin by his cardiologist. The patient develops sadness, anhedonia, sleep disturbance, decreased energy, guilty feelings, and concentration difficulties. You diagnose major depression and decide to start the patient on paroxetine. Which of the following side effects due to drug–drug interactions should you be most concerned about?

A. Increased bleeding risk.
B. Hypertension.
C. Prolonged QT interval.
D. Atrioventricular block.
E. Hypotension.

The correct response is option A.

Selective serotonin reuptake inhibitors and warfarin interactions can result in increased bleeding risks (see Table 18–3). **(p. 427)**

Table 18–3.   Selected psychotropic drug interactions with cardiovascular drugs

Psychotropic agent	Cardiovascular agent	Effect
SSRIs	Beta-blockers	Additive bradycardic effects
	Warfarin	Increased bleeding risk, especially with paroxetine and fluoxetine, despite little effect on INR
MAOIs	Epinephrine, dopamine	Hypertension
Lithium	Thiazide diuretics	Increased lithium level
TCAs	Type IA antiarrhythmic agents, amiodarone	Prolonged QT interval, increased AV block
Lithium	ACE inhibitors, angiotensin II receptor blockers	Increased lithium level
Phenothiazines	Beta-blockers	Hypotension

Note.   ACE = angiotensin-converting enzyme; AV = atrioventricular; INR = international normalized ratio; MAOIs = monoamine oxidase inhibitors; SSRIs = selective serotonin reuptake inhibitors; TCAs = tricyclic antidepressants.

18.7   Which of the following antidepressants or antidepressant classes may cause cardiac conduction delay as a side effect and ventricular arrhythmias in overdose?

A. Monoamine oxidase inhibitors (MAOIs).
B. Selective serotonin reuptake inhibitors (SSRIs).
C. Tricyclic antidepressants (TCAs).
D. Bupropion.
E. Mirtazapine.

The correct response is option C.

TCAs cause orthostatic hypotension, cardiac conduction delay (bundle branch block or complete atrioventricular nodal block), and, in overdose, ventricular arrhythmias (ventricular premature depolarization, ventricular tachycardia, and ventricular fibrillation).

MAOIs cause hypotension and orthostatic hypotension; dietary indiscretions resulting in high circulating levels of tyramine cause hypertensive crises. Consequently, there has been little interest in the use of MAOIs in patients with heart disease.

SSRIs have little to no cardiac effect in healthy subjects. The most commonly observed effect is slowing of heart rate, generally by a clinically insignificant 1–2 beats/minute. The combination of beta-adrenergic blockade and serotonin reuptake inhibitors may result in additive slowing of heart rate with increased risk of symptoms.

Bupropion appears to have few cardiovascular effects in small studies but may increase blood pressure occasionally (Roose et al. 1991).

Mirtazapine treatment (30–45 mg/day) of depression in patients who had had an acute coronary syndrome was evaluated in a randomized placebo-controlled trial as a part of the MIND-IT trial (Honig et al. 2007). Mirtazapine was well tolerated by the patients in this trial, with no effects on heart rate, blood pressure, or electrocardiographic parameters, and no difference from placebo in the rate of major adverse cardiac events. **(pp. 423–425; Table 18–2)**

Honig A, Kuyper AMG, Schene AH, et al: Treatment of post-myocardial infarction depressive disorder: a randomized, placebo-controlled trial with mirtazapine. Psychosom Med 69:606–613, 2007

Roose SP, Dalack GW, Glassman AH, et al: Cardiovascular effects of bupropion in depressed patients with heart disease. Am J Psychiatry 148:512–516, 1991

Chapter 19

Lung Disease

Select the single best response for each question.

19.1   Asthma is well known to be associated with mood and anxiety symptoms, and diagnosis is complicated by the overlap between anxiety symptoms and the hyperadrenergic symptoms characteristic of an asthma exacerbation. Which of the following features is more suggestive of a diagnosis of panic than of asthma?

   A. Shortness of breath.
   B. Palpitations.
   C. Sweating.
   D. Lightheadedness.
   E. Negative methacholine inhalation challenge test.

The correct response is option E.

Asthma may sometimes be mistakenly diagnosed as an anxiety disorder, especially panic disorder, and some anxiety disorders (panic, social anxiety) may be mislabeled as asthma. This differentiation can be difficult because shortness of breath, palpitations, sweating, chest pain, light-headedness, fear of losing control, and even fear of dying can represent either asthma or panic anxiety. When the diagnosis is unclear, a negative methacholine inhalation challenge test indicates no airway hyperresponsiveness and therefore a diagnosis other than asthma (Schmaling et al. 1999). **(p. 441)**

> Schmaling KB, Niloofar A, Barnhart S, et al: Medical and psychiatric predictors of airway reactivity. Respir Care 44:1452–1457, 1999

19.2   Sarcoidosis, even without direct central nervous system involvement, is associated with psychiatric comorbidity. According to the study by Goracci et al. (2008), which of the following comorbidities was most common in sarcoidosis?

   A. Obsessive-compulsive disorder.
   B. Generalized anxiety disorder.
   C. Major depressive disorder.
   D. Panic disorder.
   E. Bipolar disorder.

The correct response is option C.

Psychiatric comorbidity was reported in 44% of Italian sarcoidosis patients, with major depressive disorder in 25%, panic disorder in 6.3%, bipolar disorder in 6.3%, generalized anxiety disorder in 5%, and obsessive-compulsive disorder in 1.3% (Goracci et al. 2008). **(p. 446)**

> Goracci A, Fagliolini A, Martinucci M, et al: Quality of life, anxiety and depression in sarcoidosis. Gen Hosp Psychiatry 30:441–445, 2008

19.3 Tuberculosis treatment with isoniazid has been associated with mania and psychosis as a drug side effect. Risk factors for this side effect include all of the following *except*

  A. Rapid acetylation.
  B. Alcoholism.
  C. Diabetes mellitus.
  D. Liver disease.
  E. Pyridoxine deficiency.

The correct response is option A.

Rapid acetylation is not a predisposing factor for psychiatric symptoms in tuberculosis patients treated with isoniazid.

Psychiatrists must be attuned to neuropsychiatric symptoms such as mania and psychosis during treatment with isoniazid (Alao and Yolles 1998), probably related to its being a weak but irreversible inhibitor of monoamine oxidase. No dietary restrictions are required, but isoniazid can interact with other drugs. Predisposing factors for psychiatric side effects of isoniazid include alcoholism, diabetes, hepatic insufficiency, old age, slow acetylation, and family and personal history of mental illness (Djibo and Lawan 2001). Pyridoxine deficiency may also play a role in the etiology of isoniazid-related psychosis. **(p. 447)**

Alao AO, Yolles JC: Isoniazid-induced psychosis. Ann Pharmacother 32:889–891, 1998
Djibo A, Lawan A: Behavioral disorders after treatment with isoniazid [in French]. Bull Soc Pathol Exot 94(2):112–114, 2001

19.4 Lung cancer, a leading cause of cancer death and most often the consequence of smoking, is well known to be associated with mood and anxiety symptoms. Which of the following statements regarding psychopathology in lung cancer is *false?*

  A. Depression is more common in lung cancer than in breast cancer.
  B. Anxiety is less common in lung cancer than in breast cancer.
  C. Suicide in lung cancer occurs at twice the rate in the U.S. general population.
  D. Lung cancer has the highest standardized mortality ratio among organ cancers.
  E. Suicide risk peaks in the first 5 years after diagnosis.

The correct response is option B.

Depression and anxiety are more frequent in patients with lung cancer than in those with breast cancer (Brintzenhofe-Szoc et al. 2009). In one study, type of lung cancer influenced the rate of depression (i.e., more frequent in small-cell cancer than non-small-cell cancer); however, the most important risk factor was functional impairment (Hopwood and Stephens 2000). Suicide rates in cancer patients are twice that of the general population in the United States, with lung cancer having the highest standardized mortality ratio among cancers of various organs. Risk is highest in the first 5 years after diagnosis (Misono et al. 2008). **(p. 449)**

Brintzenhofe-Szoc KM, Levin TT, Li Y, et al: Mixed anxiety/depression symptoms in a large cancer cohort: prevalence by cancer type. Psychosomatics 50:383–391, 2009
Hopwood P, Stephens RJ: Depression in patients with lung cancer: prevalence and risk factors derived from quality-of-life data. J Clin Oncol 18:893–903, 2000
Misono S, Weiss NS, Fann JR, et al: Incidence of suicide in persons with cancer. J Clin Oncol 26:4731–4738, 2008

19.5 The use of benzodiazepines, with appropriate caution, may be considered for anxiety-spectrum symptoms in chronic obstructive pulmonary disease (COPD). Which of the following benzodiazepines would be safest in elderly and/or debilitated COPD patients?

    A. Chlordiazepoxide.
    B. Diazepam.
    C. Clonazepam.
    D. Lorazepam.
    E. Tranxene.

The correct response is option D.

In COPD patients who do not retain carbon dioxide, prudent doses of benzodiazepines may decrease breathlessness. In elderly or debilitated patients, shorter-acting benzodiazepines with no active metabolites, such as alprazolam, lorazepam, and oxazepam, are preferred. **(p. 452)**

19.6 Given the risk of cytochrome P450 (CYP) interactions with pulmonary drugs, which of the following selective serotonin reuptake inhibitors (SSRIs) would be preferred for management of mood disorders in pulmonary patients?

    A. Fluvoxamine.
    B. Paroxetine.
    C. Fluoxetine.
    D. Citalopram.
    E. Norfluoxetine.

The correct response is option D.

When choosing an antidepressant, the side-effect profile and CYP interactions with pulmonary drugs should be considered. Among the SSRIs, sertraline, citalopram, and escitalopram have the lowest risk of interactions with pulmonary drugs, and SSRIs may decrease dyspnea and even increase arterial oxygen concentration in some patients (Ciraulo and Shader 1990; Smoller et al. 1998). **(p. 452)**

Ciraulo DA, Shader RI: Fluoxetine drug-drug interactions, II. J Clin Psychopharmacol 10:213–217, 1990

Smoller JW, Pollack MH, Systrom D, et al: Sertraline effects on dyspnea in patients with obstructive airways disease. Psychosomatics 39:24–29, 1998

Chapter 20

Gastrointestinal Disorders

Select the single best response for each question.

20.1 An oropharyngeal disorder characterized by subjective complaint of dry mouth that may be associated with reduced saliva production is

    A. Burning mouth syndrome.
    B. Dysphagia.
    C. Globus hystericus.
    D. Rumination syndrome.
    E. Xerostomia.

The correct response is option E.

Xerostomia represents a subjective complaint of dry mouth that may be associated with reduced saliva production. Among sampled populations, xerostomia has been found to be present in up to 30%; its presence predisposes patients to dental caries and oropharyngeal *Candida albicans* infections (Guggenheimer and Moore 2003).

Burning mouth syndrome is a chronic pain condition characterized by a persistent oral burning sensation without accompanying evidence of mucosal disturbance (Sardella 2007; Scala et al. 2003). Symptoms typically persist throughout the day, intensify late in the day, and may be relieved by eating or drinking.

Successful swallowing of liquids or foodstuffs requires a coordinated sequence of voluntary and involuntary neuromuscular contractions that moves a bolus from mouth to pharynx, to esophagus, and finally the stomach. Circumstances that interfere with this series of movements lead to *dysphagia*, which is estimated to affect 7%–10% of adults older than 50 years, with higher rates in hospitalized and nursing home patients (Spieker 2000).

Globus is the sensation of having a lump or mass in the throat that does not interfere with actual swallowing. *Globus pharyngeus* or *hystericus* represents a common benign disorder responsible for 4% of ear, nose, and throat referrals (Caylakli et al. 2006).

Rumination syndrome involves repeated and effortless regurgitation of small amounts of food from the stomach, which is subsequently rechewed, reswallowed, or expelled (Papadopoulos and Mimidis 2007). This behavior is common among infants and developmentally disabled individuals, but also can appear in children and adults of normal intelligence (Olden 2001). **(pp. 463–465)**

Caylakli F, Yavuz H, Erkan AN, et al: Evaluation of patients with globus pharyngeus with barium swallow pharyngoesophagography. Laryngoscope 116:37–39, 2006

Guggenheimer J, Moore PA: Xerostomia: etiology, recognition and treatment. J Am Dent Assoc 134:61–69, 2003

Olden KW: Rumination. Curr Treat Options Gastroenterol 4:351–358, 2001

Papadopoulos V, Mimidis K: The rumination syndrome in adults: a review of the pathophysiology, diagnosis and treatment. J Postgrad Med 53:203–206, 2007

Sardella A: An up-to-date view on burning mouth syndrome. Minerva Stomatol 56:327–340, 2007

Scala A, Checci L, Montevecchi M, et al: Update on burning mouth syndrome: overview and patient management. Crit Rev Oral Biol Med 14:275–291, 2003

Spieker MR: Evaluating dysphagia. Am Fam Physician 61:3639–3648, 2000

20.2 A gastroenterologist evaluates a patient who presents with troublesome symptoms due to the efflux of stomach contents. Endoscopically, no reflux esophagitis is seen, but the patient is still symptomatic. What is the likely diagnosis?

    A. Dysphagia.
    B. Functional heartburn.
    C. Gastroesophageal reflux disorder.
    D. Noncardiac chest pain.
    E. Nonerosive reflux disorder.

The correct response is option E.

Gastroesophageal reflux disorder (GERD) is defined as "a condition which develops when the reflux of stomach contents causes troublesome symptoms and/or complications" (Vakil et al. 2006, p. 1903). When no reflux esophagitis is seen endoscopically but the patient is still symptomatic, the condition is called *nonerosive reflux disorder (NERD)*.

Dysphagia typically refers to difficulty swallowing, resulting from impeded transport of liquids and/or solids from the pharynx to the stomach. Dysphagia is considered an oropharyngeal disorder rather than an upper gastrointestinal disorder.

Functional heartburn has been defined as burning retrosternal discomfort or pain in the absence of evidence that gastroesophageal acid reflux is the cause of the symptom and absence of histopathology-based esophageal motility disorder (Drossman 2006).

Chest pain identical to myocardial ischemia can be caused by GERD and is referred to as reflux chest pain syndrome, the most common cause of *noncardiac chest pain (NCCP)* (Cannon et al. 1994; Vakil et al. 2006). GERD can cause chest pain indistinguishable from cardiac ischemia and is the most common cause of NCCP (Cannon et al. 1994; Fass and Dickman 2006; Vakil et al. 2006). **(pp. 465–466)**

Cannon RO, Quyyumi AA, Mincemoyer R, et al: Imipramine in patients with chest pain despite normal coronary angiograms. N Engl J Med 330:1411–1417, 1994

Drossman DA (ed): Rome III: The Functional Gastrointestinal Disorders, 3rd Edition. McLean, VA, Degnon Associates, 2006

Fass R, Dickman R: Non-cardiac chest pain: an update. Neurogastroenterol Motil 18:408–417, 2006

Vakil N, van Zanten SV, Kahrilas P, et al: The Montreal definition and classification of gastroesophageal reflux disease: a global evidence-based consensus. Am J Gastroenterol 101:1900–1920, 2006

20.3 The term *functional nausea and vomiting* refers to chronic nausea and vomiting without apparent cause. Several specific conditions are encompassed in this category. One of these, a condition characterized by recurrent, stereotypical bouts of severe nausea and vomiting, is called

    A. Cyclic vomiting syndrome.
    B. Functional vomiting.
    C. Chronic idiopathic nausea.
    D. Anticipatory nausea and vomiting.
    E. Gastroparesis.

The correct response is option A.

Cyclic vomiting syndrome (CVS) is characterized by recurrent, stereotypical bouts of severe nausea and vomiting. CVS consists of four phases: prodromal, emetic, recovery, and interepisode or well. For many, certain triggers can set off an episode, including infections, lack of sleep, psychologically stressful events (positive and negative), menstrual period, fasting, and certain foods.

Functional nausea and vomiting was once referred to as "psychogenic" vomiting, but there is no evidence showing a direct link between psychiatric disorders and chronic unexplained nausea and vomiting (Olden and Chepyala 2008; Talley 2007). According to Rome III criteria, functional nausea and vomiting is divided into three specific conditions: chronic idiopathic nausea (CIN), functional vomiting (FV), and cyclic vomiting syndrome (CVS) (Olden and Chepyala 2008; Talley 2007). *Chronic idiopathic nausea* involves nausea that occurs several times a week, which is not usually accompanied by vomiting. *Functional vomiting* refers to unexplained vomiting that occurs at least once a week, is not cyclical, and lacks an organic basis. The epidemiology and pathophysiology of CIN and FV are presently unknown (Olden and Chepyala 2008).

Anticipatory nausea and vomiting (ANV) are conditioned responses to settings and circumstances primarily associated with actual episodes of nausea and vomiting. This condition is well recognized in the oncology literature, in which 10%–44% of patients may be affected, but anticipatory nausea and vomiting can develop with other causes of nausea and vomiting, such as pregnancy, gastroparesis, or cyclic vomiting syndrome (Aapro 2005).

Gastroparesis is a clinical disorder of delayed gastric emptying without evidence of mechanical obstruction. Symptoms are variable but often include nausea, vomiting, early satiety, abdominal bloating, and pain. Symptom severity does not necessarily correlate with the magnitude of delayed gastric emptying present (Khoo et al. 2009; Stapleton and Wo 2009). **(pp. 467–468)**

Aapro MS, Molassiotis A, Olver I: Anticipatory nausea and vomiting. Support Care Cancer 13:117–121, 2005

Khoo J, Rayner CK, Jones KL, et al: Pathophysiology and management of gastroparesis. Expert Rev Gastroenterol Hepatol 3:167–181, 2009

Olden KW, Chepyala P: Functional nausea and vomiting. Nat Clin Pract Gastroenterol Hepatol 5:202–208, 2008

Stapleton J, Wo JM: Current treatment of nausea and vomiting associated with gastroparesis: antiemetics, prokinetics, tricyclics. Gastrointest Endosc Clin N Am 19:57–72, vi, 2009

Talley NJ: Functional nausea and vomiting. Aust Fam Physician 36:694–697, 2007

20.4   Which of the following is the most common cause of dyspepsia?

    A. Gastroesophageal reflux disorder.
    B. Functional dyspepsia.
    C. Peptic ulcer disease.
    D. Gastric malignancy.
    E. Nonerosive reflux disorder.

The correct response is option B.

Dyspepsia is characterized by chronic or recurrent pain or discomfort centered in the upper abdomen and may include early satiety and upper abdominal fullness (Talley et al. 2005a). Bloating and nausea may also occur, but do not make the diagnosis by themselves (Talley et al. 2005a). The four major causes of dyspepsia are peptic ulcer disease (PUD), gastroesophageal reflux disorder (GERD), gastric malignancy, and functional dyspepsia (FD).

Up to 70% of patients with dyspepsia have FD, which negatively affects quality of life (Talley et al. 2005b). The underlying pathophysiology remains unclear, but several possible mechanisms have been considered, one of which is hypersensitivity to gastric distension or acid exposure (Talley et al. 2005a). Many studies have shown that comorbidity between FD and psychiatric disorders, especially anxiety disorders, is high.

PUD is the cause of approximately 10% of all upper gastrointestinal symptoms, and *Helicobacter pylori* is the main cause of PUD not induced by nonsteroidal anti-inflammatory drugs (American Gastroenterological Association 2005). As the prevalence of *H. pylori* has dramatically declined in most of the Western world, so has the prevalence of PUD and gastric adenocarcinoma (Talley et al. 2005b). **(pp. 469–470)**

American Gastroenterological Association: American Gastroenterological Association medical position statement: evaluation of dyspepsia. Gastroenterology 129:1753–1755, 2005

Talley NJ, Vakil N, Practice Parameters Committee of the American College of Gastroenterology: Guidelines for management of dyspepsia. Am J Gastroenterol 100:2324–2337, 2005a

Talley NJ, Vakil N, Moayyedi P: American Gastroenterological Association technical review on the evaluation of dyspepsia. Gastroenterology 129:1756–1780, 2005b

20.5 The psychiatric disorder most commonly found in patients with irritable bowel syndrome (IBS) is

    A. Anxiety.
    B. Personality disorder.
    C. Depression.
    D. Substance use disorder.
    E. Somatization disorder.

The correct response is option C.

The prevalence of comorbid Axis I disorders is estimated to range from 40% to 94% among IBS patients primarily seen in tertiary care centers. Depression is the most common disorder, followed by anxiety and somatization disorders (Palsson and Drossman 2005). Bidirectional comorbidity exists between anxiety or depression and IBS, as elevated rates of IBS have been detected among patients with anxiety and depressive disorders (Karling et al. 2007). Frequently, however, psychiatric disorders predate the onset of IBS symptoms. The presence of anxiety or depression among IBS patients is associated with more severe gastrointestinal symptoms, greater functional impairment, and worse prognosis (Karling et al. 2007; Lee et al. 2009). Differences in coping mechanisms or personality styles have also been noted, with elevated levels of catastrophizing and neuroticism (Palsson and Drossman 2005). **(pp. 474–475)**

    Karling P, Danielsson A, Adolfsson R, et al: No difference in symptoms of irritable bowel syndrome between healthy subjects and patients with recurrent depression in remission. Neurogastroenterol Motil 19:896–904, 2007
    Lee KJ, Kwon HC, Cheong JY, et al: Demographic, clinical, and psychological characteristics of the heartburn groups classified using the Rome III criteria and factors associated with the responsiveness to proton pump inhibitors in the gastroesophageal reflux disease group. Digestion 79:131–136, 2009
    Palsson OS, Drossman DA: Psychiatric and psychological dysfunction in irritable bowel syndrome and the role of psychological treatments. Gastroenterol Clin N Am 34:281–303, 2005

20.6 Which of the following is the greatest risk factor for hepatitis C virus (HCV) infection?

    A. Hemodialysis.
    B. Blood transfusion.
    C. Sexual contact.
    D. Intravenous drug use.
    E. Tattooing.

The correct response is option D.

Intravenous drug use remains the greatest risk factor for HCV infection. Less commonly, transmission occurs by hemodialysis, blood transfusion, perinatal exposure, intranasal drug use, body piercing, tattooing, sexual contact, and receipt of an organ transplant from an HCV-positive donor (Ghany et al. 2009). Transmission via transfusion declined markedly following routine screening for HCV antibodies beginning in 1992.

HCV, the second most common bloodborne disease in the world, affects up to 2% of the world's population (Perry et al. 2008). Acute infection is often asymptomatic; therefore, many patients are unaware of being infected until they develop long-term consequences. The surreptitious nature of the disease makes screening patients at high risk for infection especially important. **(p. 476)**

    Ghany MG, Strader DB, Thomas DL, et al: Diagnosis, management, and treatment of hepatitis C: an update. Hepatology 49:1335–1374, 2009

Perry W, Hilsabeck RC, Hassanein TI: Cognitive dysfunction in chronic hepatitis C: a review. Dig Dis Sci 53:307–321, 2008

20.7   Standard treatment for hepatitis C virus (HCV) infection involves the use of pegylated interferon-alpha and ribavirin (IFN therapy) for 24–48 weeks. Which of the following drug-induced psychiatric symptoms is most likely to occur with IFN therapy?

    A. Cognitive impairment.
    B. Hypomania/mania.
    C. Psychosis.
    D. Depression.
    E. Delirium.

The correct response is option D.

IFN-induced depression has been reported to occur in 10%–40% of patients, depending on study design, diagnostic criteria, assessment methods, and study population (Schäfer et al. 2007). The incidence of depression is also influenced by the dose and duration of IFN therapy. Depressive symptoms usually develop within the first 12 weeks of treatment and are often accompanied by irritability rather than dysphoria.

Patients often report cognitive problems during IFN therapy, including difficulties with memory, concentration, and problem solving. IFN affects the frontal-subcortical system, producing problems with working memory and complex attention (Kraus et al. 2005; Pawelczk et al. 2008; Perry et al. 2008). The effect depends on the dosage, duration, and route of administration of IFN. Frank delirium is rare.

Reports of mood lability and irritability are not uncommon with IFN therapy, but frank mania is infrequent and usually requires treatment termination. Most often, hypomania or mania appears to develop after weeks or months of treatment, but cases have been reported of mania appearing after marked dose reduction or abrupt discontinuation of IFN (Constant et al. 2005; Malik and Ravasia 2004; Onyike et al. 2004). The course of IFN-induced hypomania or mania is unclear, although most cases report resolution of symptoms after psychotropic medications are started and IFN therapy stopped. Reports of IFN-induced psychosis are rare (Bozikas et al. 2001; Hoffman et al. 2003; Tamam et al. 2003). **(pp. 476–477)**

Bozikas V, Petrikis P, Balla A, et al: An interferon-alpha-induced psychotic disorder in a patient with chronic hepatitis C. Eur Psychiatry 16:136–137, 2001

Constant A, Castera L, Dantzer R, et al: Mood alterations during interferon-alfa therapy in patients with chronic hepatitis C: evidence for an overlap between manic/hypomanic and depressive symptoms. J Clin Psychiatry 66:1050–1057, 2005

Hoffman RG, Cohen MA, Alfonso CA, et al: Treatment of interferon-induced psychosis in patients with comorbid hepatitis C and HIV. Psychosomatics 44:417–420, 2003

Kraus MR, Schäfer A, Wibmann S, et al: Neurocognitive changes in patients with hepatitis C receiving interferon alfa-2b and ribavirin. Clin Pharmacol Ther 77:90–100, 2005

Malik AR, Ravasia S: Interferon-induced mania. Can J Psychiatry 49:867–868, 2004

Onyike CU, Bonner JO, Lyketsos CG, et al: Mania during treatment of chronic hepatitis C with pegylated interferon and ribavirin. Am J Psychiatry 161:429–435, 2004

Pawelczk T, Pawelczk A, Strzelecki D, et al: Pegylated interferon a and ribavirin therapy may induce working memory disturbances in chronic hepatitis C patients. Gen Hosp Psychiatry 30:501–508, 2008

Perry W, Hilsabeck RC, Hassanein TI: Cognitive dysfunction in chronic hepatitis C: a review. Dig Dis Sci 53:307–321, 2008

Schäfer A, Wittchen HU, Seufert J, et al: Methodological approaches in the assessment of interferon-alfa-induced depression in patients with chronic hepatitis C: a critical review. Int J Methods Psychiatr Res 16:186–201, 2007

Tamam L, Yerdelen D, Ozpoyraz N: Psychosis associated with interferon alfa therapy for chronic hepatitis B. Ann Pharmacother 37:384–387, 2003

20.8   Which of the following mood stabilizers is most often associated with cases of drug-induced pancreatitis?

   A. Gabapentin.
   B. Carbamazepine.
   C. Valproic acid.
   D. Lamotrigine.
   E. Topiramate.

The correct response is option C.

The mechanism behind drug-induced pancreatitis is unclear (Kaurich 2008). Valproic acid is the psychotropic drug most often reported in cases of drug-induced pancreatitis, although the true incidence is 1 in 40,000 (Ben Salem et al. 2007; Gerstner et al. 2007; Zaccara et al. 2007).

Rarely, pancreatitis has occurred with other anticonvulsants, including carbamazepine, gabapentin, lamotrigine, and topiramate (Jadresic 1994; Kaurich 2008; Soman and Swenson 1985; Zaccara et al. 2007). **(p. 479)**

Ben Salem C, Biour M, Hmouda H, et al: Valproic acid-induced pancreatitis. J Gastroenterol 42:598–599, 2007
Gerstner T, Busing D, Bell N, et al: Valproic acid-induced pancreatitis: 16 new cases and a review of the literature. J Gastroenterol 42:38–48, 2007
Jadresic D: Acute pancreatitis associated with dual vigabatrin and lamotrigine therapy. Seizure 3:319, 1994
Kaurich T: Drug-induced acute pancreatitis. Proc (Bayl Univ Med Cent) 21:77–81, 2008
Soman M, Swenson C: A possible case of carbamazepine-induced pancreatitis. Drug Intell Clin Pharm 19:925–927, 1985
Zaccara G, Franciotta D, Perucca E: Idiosyncratic adverse reactions to antiepileptic drugs. Epilepsia 48:1223–1244, 2007

Chapter 21

Renal Disease

Select the single best response for each question.

21.1   Psychiatric illness is extremely common in renal disease and is the source of much of the caseload on psychosomatic medicine services. In the study by Kimmel et al. (1998) of psychiatric illness in renal dialysis patients, the most common psychiatric diagnoses were

    A. Mood disorders.
    B. Delirium and dementia.
    C. Anxiety disorders.
    D. Psychotic disorders.
    E. Eating disorders.

The correct response is option A.

In a study of psychiatric illness involving 200,000 U.S. dialysis patients, almost 10% had been hospitalized with a psychiatric diagnosis. A psychiatric syndrome was the primary reason for hospitalization of 25% of the subgroup (Kimmel et al. 1998). Depression and other affective disorders were the most common diagnoses, followed by delirium and dementia. **(p. 492)**

> Kimmel PL, Thamer M, Richard CM, et al: Psychiatric illness in patients with end-stage renal disease. Am J Med 105:214–221, 1998

21.2   In the study by Cukor et al. (2008a) of anxiety disorders in end-stage renal disease (ESRD) patients, the most common anxiety disorder diagnoses in this population were

    A. Acute stress disorder (ASD) and posttraumatic stress disorder (PTSD).
    B. Generalized anxiety disorder and agoraphobia without panic disorder.
    C. Phobias and panic disorder.
    D. GAD and PTSD.
    E. Anxiety disorder due to a general medical condition and panic disorder.

The correct response is option C.

In a study that assessed psychiatric diagnoses in a sample of 70 predominantly African American ESRD patients, about 45% had at least one anxiety disorder. The most common diagnoses identified were phobias and panic disorder (Cukor et al. 2008). The prevalence of panic disorder was much higher than in community samples, and may be related to hypervigilance to bodily sensations associated with hemodialysis or fears about the outcome of ESRD treatment. **(p. 493)**

> Cukor D, Coplan J, Brown C, et al: Anxiety disorders in adults treated by hemodialysis: a single-center study. Am J Kidney Dis 52:128–136, 2008

21.3   Cognitive disorders are common in dialysis patients and may complicate the management of this severe chronic illness. Although uremic symptoms may vary among patients, which of the following is *not* a usual behavioral symptom with progression of uremia?

A. Mild cognitive dysfunction.
B. Fatigue.
C. Hyperactive delirium.
D. Hypoactive delirium.
E. Coma.

The correct response is option C.

Uremia refers to the clinical syndrome resulting from profound loss of renal function and has been associated with cognitive impairment, including difficulty with concentration, memory, and intellectual functioning (Pliskin et al. 1996; Souheaver et al. 1982; Williams et al. 2004). Signs and symptoms of uremia vary considerably, with severity presumably depending on both the magnitude and speed with which renal function is lost. Central nervous system symptoms may begin with mild cognitive dysfunction, fatigue, and headache, progressing to hypoactive delirium and, if untreated, coma. **(p. 494)**

> Pliskin NH, Yurk HM, Ho LT, et al: Neurocognitive function in chronic hemodialysis patients. Kidney Int 49:1435–1440, 1996
> Souheaver GT, Ryan JJ, DeWolfe AS: Neuropsychological patterns in uremia. J Clin Psychol 38:490–496, 1982
> Williams MA, Sklar AH, Burright RG, et al: Temporal effects of dialysis on cognitive functioning in patients with ESRD. Am J Kidney Dis 43:705–711, 2004

21.4   The decision to withdraw dialysis and accept hastened death may be a controversial one. Which of the following demographic factors is *not* associated with an increased likelihood of a dialysis withdrawal decision?

A. Female gender.
B. Increased age.
C. Asian ethnicity.
D. Cognitive impairment.
E. Caucasian ethnicity.

The correct response is option C.

In the United States, dialysis withdrawal has been more common among women and more elderly patients, and less common among African American and Asian patients (Kurella Tamura et al. 2010; Leggat et al. 1997; Munshi et al. 2001). Cognitive impairment has also been associated with the decision to withdraw (Chater et al. 2006). **(p. 496)**

> Chater S, Davison SN, Germain MJ, et al: Withdrawal from dialysis: a palliative care perspective. Clin Nephrol 66:364–372, 2006
> Kurella Tamura M, Goldstein M, Perez-Stable E: Preferences for dialysis withdrawal and engagement in advance care planning within a diverse sample of dialysis patients. Nephrol Dial Transplant 25:237–242, 2010
> Leggat JE Jr, Bloembergen WE, Levine G, et al: An analysis of risk factors for withdrawal from dialysis before death. J Am Soc Nephrol 8:1755–1763, 1997
> Munshi SK, Vijayakumar N, Taub NA, et al: Outcome of renal replacement therapy in the very elderly. Nephrol Dial Transplant 16:128–133, 2001

21.5 Depression in renal disease will often require medication management. Among the selective serotonin reuptake inhibitors (SSRIs) in common use, which of the following is associated with reduced clearance in renal disease?

    A. Escitalopram.
    B. Citalopram.
    C. Fluoxetine.
    D. Paroxetine.
    E. Sertraline.

The correct response is option D.

Paroxetine clearance is reduced in patients with renal insufficiency (Doyle et al. 1989). Among the SSRIs, citalopram and sertraline would be expected to have the fewest potential interactions with other medications taken by patients with renal impairment. Some evidence suggests that dosage adjustments may not be needed for citalopram (Spigset et al. 2000) and fluoxetine (Finkelstein and Finkelstein 2000) in patients with renal insufficiency. **(p. 497)**

> Doyle GD, Laher M, Kelly JG, et al: The pharmacokinetics of paroxetine in renal impairment. Acta Psychiatr Scand Suppl 350:89–90, 1989
> Finkelstein FO, Finkelstein SH: Depression in chronic dialysis patients: assessment and treatment. Nephrol Dial Transplant 15:1911–1913, 2000
> Spigset O, Hagg S, Stegmayr B, et al: Citalopram pharmacokinetics in patients with chronic renal failure and the effect of haemodialysis. Eur J Clin Pharmacol 56:699–703, 2000

21.6 Although antipsychotic medication typically can be maintained in renal failure, which of the following antipsychotics may require dosage reduction in patients with renal disease?

    A. Olanzapine.
    B. Ziprasidone.
    C. Aripiprazole.
    D. Quetiapine.
    E. Paliperidone.

The correct response is option E.

Antipsychotics typically do not depend on renal elimination, with the exception of paliperidone, which is largely excreted unchanged in urine and thus requires dose reduction in patients with renal insufficiency (Vermeir et al. 2008). As with tricyclic antidepressants, adverse effects of antipsychotics may be amplified by medical comorbidities in end-stage renal disease patients, such as diabetes, hyperlipidemia, and cerebrovascular disease. **(p. 497)**

> Vermeir M, Naessens I, Remmerie B, et al: Absorption, metabolism, and excretion of paliperidone, a new monoaminergic antagonist, in humans. Drug Metab Dispos 36:769–779, 2008

21.7 Dementia is common in renal disease patients, and many of these patients will be on pharmacotherapy for cognitive enhancement. Which of the following antidementia medications is *not* recommended in severe renal insufficiency?

    A. Memantine.
    B. Donepezil.
    C. Rivastigmine.
    D. Galantamine.
    E. None of the above.

The correct response is option D.

Galantamine should be used cautiously in patients with moderate renal insufficiency and is not recommended in patients with severe renal insufficiency.

Memantine requires dosage reduction in patients with severe renal insufficiency (Ferrando et al. 2010). While the data are limited, dosage adjustment of donepezil and rivastigmine is probably unnecessary. **(p. 498)**

Ferrando SJ, Levenson JL, Owen JA: Renal and urological disorders, in Clinical Manual of Psychopharmacology in the Medically Ill. Edited by Ferrando SJ, Levenson JL, Owen JA. Arlington, VA, American Psychiatric Publishing, 2010, pp 149–180

21.8 Several psychotropic agents are known to cause disorders of sodium metabolism. Among these agents, which of the following medications is more typically associated with *hyper*natremia, as opposed to *hypo*natremia?

    A. Carbamazepine.
    B. Oxcarbazepine.
    C. Selective serotonin reuptake inhibitors (SSRIs).
    D. Atypical antipsychotics.
    E. Lithium.

The correct response is option E.

Hypernatremia due to nephrogenic diabetes insipidus (NDI) may be caused by lithium through inhibition of renal tubular water reabsorption. Most patients receiving lithium have polydipsia and polyuria, reflecting NDI. Lithium-induced NDI varies from mild polyuria to hyperosmolar coma, and sometimes has persisted long after lithium discontinuation. Amiloride is considered the treatment of choice for lithium-induced NDI, but it also has been treated with nonsteroidal anti-inflammatory drugs, thiazides, and sodium restriction (Grünfeld and Rossier 2009).

The syndrome of inappropriate antidiuretic hormone secretion, resulting in hyponatremia, may be caused by many psychotropic drugs, especially carbamazepine and oxcarbazepine, but also SSRIs, tricyclic antidepressants, and antipsychotics. **(p. 498)**

Grünfeld JP, Rossier BC: Lithium nephrotoxicity revisited. Nat Rev Nephrol 5:270–276, 2009

Chapter 22

Endocrine and Metabolic Disorders

Select the single best response for each question.

22.1 Female patients with type 1 diabetes

    A. Frequently lose weight when their diabetes is intensively controlled.
    B. May use insulin manipulation as a means of caloric purging.
    C. Are less likely than their nondiabetic peers to have disturbed eating behaviors.
    D. Are less likely than their nondiabetic peers to develop an eating disorder.
    E. Do not develop higher hemoglobin A_{1c} values with intermittent insulin omission.

The correct response is option B.

Women with type 1 diabetes may use insulin manipulation (e.g., administering reduced insulin doses or omitting necessary doses altogether) as a means of caloric purging. Intentionally induced glycosuria is a powerful weight loss behavior and a symptom of eating disorders unique to type 1 diabetes. Questions such as "Do you ever change your insulin dose or skip insulin doses to influence your weight?" or "How often do you take less insulin than prescribed?" can be helpful in screening for insulin omission, especially when patients present with persistently elevated hemoglobin A_{1c} levels or unexplained diabetic ketoacidosis.

Despite its promise of reducing long-term complications of type 1 diabetes, a negative side effect of intensive diabetes management is weight gain. During the first 6 years of the Diabetes Control and Complications Trial (DCCT) Research Group, patients in the intensively treated group gained an average of 10.45 pounds more than the patients in the standard treatment cohort, and 9-year follow-up data showed that this weight was hard to lose.

Disturbed eating behavior, usually mild in severity, is common among adolescent girls and young women in the general population; however, those with type 1 diabetes are more likely to have two or more disturbed eating behaviors than are their peers without diabetes (Colton et al. 2004). Olmsted et al. (2008) defined disturbed eating behavior as eating disorder symptoms not yet at the level of frequency or severity to merit a formal diagnosis, including dieting for weight loss, binge eating, or calorie purging through self-induced vomiting, laxative or diuretic use, excessive exercise, or insulin restriction in the case of type 1 diabetes. Studies of the natural history of disturbed eating behaviors in type 1 diabetes indicate that these behaviors persist and increase in severity over time as well as become more common into young adulthood (Colton et al. 2004; Peveler et al. 2005). Evidence suggests that women with type 1 diabetes are 2.4 times more at risk for developing an eating disorder and 1.9 times more at risk for developing subthreshold eating disorders than are women without diabetes (Jones et al. 2000).

Although intermittent insulin omission or dose reduction for weight loss purposes has been found to be a common practice among women with type 1 diabetes, this behavior, even at a subclinical level of severity, places women at heightened risk for medical complications of diabetes. Women reporting intentional insulin misuse had higher hemoglobin A_{1c} values (approximately 2 or more percentage points higher than those in similarly aged women without eating disorders), higher rates of hospital and emergency department visits, and higher rates of neuropathy and retinopathy than women who did not report insulin omission (Bryden et al. 1999; Polonsky et al. 1994; Rydall et al. 1997). **(p. 507)**

Bryden KS, Neil A, Mayou RA, et al: Eating habits, body weight, and insulin misuse: a longitudinal study of teenagers and young adults with type 1 diabetes. Diabetes Care 22:1956–1960, 1999

Colton P, Olmsted M, Daneman D, et al: Disturbed eating behavior and eating disorders in preteen and early teenage girls with type 1 diabetes: a case-controlled study. Diabetes Care 27:1654–1659, 2004

Jones JM, Lawson ML, Daneman D, et al: Eating disorders in adolescent females with and without type 1 diabetes: cross sectional study. BMJ 320:1563–1566, 2000

Olmsted MP, Colton PA, Daneman D, et al: Prediction of the onset of disturbed eating behavior in adolescent girls with type 1 diabetes. Diabetes Care 31:1978–1982, 2008

Peveler RC, Bryden KS, Neil HA, et al: The relationship of disordered eating habits and attitudes to clinical outcomes in young adult females with type 1 diabetes. Diabetes Care 28:84–88, 2005

Polonsky WH, Anderson BJ, Lohrer PA, et al: Insulin omission in women with IDDM. Diabetes Care 17:1178–1185, 1994

Rydall AC, Rodin GM, Olmsted MP, et al: Disordered eating behavior and microvascular complications in young women with insulin-dependent diabetes mellitus. N Engl J Med 336:1849–1854, 1997

22.2   The most common cause of hyperthyroidism is

   A. Hashimoto's thyroiditis.
   B. Cushing's syndrome.
   C. Addison's disease.
   D. Pheochromocytomas.
   E. Graves' disease.

The correct response is option E.

Hyperthyroidism is accompanied by a host of physiological symptoms, including nervousness, sweating, fatigue, heat intolerance, weight loss, and muscle weakness (Kornstein et al. 2000). The most common cause of hyperthyroidism (or thyrotoxicosis) is Graves' disease. Graves' disease is an autoimmune disorder that results in hyperthyroidism when thyroid-stimulating immunoglobulins bind to thyrotropin receptors and mimic thyrotropin.

Autoimmune thyroiditis, or Hashimoto's thyroiditis, is the most common cause of *hypo*thyroidism, not hyperthyroidism.

Cushing's syndrome and Addison's disease are disorders not of the thyroid but rather of the adrenal glands. Cushing's syndrome results from abnormally high levels of cortisol and other glucocorticoids. Primary adrenal insufficiency, or Addison's disease, results from deficient secretion of mineralocorticoids and glucocorticoids.

Pheochromocytomas are rare catecholamine-secreting tumors derived from the adrenal medulla and sympathetic ganglia. They are not a common cause of hyperthyroidism. **(pp. 508–509, 511–513)**

Kornstein SG, Sholar EF, Gardner DG: Endocrine disorders, in Psychiatric Care of the Medical Patient, 2nd Edition. Edited by Stoudemire A, Fogel BS, Greenberg D. New York, Oxford University Press, 2000, pp 801–819

22.3   Hypoparathyroidism is common in which of the following disorders?

   A. Autism.
   B. Tourette's syndrome.
   C. Fragile X syndrome.
   D. Velocardiofacial syndrome (22q11.2)
   E. Asperger's syndrome.

The correct response is option D.

Hypoparathyroidism is common in the 22q11.2 deletion syndrome (velocardiofacial syndrome), in which schizophrenia and bipolar disorder are common in adults and mood, anxiety, attentional, and behavior disorders are common in children (Jolin et al. 2009).

Patients with hypoparathyroidism present with hypocalcemia causing increased neuromuscular irritability. Typical symptoms include paresthesias, muscle cramps, carpopedal spasm, and (less commonly) facial grimacing and seizures. Complications include calcification of the basal ganglia and pseudotumor cerebri. Psychiatric symptoms may include anxiety and emotional irritability and lability. Severe hypocalcemia causes tetany and seizures. Hypoparathyroidism is caused by inadequate parathyroid hormone secretion, most often as a result of parathyroid or thyroid surgery. **(p. 511)**

Jolin EM, Weller RA, Jessani NR, et al: Affective disorders and other psychiatric diagnoses in children and adolescents with 22q11.2 deletion syndrome. J Affect Disord 119:177–180, 2009

22.4   The most common psychiatric symptom in patients with Cushing's syndrome is

    A. Anxiety.
    B. Depression.
    C. Psychosis.
    D. Hypomania.
    E. Cognitive dysfunction.

The correct response is option B.

Cushing's syndrome patients commonly experience a range of psychiatric symptoms, including depression, anxiety, hypomania or frank mania, psychosis, and cognitive dysfunction (Arnaldi et al. 2003; Sonino et al. 2006), with rates varying widely across studies. Depression is the most prevalent psychiatric disturbance in Cushing's syndrome. A full depressive syndrome has been reported in 50%–80% of cases, accompanied by irritability, insomnia, crying, decreased energy and libido, poor concentration and memory, and suicidal ideation (Arnaldi et al. 2003). Although antidepressants are less effective than in regular major depressive disorder, they are helpful until definitive treatment of Cushing's syndrome can be provided. Mood symptoms generally improve with resolution of hypercortisolemia (Arnaldi et al. 2003). **(p. 512)**

Arnaldi G, Angeli A, Atkinson AB, et al: Diagnosis and complications of Cushing's syndrome: a consensus statement. J Clin Endocrinol Metab 88:5593–5602, 2003
Sonino N, Bonnini S, Fallo F, et al: Personality characteristics and quality of life in patients treated for Cushing's syndrome. Clin Endocrinol (Oxf) 64:314–318, 2006

22.5   Which of the following antipsychotics has most often been associated with cases of sustained hyperprolactinemia?

    A. Aripiprazole.
    B. Clozapine.
    C. Olanzapine.
    D. Quetiapine.
    E. Risperidone.

The correct response is option E.

Atypical antipsychotics vary with respect to their effects on prolactin. In most reports, clozapine, quetiapine, olanzapine, and ziprasidone either cause no increase in prolactin secretion or increase prolactin transiently, but sustained hyperprolactinemia can occur in patients taking risperidone and paliperidone. Haloperidol raises the serum prolactin concentration by an average of 17 ng/mL, whereas risperidone may raise it by 45–80 ng/mL, with larger increases in women than in men (David et al. 2000). Women taking prolactin-elevating antipsychotics and not receiving specific interventions to improve bone density had evidence of ongoing bone demineralization over a year, whereas women taking prolactin-sparing antipsychotics had a modest overall increase in bone mineral density (Meaney and O'Keane 2007). A study of patients switched from risperidone to aripiprazole reported that previously elevated prolactin levels were reduced to within normal range in 1 week (Byerly et al. 2009), and hyperprolactinemia in patients taking haloperidol was reversed by the addition of adjunctive aripiprazole (Shim et al. 2007). **(p. 514)**

Byerly MJ, Marcus RN, Tran QV, et al: Effects of aripiprazole on prolactin levels in subjects with schizophrenia during cross-titration with risperidone or olanzapine: analysis of a randomized, open-label study. Schizophr Res 107:218–222, 2009

David SR, Taylor CC, Kinon BJ, et al: The effects of olanzapine, risperidone, and haloperidol on plasma prolactin levels in patients with schizophrenia. Clin Ther 22:1085–1096, 2000

Meaney AM, O'Keane V: Bone mineral density changes over a year in young females with schizophrenia: relationship to medication and endocrine variables. Schizophr Res 93:136–143, 2007

Shim JC, Shin JG, Kelly DL, et al: Adjunctive treatment with a dopamine partial agonist, aripiprazole, for antipsychotic-induced hyperprolactinemia: a placebo-controlled trial. Am J Psychiatry 164:1404–1410, 2007

22.6   The classic symptom triad of dermatitis, dementia, and diarrhea is indicative of which of the following vitamin deficiencies?

    A. Thiamine.
    B. Pyridoxine.
    C. Niacin (among other vitamins and amino acids).
    D. Vitamin E.
    E. None of the above.

The correct response is option C.

Pellagra, originally thought to be a deficiency of niacin only, is now recognized as a complex deficiency of multiple vitamins and amino acids. The classic triad of symptoms is dermatitis, dementia, and diarrhea, but irritability, anxiety, depression, apathy, and psychosis all have been reported (Prakash et al. 2008).

Thiamine deficiency (beriberi) causes cardiac and neuropsychiatric syndromes, including peripheral neuropathy and Wernicke-Korsakoff encephalopathy. Wernicke's consists of vomiting, nystagmus, ophthalmoplegia, fever, ataxia, and confusion that can progress to coma and death. Korsakoff's is a dementia with amnesia, impaired ability to learn, confabulation, and often psychosis.

Pyridoxine (vitamin B_6) deficiency causes peripheral neuropathy and neuropsychiatric disorders, including reports of seizures, migraine, chronic pain, depression, and psychosis. Homocysteine is elevated in B_6 deficiency and may play a role in accelerating vascular disease and dementia.

Vitamin E deficiency can cause areflexia, ataxia, and decreased vibratory and proprioceptive sensation. **(pp. 516–517)**

Prakash R, Gandotra S, Singh LK, et al: Rapid resolution of delusional parasitosis in pellagra with niacin augmentation therapy. Gen Hosp Psychiatry 30:581–584, 2008

Chapter 23

Oncology

Select the single best response for each question.

23.1 Depression is commonly comorbid with cancer, yet the symptomatic overlap between the neurovegetative signs of a mood disorder and the physical symptoms of cancer can create ambiguity. Which of the following symptoms is more specific for a mood disorder, as opposed to a symptom of the comorbid cancer?

 A. Insomnia.
 B. Decreased appetite.
 C. Poor concentration.
 D. Hopelessness.
 E. Psychomotor slowing.

The correct response is option D.

Many of the somatic symptoms caused by cancer or its treatment overlap with the diagnostic criteria for major depression, including disturbances in sleep, appetite, energy, psychomotor activity, and concentration. Emphasis on exploring the psychological symptoms of depression (depressed mood, anhedonia, guilt, worthlessness, hopelessness, helplessness, and suicidal ideation) may be a helpful clinical approach. **(p. 527)**

23.2 In the Bardwell et al. (2006) study of depression in women with breast cancer, risk for depression was predicted by all of the following *except*

 A. Cancer diagnosis date and stage.
 B. Stressful life events.
 C. Less optimism.
 D. Ambivalence over expressing negative emotions.
 E. Sleep disturbance.

The correct response is option A.

A study in 2,595 early-stage breast cancer patients found that stressful life events, less optimism, ambivalence over expressing negative emotions, sleep disturbance, and poorer social functioning better predicted risk for depression than cancer-related variables (Bardwell et al. 2006). **(p. 527)**

> Bardwell WA, Natarajan L, Dimsdale JE, et al: Objective cancer-related variables are not associated with depressive symptoms in women treated for early stage breast cancer. J Clin Oncol 24:2420–2427, 2006

23.3 Although suicide accounts for a very low number of deaths in cancer patients, an elevated risk has been consistently reported. In the Misono et al. (2008) study of suicide risk in cancer patients, which of the following findings was reported?

 A. The risk of suicide in cancer patients was five times that in the general population.
 B. Female cancer patients had a higher suicide rate than male patients.

C. Caucasians had a lower rate of suicide than other racial groups.

D. Young age at cancer diagnosis predicted suicide risk.

E. Head and neck cancers were associated with a notably high suicide risk.

The correct response is option E.

In the United States, a large retrospective cohort study comparing cancer patients with the general population reported that patients with cancer had nearly twice the incidence of suicide (Misono et al. 2008). Higher suicide rates were associated with male gender, white race, and older age at diagnosis. The highest suicide rates were observed in cancers of the respiratory system, stomach, and head and neck. **(p. 528)**

Misono S, Weiss NS, Fann JR, et al: Incidence of suicide in persons with cancer. J Clin Oncol 26:4731–4738, 2008

23.4   Anxiety may be a clinically significant comorbidity in cancer. Which of the following conditions should be considered in the differential diagnosis of anxiety in a cancer patient?

A. Use of antipsychotics and antiemetics.

B. Pulmonary emboli.

C. Hypoxia from primary lung cancers.

D. Uncontrolled pain.

E. All of the above.

The correct response is option E.

Evaluation of acute anxiety in cancer patients includes consideration of conditions that mimic anxiety disorders. Antipsychotics, as well as antiemetic phenothiazines (prochlorperazine, perphenazine, promethazine) or metoclopramide, may cause akathisia. Akathisia's inner feeling of restlessness is frequently misperceived by patients and misdiagnosed by caregivers as anxiety. The abrupt onset of anxiety and dyspnea may signal pulmonary emboli, which are common among cancer patients. Hypoxia related to primary or secondary lung cancer may cause significant anxiety. The experience of severe, intermittent, or uncontrolled pain is associated with acute and chronic anxiety, and the patient's confidence that he or she has the analgesics to control pain alleviates anxiety. Furthermore, anxiety amplifies pain, and the drive behind additional requests for analgesia may be anxiety, rather than somatic pain. **(p. 529)**

23.5   Limbic encephalopathy is an autoimmune phenomenon associated with altered mental status, including cognitive impairment in many cases. This syndrome is most commonly associated with which type of malignancy?

A. Non-small-cell lung carcinoma.

B. Small-cell lung carcinoma.

C. Melanoma.

D. Breast cancer.

E. Head and neck cancer.

The correct response is option B.

Limbic encephalopathy (or encephalitis) is a specific type of autoimmune encephalopathy most often reported with small-cell carcinoma of the lung but uncommonly with many other malignancies. Limbic encephalopathy may present with impaired memory, fluctuating mood, and seizures (Kung et al. 2002), as well as a wide variety of psychiatric symptoms including anxiety, depression, schizophreniform or manic psychosis, and personality change (Foster and Caplan 2009). **(p. 530)**

Foster AR, Caplan JP: Paraneoplastic limbic encephalitis. Psychosomatics 50:108–113, 2009

Kung S, Mueller PS, Yonas EG, et al: Delirium resulting from paraneoplastic limbic encephalitis caused by Hodgkin's disease. Psychosomatics 43:498–501, 2002

23.6 Melanoma, a dermatological cancer with a propensity for central nervous system involvement, may be treated with interferon-alpha. Which of the following is a rare, rather than common, psychiatric complication of interferon-alpha treatment?

A. Mania.
B. Fatigue.
C. Anxiety.
D. Insomnia.
E. Depression.

The correct response is option A.

Patients with advanced melanoma may be treated with interferon-alpha, the side effects of which include fatigue, anxiety, insomnia, depression, and rarely mania (Kirkwood et al. 2002). **(p. 537)**

Kirkwood JM, Bender C, Agarwala S, et al: Mechanisms and management of toxicities associated with high-dose interferon alfa-2b therapy. J Clin Oncol 20:3703–3718, 2002

23.7 The antidepressant mirtazapine has properties that may render it particularly helpful in cancer patients with anorexia-cachexia or insomnia. Which of the following statements regarding mirtazapine is *false*?

A. It has high affinity for H_1 receptors.
B. It blocks $5-HT_2$ receptors.
C. It blocks $5-HT_3$ receptors.
D. Its side effects include constipation and drowsiness.
E. It is commonly associated with neutropenia.

The correct response is option E.

Reversible neutropenia is a rare side effect of mirtazapine, not a common one.

Mirtazapine has a high affinity for H_1 histaminic receptors and antagonizes $5-HT_2$ and $5-HT_3$ receptors, possibly contributing to its properties of anxiolysis, sedation, appetite stimulation, and antiemesis. These properties may be advantageous in anorexic–cachectic depressed cancer patients or those experiencing nausea or vomiting from chemotherapy but are less desirable in patients who are gaining weight from steroids or chemotherapy or those with significant fatigue or sedation. Small studies in which mirtazapine was used have shown improvement in anxiety, depression, and insomnia, with mixed results in nausea (Cankurtaran et al. 2008; Kim et al. 2008). Side effects include constipation, drowsiness, and, rarely, reversible neutropenia, all considerations when treating the depressed cancer patient. **(p. 541)**

Cankurtaran ES, Ozlap E, Soygur H, et al: Mirtazapine improves sleep and lowers anxiety and depression in cancer patients: superiority over imipramine. Support Care Cancer 16:1291–1298, 2008

Kim SW, Shin IL, Kim JM, et al: Effectiveness of mirtazapine for nausea and insomnia in cancer patients with depression. Psychiatry Clin Neurosci 62:75–83, 2008

Chapter 24

Hematology

Select the single best response for each question.

24.1 What is the most common cause of iron deficiency anemia (IDA)?

    A. Malnutrition.
    B. Unsupplemented milk diets.
    C. Blood loss.
    D. Pregnancy.
    E. Intestinal malabsorption of iron.

The correct response is option C.

The most common etiology of IDA is blood loss. In men and in postmenopausal women, chronic bleeding from the gastrointestinal tract is the most common cause. Peptic ulcer, hiatal hernia, gastritis, hemorrhoids, vascular anomalies, and neoplasms are the most common causes of gastrointestinal bleeding in adults.

Unsupplemented milk diets do not contain adequate amounts of iron for infants. During the first year of life, iron demands are increased and milk products are poor sources of iron; prolonged breast-feeding or bottle feeding of infants frequently leads to IDA unless there is iron supplementation. Premature infants are at even great risk of IDA.

IDA is highly prevalent in pregnant women as the result of iron loss from diversion of iron to the fetus and from blood loss during delivery. Daily iron demand dramatically increases during pregnancy and continues through to term. Breast-feeding leads to additional iron diversion to the baby.

Intestinal malabsorption of iron is an uncommon cause of iron deficiency except after gastrointestinal surgery and in malabsorption syndromes such as celiac disease (Annibale et al. 2003). In malabsorption syndromes, IDA may take years to develop due to the indolent nature of iron loss. **(pp. 551–552)**

> Annibale B, Capurso G, Delle Fave G: The stomach and iron deficiency anaemia: a forgotten link. Dig Liver Dis 35:288–295, 2003

24.2 A deficiency in which of the following has been associated with neural tube defects (NTDs) in newborns?

    A. Vitamin B_{12}.
    B. Vitamin B_6.
    C. Iron.
    D. Folate.
    E. Thiamine.

The correct response is option D.

Insufficient folate during conception and early pregnancy may result in NTDs. Since 1998, the U.S. Food and Drug Administration has mandated fortification of grains with folate to help lower women's risk of having a pregnancy affected by NTDs. This action has led to a reduction in NTDs and an improvement of blood folate status and homocysteine levels in adults in the United States (Choumenkovitch 2001, 2002; Dietrich 2005; Jacques 1999). **(p. 554)**

> Choumenkovitch SF, Jacques PF, Nadeau MR, et al: Folic acid fortification increases red blood cell folate concentrations in the Framingham study. J Nutr 131:3277–3280, 2001
>
> Choumenkovitch SF, Selhub J, Wilson PW, et al: Folic acid intake from fortification in United States exceeds predictions. J Nutr 132:2792–2798, 2002
>
> Dietrich M, Brown CJ, Block G: The effect of folate fortification of cereal-grain products on blood folate status, dietary folate intake, and dietary folate sources among adult non-supplement users in the United States. J Am Coll Nutr 24:266–274, 2005
>
> Jacques PF, Selhub J, Bostom AG, et al: The effect of folic acid fortification on plasma folate and total homocysteine concentrations. N Engl J Med 340:1449–1454, 1999

24.3 Common clinical and neuropsychiatric symptoms of vitamin B_{12} deficiency include all of the following *except*

    A. Macrocytic anemia.
    B. Symmetrical peripheral neuropathy.
    C. Intestinal metaplasia.
    D. Subacute combined degeneration of the spinal cord.
    E. Vaso-occlusive crisis.

The correct response is option E.

Vaso-occlusive crises are a hallmark of sickle cell disease, not of vitamin B_{12} deficiency.

The most common clinical manifestations of vitamin B_{12} deficiency are macrocytic anemia and neuropsychiatric symptoms. Hematological manifestations of B_{12} deficiency include megaloblastic anemia, macrocytosis with hypersegmented polymorphonuclear leukocytes, thrombocytopenia, leukopenia, pancytopenia or (rarely) hemolytic anemia, and thrombotic microangiopathy. Gastrointestinal manifestations include intestinal metaplasia, diarrhea, jaundice, and increased lactate dehydrogenase and bilirubin levels.

Neuropsychiatric manifestations are common in B_{12} deficiency, especially in the elderly (Andres et al. 2004). The hematological and neuropsychiatric symptoms of B_{12} deficiency are often disassociated, and neuropsychiatric symptoms may precede hematological signs (Reynolds 2006).

Symmetrical peripheral neuropathy occurs frequently, with paresthesias and numbness. Subacute combined degeneration of the spinal cord is less common (Reynolds 2006). Subacute combined degeneration encompasses both posterior column disruption (resulting in loss of vibration and position sense and ataxia with a positive Romberg's sign) and lateral column disruption (causing weakness, spasticity, and extensor plantar responses) (Toh et al. 1997). **(pp. 553, 555)**

> Andres E, Loukili NH, Noel E, et al: Vitamin B12 (cobalamin) deficiency in elderly patients. CMAJ 171:251–259, 2004
>
> Reynolds E: Vitamin B12, folic acid, and the nervous system. Lancet Neurol 5:949–960, 2006
>
> Toh BH, van Driel IR, Gleeson PA: Pernicious anemia. N Engl J Med 337:1441–1448, 1997

24.4 Which of the following antipsychotics has no reported hematological side effects?

    A. Olanzapine.
    B. Ziprasidone.
    C. Clozapine.
    D. Mellaril.
    E. Chlorpromazine.

The correct response is option B.

Antipsychotic agents with no reported hematological side effects include aripiprazole and ziprasidone. **(p. 561)**

24.5 The most common and serious hematological side effect of antipsychotics is

    A. Aplastic anemia.
    B. Neutropenia.
    C. Agranulocytosis.
    D. Eosinophilia.
    E. Thrombocytopenia.

The correct response is option C.

Agranulocytosis is the most common and most serious hematological side effect of antipsychotics (Buckley and Meltzer 1995; Flanagan and Dunk 2008; Gareri et al. 2008; Rajagopal 2005; Sedky et al. 2005). Low-potency antipsychotics have a higher frequency of agranulocytosis than high-potency ones. **(p. 561)**

Buckley PF, Meltzer HY: Treatment of schizophrenia, in Textbook of Psychopharmacology. Edited by Schatzberg AF, Nemeroff CB. Washington, DC, American Psychiatric Press, 1995, pp 615–639

Flanagan RJ, Dunk L: Haematological toxicity of drugs used in psychiatry. Hum Psychopharmacol 23 (suppl 1):27–41, 2008

Gareri P, De Fazio P, Russo E, et al: The safety of clozapine in the elderly. Exp Opin Drug Saf 7:525–538, 2008

Rajagopal S: Clozapine, agranulocytosis, and benign ethnic neutropenia. Postgrad Med J 81:545–546, 2005

Sedky K, Shaughnessy R, Hughes T, et al: Clozapine-induced agranulocytosis after 11 years of treatment. Am J Psychiatry 162:814, 2005

24.6 A patient who has been on an antidepressant for 8 weeks begins to experience bruising and bleeding. She reports that the only other medication she takes is low-dose aspirin to reduce the risk of myocardial infarction. Which of the following classes of antidepressants is most likely responsible for this adverse interaction effect?

    A. Tricyclic antidepressants (TCAs).
    B. Monoamine oxidase inhibitors (MAOIs).
    C. Serotonin–2 receptor antagonists with serotonin reuptake blockade.
    D. Selective serotonin reuptake inhibitors (SSRIs).
    E. Alpha-2 antagonists with serotonin-2 and serotonin-3 antagonism.

The correct response is option D.

SSRIs inhibit platelet function and have been associated with bruising and bleeding, especially with concomitant use of aspirin or nonsteroidal anti-inflammatory drugs (Andreasen et al. 2006; de Abajo et al. 2006; Goldberg 1998; Mort et al. 2006; Turner et al. 2007; Wessinger et al. 2006). SSRIs increase central nervous system 5-hydroxytryptamine (5-HT; serotonin), and reduce 5-HT in platelets (leading to reduced platelet aggregation). Platelets normally release serotonin at the site of a vascular tear, leading to further platelet aggregation and vasodilatation, and permitting the sealing of the tear without thrombosis of the vessel (Hourani and Cusack 1991). **(p. 561)**

Andreasen JJ, Riis A, Hjortdal VE, et al: Effect of selective serotonin reuptake inhibitors on requirement for allogeneic red blood cell transfusion following coronary artery bypass surgery. Am J Cardiovasc Drugs 6:243–250, 2006

de Abajo FJ, Montero D, Rodriguez LA, et al: Antidepressants and risk of upper gastrointestinal bleeding. Basic Clin Pharmacol Toxicol 98:304–310, 2006

Goldberg RJ: Selective serotonin reuptake inhibitors: infrequent medical adverse effects. Arch Fam Med 7:78–84, 1998

Hourani SM, Cusack NJ: Pharmacological receptors on blood platelets. Pharmacol Rev 43:243–298, 1991

Mort JR, Aparasu RR, Baer RK: Interaction between selective serotonin reuptake inhibitors and nonsteroidal antiinflammatory drugs: review of the literature. Pharmacotherapy 26:1307–1313, 2006

Turner MS, May DB, Arthur RR, et al: Clinical impact of selective serotonin reuptake inhibitors therapy with bleeding risks. J Intern Med 261:205–213, 2007

Wessinger S, Kaplan M, Choi L, et al: Increased use of selective serotonin reuptake inhibitors in patients admitted with gastrointestinal haemorrhage: a multicentre retrospective analysis. Aliment Pharmacol Ther 23:937–944, 2006

Chapter 25

Rheumatology

Select the single best response for each question.

25.1 Rating scales for mood disorders may overestimate the diagnosis of depression in rheumatological patients because of their focus on somatic symptoms. Among the following instruments, which is *least* reliant on somatic content and thus potentially more useful for psychiatric screening in rheumatological populations?

    A. Beck Depression Inventory (BDI).
    B. Center for Epidemiologic Studies Depression Scale (CES-D).
    C. Hamilton Rating Scale for Depression (HAM-D).
    D. Hospital Anxiety and Depression Scale (HADS).
    E. Mini-Mental State Examination (MMSE).

The correct response is option D.

Self-rated questionnaires may be used by rheumatologists or nurse specialists to screen for possible cases of psychiatric disorder, with the recognition that some questionnaires (BDI and the CES-D) tend to overestimate the prevalence of depression in medically ill populations because of their prominent inclusion of somatic symptoms that occur in medical illness, including rheumatological disorders (Callahan et al. 1991).

Scales that have little somatic content, such as the Geriatric Depression Scale (Sheikh and Yesavage 1989), the HADS (Zigmond and Snaith 1983), or disease-specific instruments (Smedstad et al. 1995), may aid accurate diagnosis of depression in such patients. **(p. 572)**

> Callahan LF, Kaplan MR, Pincus T: The Beck Depression Inventory, Center for Epidemiological Studies Depression Scale (CES-D), and General Well-Being Schedule depression subscale in rheumatoid arthritis. Criterion contamination of responses. Arthritis Care Res 4:3–11, 1991
>
> Sheikh JI, Yesavage J: Geriatric Depression Scale (GDS): recent evidence and development of a shorter version, in Clinical Gerontology: A Guide to Assessment and Intervention. Edited by Brink TL. New York, Haworth, 1986, pp 165–173
>
> Smedstad LM, Vaglum P, Kvien TK, et al: The relationship between self-reported pain and sociodemographic variables, anxiety, and depressive symptoms in rheumatoid arthritis. J Rheumatol 22:514–520, 1995
>
> Zigmond AS, Snaith RP: The Hospital Anxiety and Depression Scale. Acta Psychiatr Scand 67:361–370, 1983

25.2 Psychotherapy is a very helpful treatment for rheumatological patients with comorbid depressive symptoms. Based on reviewed evidence, which of the following psychotherapy models has proven to be the most applicable to rheumatological patients?

    A. Interpersonal therapy (IPT).
    B. Psychodynamic psychotherapy.
    C. Cognitive-behavioral therapy (CBT).
    D. Group psychotherapy.
    E. Supportive psychotherapy.

The correct response is option C.

Given the particularly strong role that cognitive appraisal mechanisms can play in rheumatological illness, it is perhaps not surprising that CBT is considered the gold standard of behavioral approaches to these conditions. CBT attempts to change maladaptive ways of thinking and feeling in response to the illness with an extensive range of strategies, including biofeedback and relaxation training, cognitive restructuring and distraction, and activity pacing. Most studies have focused on the management of pain. A recent review of 25 randomized clinical trials that tested psychosocial treatments for rheumatoid arthritis underscored the effectiveness of CBT in increasing efficacy in coping with pain and in reducing pain, physical disability, and depressive symptoms (Astin et al. 2002). **(p. 573)**

> Astin JA, Beckner W, Soeken K, et al: Psychological interventions for rheumatoid arthritis: a meta-analysis of randomized controlled trials. Arthritis Rheum 47:291–302, 2002

25.3 Antidepressant medications may be a very helpful adjunctive treatment for painful rheumatological conditions. Which of the following antidepressants has been demonstrated to have analgesic efficacy in rheumatological disorders?

    A. Mirtazapine.
    B. Venlafaxine.
    C. Bupropion.
    D. Selective serotonin reuptake inhibitors (SSRIs).
    E. Tricyclic antidepressants (TCAs).

The correct response is option E.

The only placebo-controlled randomized controlled trials reporting analgesic efficacy of antidepressants in rheumatological disorders have been of TCAs (e.g., Ash et al. 1999; Grace et al. 1985). TCAs have long been recognized to have analgesic benefits, even at low doses (e.g., 25 mg of amitriptyline) and independent of whether depression is present. In higher doses, tolerability and safety are poor, particularly in the elderly.

SSRIs have comparable antidepressant efficacy but less analgesic efficacy. Serotonin–norepinephrine reuptake inhibitors possess more analgesic potential than do SSRIs. **(p. 573)**

> Ash G, Dickens CM, Creed FH, et al: The effects of dothiepin on subjects with rheumatoid arthritis and depression. Rheumatology (Oxford) 38:959–967, 1999
> Grace EM, Bellamy N, Kassam Y, et al: Controlled, double-blind, randomized trial of amitriptyline in relieving articular pain and tenderness in patients with rheumatoid arthritis. Curr Med Res Opin 9:426–429, 1985

25.4 Systemic lupus erythematosus (SLE) is a complex rheumatological disease with notably problematic central nervous system involvement. Which of the following is the most common psychiatric comorbidity in SLE?

    A. Cognitive disorders.
    B. Mood disorders.
    C. Anxiety disorders.
    D. Psychotic disorders.
    E. Impulse-control disorders.

The correct response is option A.

Cognitive dysfunction is the most common neuropsychiatric disorder in patients with SLE, occurring in up to 80% of patients (Ainiala et al. 2001; Denburg et al. 1994). On neuropsychological testing, even patients who have never had overt neuropsychiatric symptoms are often found to have cognitive impairment. Patients with anticardiolipin antibodies have a three- to fourfold increased risk of cognitive impairment, which is often progressive (Hanly et al. 1997). Cognitive impairment may be associated with lymphocytotoxic antibodies, cerebrospinal fluid antineuronal antibodies, and pathological findings such as microinfarcts and cortical atrophy. Although cognitive dysfunction often fluctuates and is reversible (Hanly et al. 1997), presumably when attributable to edema and inflammation, it tends to be irreversible when secondary to multiple infarcts and may culminate in dementia. **(p. 581)**

Ainiala H, Hietaharju A, Loukkola J, et al: Validity of the American College of Rheumatology criteria for neuropsychiatric lupus syndromes: a population-based evaluation. Arthritis Care Res 45:419–423, 2001

Denburg SD, Carbotte RM, Denburg JA: Corticosteroids and neuropsychological functioning in patients with systemic lupus erythematosus. Arthritis Rheum 37:1311–1320, 1994

Hanly JG, Cassell K, Fisk JD: Cognitive function in systemic lupus erythematosus: results of a 5-year prospective study. Arthritis Rheum 40:1542–1543, 1997

25.5   What is the most common cause of mania in systemic lupus erythematosus (SLE)?

    A. Direct central nervous system involvement from SLE.
    B. Strokes in the right hemisphere.
    C. Strokes in the left hemisphere.
    D. Preexisting bipolar disorder.
    E. Corticosteroid treatment.

The correct response is option E.

In patients with SLE, the most common cause of mania is corticosteroid therapy. **(p. 581)**

25.6   Other rheumatological illnesses may mimic some of the clinical features of systemic lupus erythematosus (SLE). Clinical laboratory tests may be helpful in the differential diagnosis of these conditions. Which of the following rheumatological illnesses is associated with a medium to high, rather than a low or negative, antinuclear antibody (ANA) titer?

    A. Polyarteritis nodosa.
    B. Wegener's granulomatosis.
    C. Behçet's syndrome.
    D. Rheumatoid arthritis.
    E. Sjögren's syndrome.

The correct response is option E.

A wide variety of diseases can mimic neuropsychiatric SLE. One group of diseases, associated with a medium to high ANA titer (>1:160), includes Sjögren's syndrome and mixed or undifferentiated connective tissue disease. A second group of diseases, associated with a low ANA titer (<1:160), includes multiple sclerosis and, less commonly, ANA-positive rheumatoid arthritis, sarcoidosis, and hepatitis C. A third group of diseases, characterized by a negative ANA, also may be mistaken for central nervous system lupus. This group includes polyarteritis nodosa, microscopic angiitis, Wegener's granulomatosis, chronic fatigue syndrome, fibromyalgia, temporal arteritis, and Behçet's syndrome. **(p. 583)**

25.7 The most common psychiatric side effect of corticosteroid therapy is

A. Anxiety.
B. Anorexia.
C. Mood disorder, often with psychotic features.
D. Psychosis without mood symptoms.
E. Delirium.

The correct response is option C.

Mood disorders, including depression and mania, are the most common psychiatric reaction to corticosteroids. Patients may experience both mania and depression during a single course of corticosteroid therapy. Affective symptoms are often accompanied by psychotic symptoms. The psychiatric symptoms induced by corticosteroids most often resemble those of bipolar disorder, with manic symptoms most often encountered with high-dose, short-term administration and depression most often seen with chronic therapy (Bolanos et al. 2004). Delirium and psychosis (without mood symptoms) are less common. Cognitive dysfunction also has been reported. The most common symptoms in children are agitation and sleep disturbances (Tavassoli et al. 2008). Mild psychiatric side effects include insomnia, hyperexcitability, mood lability, mild euphoria, irritability, anxiety, agitation, and racing thoughts. **(pp. 586–587)**

Bolanos SH, Khan DA, Hanczyc M, et al: Assessment of mood states in patients receiving long-term corticosteroid therapy and in controls with patient-rated and clinician-rated scales. Ann Allergy Asthma Immunol 92:500–505, 2004

Tavassoli N, Montastruc-Fournier J, Montastruc JL: Psychiatric adverse drug reactions to glucocorticoids in children and adolescents: a much higher risk with elevated doses. French Association of Regional Pharmacovigilance Centres. Br J Clin Pharmacol 66:566–567, 2008

Chapter 26

Chronic Fatigue and Fibromyalgia Syndromes

Select the single best response for each question.

26.1 Which of the following is a core feature of fibromyalgia?

A. Peripheral neuropathy.
B. Headache.
C. Sore throat.
D. Postexertional malaise lasting more than 24 hours.
E. Chronic widespread pain.

The correct response is option E.

The core features of fibromyalgia are chronic widespread pain and musculoskeletal tenderness (muscles; ligaments and tendons). Pain typically occurs in all four quadrants of the body and the axial skeleton but also can be regional. Fatigue, sleep disturbance, and subjective cognitive impairment (memory and concentration) are common associations. As with chronic fatigue syndrome, the report of pain is essentially a subjective phenomenon and may not be reflected in attempts to assess physical and mental performance objectively. **(p. 595)**

26.2 Chronic fatigue syndrome (CFS) and fibromyalgia syndrome (FMS) are more common in

A. Men.
B. Individuals between 50 and 65 years of age.
C. Higher socioeconomic classes.
D. College-educated individuals.
E. Western nations.

The correct response is option E.

It is often noted that the diagnoses of CFS and FMS are almost entirely restricted to Western nations, whereas the symptoms of fatigue and pain are universal. It is unclear to what extent this reflects differing epidemiology or simply different diagnostic practice.

Both CFS and FMS are more common in women. The female-to-male ratio for CFS has been reported to be about 4:1 (Reyes et al. 2003) and for FMS, 8:1 (Wolfe et al. 1995), although this increased female preponderance in FMS may reflect a greater frequency of tender points rather than more frequent pain (Clauw and Crofford 2003).

The most common age at onset for both CFS and FMS is between 30 and 50 years, although patients who present with FMS are on average 10 years older (Reyes et al. 2003; White et al. 1999). These syndromes are also diagnosed, although controversially, in children. An epidemiological study from the United Kingdom found a prevalence of CFS of only 0.002% in 5- to 15-year-olds (Chalder et al. 2003). CFS and FMS are also diagnosed in the elderly, but the frequency of other chronic medical conditions complicates the differential diagnosis.

Both CFS and FMS are more prevalent in persons of lower socioeconomic status and in those who have received less education (Jason et al. 1999; White et al. 1999). CFS is 50% more common in semiskilled and unskilled workers than in professionals. **(p. 598)**

Chalder T, Goodman R, Wessely S, et al: Epidemiology of chronic fatigue syndrome and self reported myalgic encephalomyelitis in 5–15 year olds: cross sectional study. BMJ 327:654–655, 2003

Clauw DJ, Crofford LJ: Chronic widespread pain and fibromyalgia: what we know, and what we need to know. Best Pract Res Clin Rheumatol 17:685–701, 2003

Jason LA, Richman JA, Rademaker AW, et al: A community-based study of chronic fatigue syndrome. Arch Intern Med 159:2129–2137, 1999

Reyes M, Nisenbaum R, Hoaglin DC, et al: Prevalence and incidence of chronic fatigue syndrome in Wichita, Kansas. Arch Intern Med 163:1530–1536, 2003

White KP, Speechley M, Harth M, et al: The London Fibromyalgia Epidemiology Study: the prevalence of fibromyalgia syndrome in London, Ontario. J Rheumatol 26:1570–1576, 1999

Wolfe F, Ross K, Anderson JA, et al: The prevalence and characteristics of fibromyalgia in the general population. Arthritis Rheum 38:19–28, 1995

26.3   Etiological factors reported (and to various degrees documented) to predispose to, precipitate, or perpetuate chronic fatigue syndrome (CFS) include all of the following *except*

    A. Genetic factors.
    B. Abuse.
    C. Immunological factors.
    D. Infections.
    E. Life stress.

The correct response is option C.

Immunological factors, especially cytokines, have been much investigated in CFS and fibromyalgia syndrome (FMS). However, a systematic review found no evidence of any consistent immune abnormality in CFS (Lyall et al. 2003). The hypothesis that CFS is associated with immune activation therefore remains tantalizing but unproven.

Modest evidence from family and twin studies suggests that genetic factors play a part in predisposing individuals to CFS and to FMS. In a study of 146 female–female twins, one of whom had CFS, the concordance was 55% in monozygotic and 20% in dizygotic twins (Buchwald et al. 2001), suggesting both moderate heritability and the importance of environmental factors. In FMS, a similar familial clustering has been reported (Buskila and Neumann 1997).

Childhood and adult neglect, abuse, and maltreatment have been reported to be more common in CFS and FMS (Heim et al. 2006; Paras et al. 2009) than in comparison groups. A recent study reported that people who reported abuse had six times the risk of CFS (Paras et al. 2009). Both psychological and biological etiological mechanisms for the etiological role of trauma have been suggested.

Some evidence indicates that infection can precipitate CFS, and some, but less, evidence indicates that infection also may trigger FMS (Rea et al. 1999).

Clinical experience indicates that patients often report the onset of CFS and FMS as occurring during or after a stressful period in their lives. The evidence for life stress or life events being a precipitant of FMS and CFS is, however, both limited and retrospective (Anderberg et al. 2000; Theorell et al. 1999). **(pp. 599–600)**

Anderberg UM, Marteinsdottir I, Theorell T, et al: The impact of life events in female patients with fibromyalgia and in female healthy controls. Eur Psychiatry 15:295–301, 2000

Buchwald D, Herrell R, Ashton S, et al: A twin study of chronic fatigue. Psychosom Med 63:936–943, 2001

Buskila D, Neumann L: Fibromyalgia syndrome (FM) and nonarticular tenderness in relatives of patients with FM. J Rheumatol 24:941–944, 1997

Heim C, Wagner D, Maloney E, et al: Early adverse experience and risk for chronic fatigue syndrome: results from a population-based study. Arch Gen Psychiatry 63:1258–1266, 2006

Lyall M, Peakman M, Wessely S: A systematic review and critical evaluation of the immunology of chronic fatigue syndrome. J Psychosom Res 55:79–90, 2003

Paras ML, Murad MH, Chen LP, et al: Sexual abuse and lifetime diagnosis of somatic disorders: a systematic review and meta-analysis. JAMA 302:550–561, 2009

Rea T, Russo J, Katon W, et al: A prospective study of tender points and fibromyalgia during and after an acute viral infection. Arch Intern Med 159:865–870, 1999

Theorell T, Blomkvist V, Lindh G, et al: Critical life events, infections, and symptoms during the year preceding chronic fatigue syndrome (CFS): an examination of CFS patients and subjects with a nonspecific life crisis. Psychosom Med 61:304–310, 1999

26.4 One of the best-supported biological abnormalities reported to be associated with both chronic fatigue syndrome (CFS) and fibromyalgia syndrome (FMS) is

  A. Changes in neuroendocrine stress hormones.
  B. Sleep abnormalities.
  C. Chronic infection.
  D. Abnormalities of muscle metabolism.
  E. Structural brain abnormalities.

The correct response is option A.

One of the best-supported biological abnormalities reported to be associated with both CFS and FMS is changes in the level and response of neuroendocrine stress hormones. A repeated observation has been of a tendency to low blood levels of cortisol and a poor cortisol response to stress (Parker et al. 2001). This finding differs from what would be expected in depression (in which blood levels of cortisol are typically elevated), but is similar to that reported in other stress-induced and anxiety states.

Patients with CFS and FMS typically complain of unrefreshing and broken sleep, a symptom that has been objectively confirmed with polysomnography. Although a number of abnormalities in sleep variables have been reported in recent years in CFS and FMS, no clear and consistent differences are apparent.

There has been much interest in the potential role of ongoing infection and in associated immunological factors, especially in CFS. It was previously thought that chronic Epstein-Barr virus infection was a cause of CFS, but that hypothesis has been rejected. There have been numerous reports of evidence of chronic infection with other agents in both CFS and FMS, but none has so far been substantiated.

The bulk of evidence indicates that there are no proven pathological or biochemical abnormalities of muscle or muscle metabolism, either at rest or with exercise, other than those expected with deconditioning.

The brains of patients with CFS and FMS are probably structurally normal, although a reduction in gray matter has been reported in both CFS (de Lange et al. 2005) and FMS (Burgmer et al. 2009). However, this apparent difference in amount of gray matter has been reported to disappear after controlling for depression (Hsu et al. 2009). **(pp. 600–601)**

Burgmer M, Gaubitz M, Konrad C, et al: Decreased gray matter volumes in the cingulo-frontal cortex and the amygdala in patients with fibromyalgia. Psychosom Med 71:566–573, 2009

de Lange FP, Kalkman JS, Bleijenberg G, et al: Gray matter volume reduction in the chronic fatigue syndrome. Neuroimage 26:777–781, 2005

Hsu MC, Harris RE, Sundgren PC, et al: No consistent difference in gray matter volume between individuals with fibromyalgia and age-matched healthy subjects when controlling for affective disorder. Pain 143:262–267, 2009

Parker AJ, Wessely S, Cleare AJ: The neuroendocrinology of chronic fatigue syndrome and fibromyalgia. Psychol Med 31:1331–1345, 2001

26.5   Which of the following medical conditions has been reported to be very common (about 1 per 100) in patients with either chronic fatigue syndrome (CFS) or fibromyalgia syndrome (FMS)?

      A. Systemic lupus erythematosus.
      B. Multiple sclerosis.
      C. Narcolepsy.
      D. Thyroid disorders.
      E. Myopathy.

The correct response is option D.

Thyroid disorders (both hypo- and hyperthyroidism) are present in 1 out of 100 patients with either CFS or FMS. The medical differential diagnosis for CFS and FMS is a long one because so many diseases can present with pain and/or fatigue. **(p. 603 [Table 26–4])**

Chapter 27

Infectious Diseases

Select the single best response for each question.

27.1 Rocky Mountain spotted fever (RMSF) can include neuropsychiatric manifestations that may come to the attention of the psychosomatic medicine consultant. Which of the following statements regarding RMSF is *true*?

 A. Central nervous system (CNS) involvement is seen in more than 50% of cases.
 B. Patients may present with lethargy, confusion, or delirium.
 C. Behavioral changes typically follow the emergence of the characteristic rash.
 D. CNS symptoms are rare in the absence of focal lesions on neuroimaging.
 E. Apathy is seen only in adult cases.

The correct response is option B.

CNS involvement occurs in 25% of cases and includes lethargy, confusion, and occasionally fulminant delirium. Subtle changes such as irritability, personality changes, and apathy may occur before the rash, particularly in children.

RMSF typically (although not invariably) includes fever and a rash characterized by erythematous macules that later progress to maculopapular lesions with central petechiae. Initially appearing as a nonspecific severe febrile illness, the diagnosis is seldom suspected until the rash appears.

Abnormalities on brain imaging may show focal lesions, but 80% of RMSF patients with normal scans have symptoms of encephalopathy as well (Bonawitz et al. 1997). **(p. 617)**

> Bonawitz C, Castillo M, Mukherji SK: Comparison of CT and MR features with clinical outcome in patients with Rocky Mountain spotted fever. Am J Neuroradiol 18:459–464, 1997

27.2 Lyme disease, a systemic infection due to *Borrelia burgdorferi*, which is transmitted by a tick vector, is well known to be associated with neuropsychiatric symptoms. Which of the following is *not* a symptom of classic Lyme disease encephalopathy?

 A. Poor concentration.
 B. Poor memory performance.
 C. Fatigue.
 D. Depression.
 E. Hypochondriasis.

The correct response is option E.

Hypochondriasis is not a classic symptom of Lyme disease encephalopathy. Typical symptoms include difficulty with concentration and memory, fatigue, daytime hypersomnolence, irritability, and depression.

Many different psychiatric symptoms have been reported to be associated with Lyme disease, including depression, mania, delirium, dementia, psychosis, obsessions or compulsions, panic attacks, catatonia, and personality change (Tager and Fallon 2001). **(pp. 619–620)**

> Tager FA, Fallon BA: Psychiatric and cognitive features of Lyme disease. Psychiatric Annals 31:172–181, 2001

27.3 Because Epstein-Barr virus (EBV) may persist lifelong in a latent state following acute infection, periodic reactivation may occur. Which of the following is *not* a common symptom in patients with EBV reactivation?

    A. Fatigue.
    B. Malaise.
    C. Depression.
    D. Hypomania with excess energy.
    E. Low-grade fever.

The correct response is option D.

Hypomania is not present with reactivated EBV infection.

    Patients with reactivated EBV infection typically report overwhelming fatigue, malaise, depression, low-grade fever, lymphadenopathy, and other nonspecific symptoms, essentially the picture of the chronic fatigue syndrome. However, only a small fraction of chronic fatigue symptoms are attributable to EBV infection. In the past, patients with chronic fatigue and depression (and sometimes their physicians) pursued an explanation in chronic EBV infection, erroneously confirming this after a positive Monospot test result. It was erroneous because the test result remains positive long after complete resolution of uncomplicated infectious mononucleosis in youths, and most adults have had the infection. **(p. 622)**

27.4 Patients with acute viral encephalitis commonly present with psychiatric symptoms, even in the absence of neurological symptoms. In the review of this topic by Caroff et al. (2001), which of the following psychiatric presentations was the most common?

    A. Psychosis.
    B. Catatonia.
    C. Depression.
    D. Mania.
    E. Obsessive-compulsive disorder.

The correct response is option A.

In viral encephalitis, psychiatric symptoms are very common in the acute phase and frequent after recovery (Arciniegas and Anderson 2004; Caroff et al. 2001). Occasionally, patients with viral encephalitis may present initially with psychopathology without neurological symptoms. Caroff et al. (2001) reviewed 108 published cases of psychiatric presentation, classified as psychosis (35%), catatonia (33%), psychotic depression (16%), or mania (11%). Patients in such cases often receive misdiagnosis and inappropriate treatment, and Caroff et al. (2001) noted that patients with viral encephalitis are more vulnerable to adverse effects of neuroleptics, including extrapyramidal side effects, catatonia, and neuroleptic malignant syndrome. **(p. 623)**

Arciniegas DB, Anderson CA: Viral encephalitis: neuropsychiatric and neurobehavioral aspects. Curr Psychiatry Rep 6:372–379, 2004
Caroff SN, Mann SC, Glittoo MF, et al: Psychiatric manifestations of acute viral encephalitis. Psychiatric Annals 31:193–204, 2001

27.5 Psychiatric disorders can occur in the aftermath of acute viral encephalitis. Which of the following disorders is most commonly seen in this context?

    A. Psychosis.
    B. Anxiety disorders.
    C. Mood disorders.

D. Cognitive disorders.

E. Adjustment disorders.

The correct response is option C.

Psychiatric sequelae, especially mood disorders, are common following recovery from acute viral encephalitis and constitute a major cause of disability. Depression, hypomania, irritability, and disinhibition of anger, aggression, or sexuality have been frequently noted months after recovery, with psychosis occurring rarely. Depressive symptoms may respond to treatment with antidepressants or stimulants (Neel 2000). Hypomania, irritability, and disinhibition have benefited from neuroleptics, mood stabilizers including lithium, and electroconvulsive therapy (Ferrando et al. 2010; Monnet 2003). **(p. 623)**

Ferrando SJ, Levenson JL, Owen JA: Infectious diseases, in Clinical Manual of Psychopharmacology in the Medically Ill. Edited by Ferrando SJ, Levenson JL, Owen JA. Arlington, VA, American Psychiatric Publishing, 2010, pp 371–404

Monnet FP: Behavioural disturbances following Japanese B encephalitis. Eur Psychiatry 18:269–273, 2003

Neel JL: Neuropsychiatric sequelae in a case of St. Louis encephalitis. Gen Hosp Psychiatry 22:126–128, 2000

27.6 Even after recovery from acute herpes simplex virus (HSV) infection, patients may manifest persistent behavioral symptoms attributable to the virus. One well-known complication of HSV is Klüver-Bucy syndrome, symptoms of which include all of the following *except*

A. Oral touching compulsions.

B. Hyposexuality.

C. Hyperphagia.

D. Amnesia.

E. Agnosia.

The correct response is option B.

One possible sequela of HSV encephalitis is the Klüver-Bucy syndrome, which includes oral touching compulsions, hypersexuality, amnesia, placidity, agnosia, and hyperphagia. **(p. 624)**

27.7 Standard treatment for hepatitis C virus (HCV) infection involves the use of interferon (IFN), which is known to cause depression. In regard to the association between depression and IFN therapy, which of the following statements is *false?*

A. IFN causes depression in 20%–40% of patients treated.

B. Depression is the most common adverse effect leading to discontinuation of IFN.

C. Depression is associated with reduced adherence to IFN treatment.

D. IFN-associated depression is responsive to antidepressants.

E. Major depression is a contraindication to IFN treatment for HCV.

The correct response is option E.

Treatment with interferon causes depression itself in 20%–40% of patients and depressive symptoms in as many as two-thirds receiving long-term interferon treatment (Neri et al. 2006). Depression has been the most common adverse effect leading to cessation of interferon treatment. Depression reduces adherence to antiviral therapy (Martín-Santos et al. 2008) and is associated with a poorer antiviral response (Fontana et al. 2008). Depression associated with hepatitis or interferon is amenable to treatment with antidepressants (Kraus et al. 2008), allowing continuation of interferon in most patients. Therefore, depression should not be considered a contraindication to interferon therapy. Dosing should be adjusted downward if the patient has impaired liver function. **(p. 625)**

Fontana RJ, Kronfol Z, Lindsay KL, et al: Changes in mood states and biomarkers during peginterferon and ribavirin treatment of chronic hepatitis C. Am J Gastroenterol 103:2766–2775, 2008

Kraus MR, Schäfer A, Schöttker K, et al: Therapy of interferon-induced depression in chronic hepatitis C with citalopram: a randomised, double-blind, placebo-controlled study. Gut 57:531–536, 2008

Martín-Santos R, Díez-Quevedo C, Castellví P, et al: De novo depression and anxiety disorders and influence on adherence during peginterferon-alpha-2a and ribavirin treatment in patients with hepatitis C. Aliment Pharmacol Ther 27:257–265, 2008

Neri S, Pulvirenti D, Bertino G: Psychiatric symptoms induced by antiviral therapy in chronic hepatitis C: comparison between interferon-alpha-2a and interferon-alpha-2b. Clin Drug Investig 26:655–662, 2006

Chapter 28

HIV/AIDS

Select the single best response for each question.

28.1 The single most important factor affecting outcome of human immunodeficiency virus (HIV) treatment is

A. The source of the viral infection.
B. The age of the patient.
C. The patient's ability to adhere to the prescribed medication regimen.
D. The educational level of the patient.
E. The patient's gender.

The correct response is option C.

The single most important factor affecting outcome of HIV treatment is the patient's ability to adhere to a prescribed regimen. A study of HIV-infected prisoners reported that under directly observed therapy in a prison setting, 85% of the individuals developed undetectable viral loads, with prisoners taking approximately 93% of doses (Kirkland et al. 2002). In contrast, British community studies found that only 42% of treatment-naive patients taking antiretroviral medications attained undetectable viral loads (Lee and Monteiro 2003). Antiretroviral adherence rates between 54% and 76% have been reported in other general clinic or community samples (Liu et al. 2001; McNabb et al. 2001; Paterson et al. 2000; Wagner and Ghosh-Dastidar 2002), including groups of patients with serious mental illness (Beyer et al. 2007; Wagner et al. 2003).

Psychiatric factors associated with nonadherence include dementia, depression, psychosis, aversive life experience, personality factors, and substance use (Mellins et al. 2009). Many studies have shown decreased adherence to highly active antiretroviral therapy attributable to depression (Campos et al. 2010; Koenig et al. 2008). **(p. 640)**

Beyer JL, Taylor L, Gersing KR, et al: Prevalence of HIV infection in a general psychiatric outpatient population. Psychosomatics 48:31–37, 2007

Campos LN, Guimarães MD, Remien RH: Anxiety and depression symptoms as risk factors for non-adherence to antiretroviral therapy in Brazil. AIDS Behav 14:289–299, 2010

Kirkland LR, Fischl MA, Tashima KT, et al: Response to lamivudine-zidovudine plus abacavir twice daily in antiretroviral-naive, incarcerated patients with HIV infection taking directly observed treatment. Clin Infect Dis 34:511–518, 2002

Koenig LJ, Pals SL, Bush T, et al: Randomized controlled trial of an intervention to prevent adherence failure among HIV-infected patients initiating antiretroviral therapy. Health Psychol 27:159–169, 2008

Lee R, Monteiro EF: Third regional audit of antiretroviral prescribing in HIV patients. Yorkshire Audit Group for HIV Related Diseases. Int J STD AIDS 14:58–60, 2003

Liu H, Golin CE, Miller LG, et al: A comparison study of multiple measures of adherence to HIV protease inhibitors. Ann Intern Med 134:968–977, 2001

McNabb J, Ross JW, Abriola K, et al: Adherence to highly active antiretroviral therapy predicts outcome at an inner-city human immunodeficiency virus clinic. Clin Infect Dis 33:700–705, 2001

Mellins CA, Havens JF, McDonnell C, et al: Adherence to antiretroviral medications and medical care in HIV-infected adults diagnosed with mental and substance abuse disorders. AIDS Care 21:168–177, 2009

Paterson DL, Swindells S, Mohn J, et al: Adherence to protease inhibitor therapy and outcomes in patients with HIV infection. Ann Intern Med 133:21–30, 2000

Wagner GJ, Ghosh-Dastidar B: Electronic monitoring: adherence assessment or intervention? HIV Clin Trials 3:45–51, 2002

Wagner GJ, Kanouse DE, Koegel P, et al: Adherence to HIV antiretrovirals among persons with serious mental illness. AIDS Patient Care STDS 17:179–186, 2003

28.2   You are working in a human immunodeficiency virus (HIV) clinic, providing psychiatric care to acquired immunodeficiency syndrome (AIDS) patients. One patient whom you are treating has exhibited a change in his level of alertness, confusion, headache, fever, and focal neurological signs. You obtain a computed tomography (CT) scan, which shows multiple bilateral, ring-enhancing lesions in the basal ganglia. What is the most likely medical diagnosis for this patient?

   A. Cytomegalovirus.
   B. Cryptococcal meningitis.
   C. Progressive multifocal leukoencephalopathy.
   D. Toxoplasmosis.
   E. Central nervous system (CNS) lymphoma.

The correct response is option D.

Infection with *Toxoplasma gondii* generally occurs in 30% of patients with fewer than 100 CD4 cells/mm^3 (Kaplan et al. 2009). In AIDS patients, toxoplasmosis is the most common reason for intracranial masses, affecting between 2% and 4% of the AIDS population. Symptoms of CNS infection are fever, change in level of alertness, headache, confusion, focal neurological signs (approximately 80% of cases), and partial or generalized seizures (approximately 30% of cases). CT scanning usually shows multiple bilateral, ring-enhancing lesions in the basal ganglia or at the gray–white matter junction.

Cytomegalovirus (CMV) infection is found at autopsy in about 30%–50% of brains from HIV-infected patients (Jellinger et al. 2000). Short-term memory is especially impaired in CMV encephalitis in HIV-infected patients, mimicking Korsakoff's syndrome (Pirskanen-Matell et al. 2009).

Although meningitis caused by *Cryptococcus neoformans* is rare in immunocompetent persons, it is a devastating illness that has occurred in approximately 8%–10% of AIDS patients in the United States and in up to 30% of AIDS patients in other parts of the world (Powderly 2000). Patients generally present with fever and delirium. Meningeal signs are not universally seen. Seizures and focal neurological deficits occur in about 10% of patients, and intracranial pressure is elevated in about 50% of patients.

Progressive multifocal leukoencephalopathy is a demyelinating disease of white matter in immunocompromised patients. The clinical syndrome consists of multiple focal neurological deficits, such as mono- or hemiparetic limb weakness, dysarthria, gait disturbances, sensory deficits, and progressive dementia, with eventual coma and death. Occasionally, seizures or visual losses may occur.

Lymphoma is the most common neoplasm seen in AIDS patients, affecting between 0.6% and 3%. The patient is generally afebrile; may develop a single lesion with focal neurological signs or small, multifocal lesions; and most commonly presents with mental status change. Seizures occur in about 15% of these patients. CNS lymphoma presents late in the course of HIV infection and is associated with a very poor prognosis. CNS lymphoma is at times misdiagnosed as toxoplasmosis, HIV dementia, or other encephalopathy. CT scan of the brain may be normal or show one or multiple hypodense or patchy, nodular enhancing lesions. Magnetic resonance imaging generally shows enhanced lesions that may be difficult to differentiate from CNS toxoplasmosis, but thallium single photon emission computed tomography and positron emission tomography scanning may help differentiate the two disorders. **(pp. 641–642)**

Jellinger KA, Setinek U, Drlicek M, et al: Neuropathology and general autopsy findings in AIDS during the last 15 years. Acta Neuropathol 100:213–220, 2000

Kaplan JE, Benson C, Holmes KH, et al: Guidelines for prevention and treatment of opportunistic infections in HIV-infected adults and adolescents: recommendations from CDC, the National Institutes of Health, and the HIV Medicine Association of the Infectious Diseases Society of America. MMWR Recomm Rep 58(RR-4):1–207, 2009

Pirskanen-Matell R, Grützmeier S, Nennesmo I, et al: Impairment of short-term memory and Korsakoff syndrome are common in AIDS patients with cytomegalovirus encephalitis. Eur J Neurol 16:48–53, 2009

Powderly WG: Cryptococcal meningitis in HIV-infected patients. Curr Infect Dis Rep 2:352–357, 2000

28.3 Specific risk factors associated with acquired immunodeficiency syndrome (AIDS) dementia include all of the following *except*

    A. Illicit drug abuse.
    B. Male sex.
    C. Older age.
    D. Lower educational level.
    E. Anemia.

The correct response is option B.

With the widespread use of highly active antiretroviral therapy (HAART) in developing countries in the mid-1990s, there was a dramatic decrease in the rates of AIDS dementia (Bhaskaran et al. 2008), with cases usually associated with specific risk factors, including higher human immunodeficiency virus (HIV) RNA viral load, lower educational level, older age, anemia, illicit drug use, and female sex. In the post-HAART era, minor cognitive–motor disorder and depression are more predictive of severity of HIV-associated dementia (Dunlop et al. 2002; Sevigny et al. 2004; Stern et al. 2001). With patients living longer on HAART, there is some concern that AIDS dementia prevalence will increase in association with the length of infection, or with residual virus confined to the central nervous system (Letendre et al. 2008). However, the overall incidence and prevalence rates of HIV dementia in the post-HAART era vary greatly by geography, treatment, and risk factors studied, as well as by whether patients are sampled in the community, a clinic, or a hospital. **(p. 644)**

Bhaskaran K, Mussini C, Antinori A, et al: Changes in the incidence and predictors of human immunodeficiency virus-associated dementia in the era of highly active antiretroviral therapy. Ann Neurol 63:213–221, 2008

Dunlop O, Bjørklund R, Bruun JN, et al: Early psychomotor slowing predicts the development of HIV dementia and autopsy-verified HIV encephalitis. Acta Neurol Scand 105:270–275, 2002

Letendre S, Marquie-Beck J, Capparelli E, et al: Validation of the CNS Penetration-Effectiveness rank for quantifying antiretroviral penetration into the central nervous system. Arch Neurol 65:65–70, 2008

Sevigny JJ, Albert SM, McDermott MP, et al: Evaluation of HIV RNA and markers of immune activation as predictors of HIV-associated dementia. Neurology 63:2084–2090, 2004

Stern Y, McDermott MP, Albert S, et al: Factors associated with incident human immunodeficiency virus-dementia. Arch Neurol 58:473–479, 2001

28.4 Which of the following statements concerning major depression and its relationship to human immunodeficiency virus (HIV) infection is *false?*

    A. Major depression is a risk factor for developing HIV.
    B. HIV patients with depression rarely exhibit somatic symptoms.
    C. Patients with major depression are at increased risk for HIV disease progression.
    D. Fatigue has been found to be more associated with depression than with HIV disease progression.
    E. Certain HIV central nervous system (CNS) infections, such as toxoplasmosis, cryptococcal meningitis, and lymphoma, can cause depressive symptoms.

The correct response is option B.

HIV-infected patients with major depression frequently present to internists and family practitioners with multiple somatic symptoms, including headache, gastrointestinal disturbances, inexplicable musculoskeletal or visceral pain, cardiac symptoms, dizziness, tinnitus, weakness, and anesthesia. Neurovegetative symptoms are especially common. Patients report slowed thought processes, with impairments in concentration and short-term memory and occasionally generalized confusion. Given the burdens of HIV, the medical problems associated with the disease, and the side effects of medications, depression may be very low on the list of considered causes of the patient's complaints.

Major depression is a risk factor for HIV infection (McDermott et al. 1994) by virtue of its effect on behavior, intensification of substance abuse, exacerbation of self-destructive behaviors, and promotion of poor partner choice in relationships. Patients with major depression are at increased risk for disease progression and mortality (Alciati et al. 2007; Ickovics et al. 2001).

Fatigue has been found to be more associated with depression than with HIV disease progression. These findings support the notion that somatic symptoms generally suggestive of depression should trigger a full psychiatric evaluation.

Certain HIV-related medical conditions and medications can cause depressive symptoms. These include CNS infections, such as toxoplasmosis, cryptococcal meningitis, lymphoma, and syphilis. **(pp. 647–648)**

Alciati A, Gallo L, Monforte AD, et al: Major depression-related immunological changes and combination antiretroviral therapy in HIV-seropositive patients. Hum Psychopharmacol 22:33–40, 2007

Ickovics JR, Hamburger ME, Vlahov D, et al: Mortality, CD4 cell count decline, and depressive symptoms among HIV-seropositive women: longitudinal analysis from the HIV epidemiology research study. JAMA 285:1466–1474, 2001

McDermott BE, Sautter FJ, Winstead DK, et al: Diagnosis, health beliefs, and risk of HIV infection in psychiatric patients. Hosp Community Psychiatry 45:580–585, 1994

28.5 Among medications with demonstrated efficacy in the treatment of mania in human immunodeficiency virus (HIV) infection, which of the following, when used in combination with antiviral medications, may lower serum levels of protease inhibitors, thereby increasing the risk for bone marrow suppression?

    A. Lamotrigine.
    B. Valproic acid.
    C. Risperidone.
    D. Lithium.
    E. Carbamazepine.

The correct response is option E.

Carbamazepine was demonstrated to be effective in the treatment of HIV mania in a placebo-controlled trial (Vlassova et al. 2009). However, concerns exist regarding the potential for synergistic bone marrow suppression in combination with antiviral medications and HIV itself. It also may lower serum levels of protease inhibitors (Ferrando and Freyberg 2008).

Lamotrigine may be ideal as monotherapy because it is well tolerated in the elderly and is efficacious in treating bipolar disorder (Angelino and Treisman 2008).

A study of valproic acid in the treatment of HIV-associated mania reported that it was well tolerated and led to significant improvement in manic symptoms. Concern has been raised over hepatotoxicity in patients with HIV taking valproic acid (Cozza et al. 2000) and potential interactions with antiretroviral therapy (Sheehan et al. 2006).

The treatment of psychosis in HIV-related mania with risperidone has shown significant improvement (Singh et al. 1997). Two case reports note potential drug interactions when combined with the cytochrome P450

(CYP) 2D6 inhibitor ritonavir, including extrapyramidal symptoms (Kelly et al. 2002) and a reversible coma from risperidone toxicity (Jover et al. 2002).

One case report of lithium use in secondary HIV mania showed control of symptoms at a dose of 1,200 mg/day (Tanquary 1993). Lithium use has been problematic for several reasons, including side effects of cognitive slowing, nausea, diarrhea, and polyuria resulting in dehydration, all of which may already plague HIV-infected patients. The major problem with lithium in AIDS patients has been rapid fluctuations in blood level, especially in the hospital, despite previously stable doses. **(p. 651)**

Angelino AF, Treisman GJ: Issues in co-morbid severe mental illnesses in HIV infected individuals. Int Rev Psychiatry 20:95–101, 2008

Cozza KL, Swanton EJ, Humphreys CW: Hepatotoxicity with combination of valproic acid, ritonavir, and nevirapine: a case report. Psychosomatics 41:452–453, 2000

Ferrando SJ, Freyberg Z: Treatment of depression in HIV positive individuals: a critical review. Int Rev Psychiatry 20:61–71, 2008

Jover F, Cuadrado JM, Andreu L, et al: Reversible coma caused by risperidone-ritonavir interaction. Clin Neuropharmacol 25:251–253, 2002

Kelly DV, Béïque LC, Bowmer MI: Extrapyramidal symptoms with ritonavir/indinavir plus risperidone. Ann Pharmacother 36:827–830, 2002

Sheehan NL, Brouillette MJ, Delisle MS, et al: Possible interaction between lopinavir/ritonavir and valproic acid exacerbates bipolar disorder. Ann Pharmacother 40:147–150, 2006

Singh A, Golledge H, Catalan J: Treatment of HIV-related psychotic disorders with risperidone: a series of 21 cases. J Psychosom Res 42:489–493, 1997

Tanquary J: Lithium neurotoxicity at therapeutic levels in an AIDS patient. J Nerv Ment Dis 181:519–520, 1993

Vlassova N, Angelino AF, Treisman GJ: Update on mental health issues in patients with HIV infection. Curr Infect Dis Rep 11:163–169, 2009

28.6   The term *triple diagnosis* refers to the concurrent presence of

A. A substance use disorder, a psychiatric disorder, and human immunodeficiency virus (HIV) infection.
B. HIV, AIDS, and depression.
C. Three psychiatric disorders and HIV.
D. Two medical disorders and HIV.
E. Two substance use disorders and HIV.

The correct response is option A.

Triple diagnosis refers to a patient with a dual diagnosis (substance abuse and psychiatric disorder) who also has HIV. Such patients are overrepresented in HIV-infected populations. One study found that as many as 44% of the new entrants to the HIV medical clinic at the Johns Hopkins Hospital had an active substance use disorder. Of these patients, 24% had both a current substance use disorder and another non-substance-related Axis I diagnosis (Lyketsos et al. 1994). The Criminal Justice Drug Abuse and Treatment studies (CJDATS) show the strongest correlation between comorbid substance abuse and mental illness for risk of contracting HIV (Pearson et al. 2008; Treisman et al. 2001). **(p. 652)**

Lyketsos CG, Hanson A, Fishman M, et al: Screening for psychiatric morbidity in a medical outpatient clinic for HIV infection: the need for a psychiatric presence. Int J Psychiatry Med 24:103–113, 1994

Pearson FS, Cleland CM, Chaple M, et al: Substance use, mental health problems, and behavior at risk for HIV: evidence from CJDATS. J Psychoactive Drugs 40:459–469, 2008

Treisman GJ, Angelino AF, Hutton HE: Psychiatric issues in the management of patients with HIV infection. JAMA 286:2857–2864, 2001

28.7 People with which of the following personality characteristics have been shown to be at highest risk for human immunodeficiency virus (HIV) infection?

    A. Stable extroverts.
    B. Unstable introverts.
    C. Unstable extroverts.
    D. Stable introverts.
    E. None of the above.

The correct response is option C.

Unstable extroverts are the most prone to engage in practices that place them at risk for HIV. In the psychiatry service of the Johns Hopkins AIDS clinic (a referral-biased sample), about 60% of patients present with a blend of extroversion and emotional instability. These individuals are preoccupied by, and act on, their feelings, which are labile, leading to unpredictable and inconsistent behavior. Most striking is the inconsistency between thought and action. Regardless of intellectual ability or knowledge of HIV, unstable extroverts can engage in extremely risky behavior. Past experience and future consequences have little importance in decision making for the individual who is ruled by feeling; the present is paramount. Their primary goal is to achieve immediate pleasure or removal of pain, regardless of circumstances. Unstable extroverts are more likely to engage in behavior that places them at risk for HIV infection and are more likely to pursue sex promiscuously. They are less likely to plan and carry condoms and more likely to have unprotected vaginal or anal sex. They are more fixed on the reward of sex and remarkably inattentive to the sexually transmitted disease they may acquire if they do not use a condom. Unstable extroverts are also less likely to accept the diminution of pleasure associated with the use of condoms or, once aroused, to interrupt the "heat of the moment" to use condoms.

Stable extroverts are also present oriented and pleasure seeking; however, their emotions are not as intense, as easily provoked, or as mercurial. Hence, they are not as strongly driven to achieve pleasure. Stable extroverts may be at risk because they are too optimistic or sanguine to believe that they will become infected with HIV.

Introverted personalities appear to be less common among HIV psychiatric patients. Their focus on the future, avoidance of negative consequences, and preference for cognition over feeling render them more likely to engage in protective and preventive behaviors. HIV risk for introverts is determined by the dimension of emotional instability. Unstable introverts are anxious, moody, and pessimistic. Typically, these patients seek drugs and/or sex not for pleasure, but for relief or distraction from pain. They are concerned about the future and adverse outcomes but believe that they have little control over their fates. Stable introverts, with their controlled, even-tempered personalities, are least likely to engage in risky or hedonistic behaviors. Typically, these individuals are HIV positive as a result of a blood transfusion or an occupational needle stick. **(pp. 654–655)**

Chapter 29

Dermatology

Select the single best response for each question.

29.1 The pharmacological properties of some psychotropic drugs make them useful not only to treat psychiatric disorders but also to treat comorbid dermatological conditions. Which of the following tricyclic antidepressants has antihistaminic effects and is available in a dermatological cream preparation?

    A. Nortriptyline.
    B. Amitriptyline.
    C. Imipramine.
    D. Desipramine.
    E. Doxepin.

The correct response is option E.

Standard psychiatric therapies are used to treat psychiatric comorbidity in the dermatology patient. Psychiatric drugs are generally used for one of three purposes: 1) management of dermatological manifestations of primary psychiatric disorders, 2) management of psychiatric disorders that are comorbid with primary dermatological disorders, and 3) provision of certain desired pharmacological properties of psychotropic agents (e.g., the antihistaminic effect of doxepin), even in the absence of a comorbid psychiatric disorder. Currently, no orally administered psychotropic agents are approved by the U.S. Food and Drug Administration (FDA) for the treatment of a primary dermatological disorder; 5% topical doxepin cream is FDA-approved for short-term (up to 8 days) management of moderate pruritus in adults with conditions such as atopic dermatitis. **(p. 668)**

29.2 Patients with delusional parasitosis (a primary psychotic disorder with dermatological manifestations) typically first present to dermatologists rather than to psychiatrists. Which of the following statements regarding this illness is *true*?

    A. The mean age at onset is the 30s.
    B. In patients younger than 50 years, the male-to-female prevalence ratio is 1:3.
    C. In patients older than 50 years, the male-to-female prevalence ratio is 1:1.
    D. Tactile and olfactory hallucinations are not a prominent feature of the disorder.
    E. Patients often complain of formication or various cutaneous sensations.

The correct response is option E.

Patients with delusional parasitosis often complain of formication or cutaneous sensations of crawling, stinging, and/or biting.

Delusional parasitosis (delusions of infestation) is classified as a delusional disorder, somatic type, and is characterized by a fixed false belief that one is infested by parasites or insects that is maintained despite negative clinical and laboratory findings (Bishop 1983). Delusional parasitosis is rarely seen by general psychiatrists but is common in dermatological practice. The mean age at onset is the mid-50s to 60s, with an equal sex distribution in patients younger than 50 years and a female-to-male ratio of 3:1 in patients ages 50 years and older (Lyell

1983). Patients with delusional parasitosis typically present the doctor with alleged parasite specimens in a pill bottle, matchbox, adhesive tape, or plastic bag (Lepping and Freudenmann 2008). Such patients tend to treat their skin by scratching, and may use disinfectants, repellants, pesticides, and antimicrobials. They may consult exterminators or entomologists, repeatedly launder clothing and linens, and discard possessions and even pets (fearing them as the source). Tactile and olfactory hallucinations related to the delusional theme may be present. **(p. 669)**

Bishop ER Jr: Monosymptomatic hypochondriacal syndromes in dermatology. J Am Acad Dermatol 9:152–158, 1983

Lepping P, Freudenmann RW: Delusional parasitosis: a new pathway for diagnosis and treatment. Clin Exp Dermatol 33:113–117, 2008

Lyell A: The Michelson Lecture. Delusions of parasitosis. Br J Dermatol 108:485–499, 1983

29.3 Although delusional parasitosis may be idiopathic, some cases are associated with abuse of psychoactive substances. Abuse of which of the following is most specifically associated with delusional parasitosis?

    A. Psychostimulants.
    B. Opioids.
    C. Alcohol.
    D. Marijuana.
    E. Inhalants.

The correct response is option A.

Although most cases of delusional parasitosis appear to represent a primary delusional disorder, some have been considered secondary to other psychiatric disorders—for example, schizophrenia, obsessive-compulsive disorder, or psychotic depression—or medical disorders—for example, structural brain disease, delirium, dementia, endocrinopathy (e.g., hypothyroidism), vitamin deficiency (B_{12} deficiency and pellagra), neuropathies, uremia, hepatic encephalopathy, and other toxic states, especially abuse of amphetamines or cocaine (Lepping and Freudenmann 2008). **(p. 669)**

Lepping P, Freudenmann RW: Delusional parasitosis: a new pathway for diagnosis and treatment. Clin Exp Dermatol 33:113–117, 2008

29.4 Trichotillomania—nonscarring alopecia as a result of self-plucking of hair—has been associated with all of the following factors *except*

    A. Low dissociation scores.
    B. Psychological trauma.
    C. Posttraumatic stress disorder (PTSD).
    D. Depression.
    E. Mental retardation.

The correct response is option A.

Trichotillomania has been associated with a history of psychological trauma (e.g., bereavement) and PTSD (Gershuny et al. 2006), high dissociation scores (Gupta et al. 2000; Lochner et al. 2004), and depression. Trichotillomania may be a feature of mental retardation, eating disorders, and personality disorders in which patients tend to be highly dissociated. **(p. 672)**

Gershuny BS, Keuthen NJ, Gentes EL, et al: Current posttraumatic stress disorder and history of trauma in trichotillomania. J Clin Psychol 62:1521–1529, 2006

Gupta MA, Gupta AK, Chandarana PC, et al: Dissociative symptoms and self-induced dermatoses: a preliminary empirical study (abstract). Psychosom Med 62:116, 2000

Lochner C, Seedat S, Hemmings SMJ, et al: Dissociative experiences in obsessive-compulsive disorder and trichotillomania: clinical and genetic findings. Compr Psychiatry 45:384–391, 2004

29.5 Which tricyclic antidepressant has been shown to be superior to placebo in the management of trichotillomania?

   A. Nortriptyline.
   B. Amitriptyline.
   C. Imipramine.
   D. Desipramine.
   E. Clomipramine.

The correct response is option E.

The three major treatments studied in trichotillomania include habit-reversal therapy (HRT), selective serotonin reuptake inhibitors (SSRIs), and clomipramine (Bloch et al. 2007). A systematic review of these interventions in seven blinded, randomized clinical trials in which the primary outcome measure was mean change in trichotillomania severity revealed that HRT was superior to both SSRIs and clomipramine. Clomipramine, but not SSRIs, was more effective than placebo (Bloch et al. 2007). **(p. 672)**

Bloch MH, Landeros-Weisenberger A, Dombrowski P, et al: Systematic review: pharmacological and behavioral treatment for trichotillomania. Biol Psychiatry 62:839–846, 2007

29.6 Atopic dermatitis may be managed, in part, by the judicious use of antidepressant medications. Which of the following antidepressants, due to its anticholinergic properties, would be preferred for this condition?

   A. Paroxetine.
   B. Monoamine oxidase inhibitors.
   C. Trimipramine.
   D. Imipramine.
   E. Duloxetine.

The correct response is option C.

Sedating antidepressants may be beneficial in part through promoting sleep. The strongly antihistaminic antidepressants doxepin, trimipramine, and amitriptyline may also be effective because of their strong anticholinergic properties, as the eccrine sweat glands in atopic dermatitis have been found to be hypersensitive to acetylcholine. **(p. 676)**

29.7 Although psychiatrists may more routinely see cases of lithium-associated acne, lithium-associated psoriasis can also be a painful complication of lithium therapy. Which of the following statements regarding lithium-associated psoriasis is *true*?

   A. Lithium-associated psoriasis is very responsive to topical antipsoriatic treatment.
   B. Psoriasis usually resolves within 2 weeks of discontinuing lithium.
   C. Inositol supplements may have a beneficial effect on psoriasis.
   D. Recent population-based studies document that beta-blockers confer a significant increased risk of psoriasis when given with lithium.
   E. Psoriasis from lithium commonly occurs within the first 4 weeks of treatment.

The correct response is option C.

A small randomized clinical trial showed that inositol supplements have a significant beneficial effect on psoriasis patients taking lithium (Allan et al. 2004).

Lithium-induced psoriasis can occur within a few months, but usually occurs within the first few years of treatment. The absolute increased risk is quite small (Brauchli et al. 2009). Psoriasis precipitated or exacerbated by lithium is typically resistant to conventional antipsoriatic treatments. When the psoriasis becomes intractable, lithium must be discontinued and the psoriasis usually remits within a few months.

Beta-blockers such as propranolol (often used to treat lithium-induced tremors) have also been associated with psoriasis, but a recent population-based study does not support this (Brauchli et al. 2008). **(p. 677)**

Allan SJ, Kavanagh GM, Herd RM, et al: The effect of inositol supplements on the psoriasis of patients taking lithium: a randomized, placebo-controlled trial. Br J Dermatol 150:966–969, 2004

Brauchli YB, Jick SS, Curtin F, et al: Association between beta-blockers, other antihypertensive drugs and psoriasis: population-based case-control study. Br J Dermatol 158:1299–1307, 2008

Brauchli YB, Jick SS, Curtin F, et al: Lithium, antipsychotics, and risk of psoriasis. J Clin Psychopharmacol 29:134–140, 2009

29.8   Isotretinoin is used in dermatology for the management of problematic acne vulgaris. Which of the following psychiatric complications is associated with isotretinoin?

    A. Depression.
    B. Psychosis.
    C. Suicide.
    D. Aggression.
    E. All of the above.

The correct response is option E.

Isotretinoin, which is generally used to treat severe acne, has been associated with depression, psychosis, suicide, and aggressive behaviors (Physicians' Desk Reference 2008). **(p. 682)**

Physicians' Desk Reference: Physicians' Desk Reference 2009, 63rd Edition. New York, Thomson Reuters, 2008

29.9   Erythema multiforme, a dangerous dermatological reaction, is associated with which of the following psychotropic agents?

    A. Carbamazepine.
    B. Valproate.
    C. Lamotrigine.
    D. Gabapentin.
    E. All of the above.

The correct response is option E.

Although rarely associated with antipsychotics and antidepressants, erythema multiforme is most commonly associated with carbamazepine, valproic acid, lamotrigine, gabapentin, and oxcarbazepine. It may occur within days of starting these drugs and may present as a polymorphous eruption, with pathognomonic "target lesions" typically involving the extremities and palmoplantar surfaces. Evolution to more serious Stevens-Johnson syndrome and toxic epidermal necrolysis should always be considered. **(p. 683)**

Chapter 30

Surgery

Select the single best response for each question.

30.1 General surgical units and specialized surgical units have different operational styles. According to systems theory, burn units exemplify which of the following system types?

    A. Closed.
    B. Partial.
    C. Random.
    D. Open.
    E. Incomplete.

The correct response is option A.

Most general surgical units are open systems, and some poorly functioning ones are random systems. Specialized units, such as burn units, are often closed systems with very rigid rules about entering or leaving the system.

The general surgical unit and specialized units often have significant differences in operational style. Systems theory can be helpful in understanding these differences (Luhmann and Knodt 1995). An *open system* has regular members who belong to the system and flexible rules about entering and leaving the system. In a *closed system*, only certain individuals can come into and go out of the system, and "outsiders" are excluded from the system. In a *random system*, individuals move into and out of the system at random, with few rules about how entry and exit occur. **(p. 691)**

> Luhmann N, Knodt EM: Social Systems (Writing Science). Translated by Bedrara J, Baeder D. Stanford, CA, Stanford University Press, 1995

30.2 Valid informed surgical consent includes all of the following principles *except*

    A. Capacity for decision making.
    B. Disclosure.
    C. Acceptance of the procedure.
    D. Understanding.
    E. Volunteerism.

The correct response is option C.

Informed consent is required prior to the performance of any surgical procedure. In this process, surgeons provide patients with information necessary to make an autonomous decision about whether to have surgery and ensure that patients are aware of the risks, benefits, and alternatives. The ethical practice of surgery requires a patient's voluntary informed consent. Valid informed surgical consent includes principles of volunteerism, disclosure, understanding, and capacity for decision making (del Carmen and Joffe 2005). In some instances, however, direct consent is impossible, and surgeons seek permission from surrogates or guidance from written advance directives. Informed consent and decision making are at the core of the preoperative period. The communication of factual information understandable to the patient is the responsibility of the surgeon. It should include diagnosis, reasons that the operation is thought to be the treatment of choice, and expected risks and benefits and their probabilities. Alternatives and their consequences, as well as financial costs, also should be discussed. Informed consent is not merely the provision of information; it also involves ascertaining that patients have an adequate understanding of the procedure they are to undergo. Asking patients to describe, in their own words, the procedure they are about to have is a way the surgeon can assess whether patients have sufficient health literacy to understand the procedures to be performed and the risks, benefits, and alternatives to surgery. (pp. 693–694)

del Carmen MG, Joffe S: Informed consent for medical treatment and research: a review. Oncologist 10:636–641, 2005

30.3   Which of the following psychiatric disorders is viewed as a risk factor for development of chronic postsurgical pain?

    A. Posttraumatic stress disorder.
    B. Schizophrenia.
    C. Bipolar disorder.
    D. Depression.
    E. Dementia.

The correct response is option D.

The proportion of patients taking antidepressants who undergo surgery is reported to be 35% (Scher and Anwar 1999). Preoperative executive dysfunction and depressive symptoms are predictive of postoperative delirium among noncardiac surgical patients (Smith et al. 2009). Brander et al. (2003) found that the most severe cases of chronic postsurgical pain after 1 year appeared in those patients with the most severe levels of preoperative depression. Undoubtedly, depression can emerge from the experience of pain. However, in the study of Hinrichs-Rocker et al. (2009) it is suggested that depression, at least in severe cases, represents a risk factor for the development of chronic postsurgical pain. (p. 694)

Brander VA, Stulberg SD, Adams AD, et al: Predicting total knee replacement pain: a prospective, observational study. Clin Orthop Relat Res 416:27–36, 2003

Hinrichs-Rocker A, Schulz K, Järvinen I, et al: Psychosocial predictors and correlates for chronic post-surgical pain (CPSP)—a systemic review. Eur J Pain 13:719–730, 2009

Scher CS, Anwar M: The self-reporting of psychiatric medications in patients scheduled for elective surgery. J Clin Anesth 11:619–621, 1999

Smith PJ, Attix DK, Weldon BC, et al: Executive function and depression as independent risk factors for postoperative delirium. Anesthesiology 110:781–787, 2009

30.4   Which of the following factors is associated with an increased likelihood of developing posttraumatic stress disorder (PTSD) after trauma?

    A. Concussion.
    B. PTSD symptoms during the acute hospitalization period.
    C. Alcohol intoxication.
    D. Severity of the injury.
    E. Better prior emotional adjustment.

The correct response is option B.

In the surgical arena, PTSD has been best studied in trauma patients (especially burn patients) and motor vehicle accident victims (Klein et al. 2003), but several studies have shown that a significant percentage of patients also develop PTSD following cardiac surgery or neurosurgery (Powell et al. 2002; Stoll et al. 2000). Although full syndromal PTSD develops in 18%–40% of adult patients after trauma, many more develop some of the symptoms of PTSD. Several studies have tried to identify factors that predict the emergence of PTSD (Tedstone and Tarrier 2003). As expected, better prior emotional adjustment and social support are relatively protective. However, contrary to expectation, the severity of the injury, or the severity of the illness requiring surgery, is not clearly correlated with the emergence of PTSD. Also, alcohol intoxication or concussion at the time of the trauma seems to decrease the likelihood of PTSD (perhaps because memory for the event is impaired). Furthermore, some patients with no apparent predisposing factors develop PTSD. The course of PTSD is not completely clear, but symptoms usually appear within the first week after a trauma and increase in intensity over the next 3 months. Perhaps the best predictor of PTSD at 1 year is the presence of symptoms during the acute hospitalization after a trauma (McKibben et al. 2008; Zatzick et al. 2002). **(p. 700)**

Klein E, Koren D, Arnon I, et al: Sleep complaints are not corroborated by objective sleep measures in post-traumatic stress disorder: a 1-year prospective study in survivors of motor vehicle crashes. J Sleep Res 12:35–41, 2003

McKibben JB, Bresnick MG, Wiechman Askay SA, et al: Acute stress disorder and posttraumatic stress disorder: a prospective study of prevalence, course, and predictors in a sample with major burn injuries. J Burn Care Res 29:22–35, 2008

Powell J, Kitchen N, Heslin J, et al: Psychosocial outcomes at three and nine months after good neurological recovery from aneurysmal subarachnoid haemorrhage: predictors and prognosis. J Neurol Neurosurg Psychiatry 72:772–781, 2002

Stoll C, Schelling G, Goetz AE, et al: Health-related quality of life and post-traumatic stress disorder in patients after cardiac surgery and intensive care treatment. J Thorac Cardiovasc Surg 120:505–512, 2000

Tedstone JE, Tarrier N: Posttraumatic stress disorder following medical illness and treatment. Clin Psychol Rev 23:409–448, 2003

Zatzick DF, Jurkovich GJ, Gentilello L, et al: Posttraumatic stress, problem drinking, and functional outcomes after injury. Arch Surg 137:200–205, 2002

30.5   Which of the following factors is *not* associated with improved functional outcome following surgery?

    A. Appropriate pain management.
    B. Management of postsurgical psychiatric problems.
    C. Preparation of the patient for surgery.
    D. Management of preoperative fears.
    E. Actual severity of the trauma or surgery.

The correct response is option E.

Functional outcome includes the ability to carry out the activities of daily living, the ability to function in one's usual role, and satisfaction with life. The actual severity of the underlying trauma or surgery does not necessarily appear to determine quality of life. For example, the total body surface area burned does not directly correlate with the likelihood of posttraumatic stress disorder (PTSD), nor does the size of a scar necessarily correlate with posttrauma adjustment. It has been repeatedly reported that an adequate social support system is positively correlated with postsurgical and posttrauma adaptation.

A confluence of factors determines functional outcome. These factors include the condition requiring surgical intervention, presurgical psychiatric status, and surgical strategy. Other factors that may improve outcome include preparation of the patient and family for surgery, detection and management of preoperative fears, respectful attitude of the surgeon and operating room personnel during surgery, detection and appropriate treatment of pain, and detection and management of various psychiatric problems following surgery, including delirium and PTSD. (p. 702)

30.6 Which of the following psychiatric disorders is most common and problematic in burn patients?

A. Depression.
B. Dementia.
C. Alcohol abuse or dependence.
D. Bipolar disorder.
E. Schizophrenia.

The correct response is option C.

Preinjury substance use disorders are common among burn victims. One study found that among 727 deaths from fires, blood alcohol assays were positive in 29%, with a mean blood ethanol level of 193.9 mg/dL.

Among patients who survive to be treated, several studies have attempted to identify the prevalence of alcohol intoxication, alcohol abuse, or alcohol dependence. One study (Jones et al. 1991) found that 27% were intoxicated at the time of the burn, and 90% of these were then identified as having an alcohol abuse diagnosis compared with 11% of the nonintoxicated burn patients. Other reports estimated the prevalence of alcohol abuse and dependence in patients with burn injuries as between 6% and 11% (Powers et al. 1994; Tabares and Peck 1997). The Alcohol Use Disorders Identification Test (developed by the World Health Organization) was more effective in identifying at-risk drinkers than the blood alcohol level among a group of 123 burn patients (Albright et al. 2009). Steenkamp et al. (1994) found that 57% of the patients had evidence of alcohol problems on the Michigan Alcoholism Screening Test, and of these patients, 57% thought that the use of alcohol had contributed to the accident.

Among burn patients who are identified as having alcohol or drug problems, referral for treatment occurs in fewer than half of the patients (Powers et al. 1994), and among those who are referred, fewer than half accept treatment (Tabares and Peck 1997). (pp. 703–704)

Albright JM, Kovacs EJ, Gamelli RL, et al: Implications of formal alcohol screening in burn patients. J Burn Care Res 30:62–69, 2009
Jones JD, Barber B, Engrav L, et al: Alcohol use and burn injury. J Burn Care Rehabil 12:148–152, 1991
Powers PS, Stevens B, Arias F, et al: Alcohol disorders among patients with burns: crisis and opportunity. J Burn Care Rehabil 15:386–391, 1994
Steenkamp WC, Botha NJ, Van der Merwe AE: The prevalence of alcohol dependence in burned adult patients. Burns 20:522–525, 1994
Tabares R, Peck MD: Chemical dependency in patients with burn injuries: a fortress of denial. J Burn Care Rehabil 18:283–286, 1997

30.7 Which of the following psychiatric disorders has been found to be most prevalent in obese patients being evaluated for bariatric surgery?

A. Eating disorder.
B. Mood disorder.
C. Anxiety disorder.
D. Alcohol abuse or dependence.
E. Substance use disorder.

The correct response is option B.

Recent studies have documented a high prevalence of psychiatric disorders among extremely obese patients who present for bariatric surgery. The prevalence of Axis I diagnoses among candidates for bariatric surgery is high. Two recent relatively large studies (Mauri et al. 2008; Rosenberger et al. 2006) utilized the well-validated Structured Clinical Interview for DSM-IV Axis I Diagnoses (SCID) to examine the prevalence of Axis I psychiatric disorders in severely obese bariatric surgery candidates. The lifetime prevalence of Axis I diagnoses was very similar in the two studies (36.8% in Rosenberger et al. [2006] vs. 37.6% in Mauri et al. [2008]), and current Axis I diagnosis rate was also very similar (24.1% vs. 20.9%). In both studies, the most common Axis I diagnoses were affective disorders, followed by anxiety disorders and then eating disorders. Interestingly, alcohol and other substance use disorders were uncommon in the two studies. This may be because physicians identify patients with substance use disorders and do not refer them for surgery, or it may be that patients do not reveal substance use disorders during the initial evaluation. **(pp. 712–713)**

Mauri M, Rucci P, Calderone A, et al: Axis I and II disorders and quality of life in bariatric surgery candidates. J Clin Psychiatry 69:295–301, 2008

Rosenberger PH, Henderson KE, Grilo CM: Psychiatric disorder comorbidity and association with eating disorders in bariatric surgery patients: a cross-sectional study using structured interview-based diagnosis. J Clin Psychiatry 67:1080–1085, 2006

Chapter 3 1

Organ Transplantation

Select the single best response for each question.

31.1   Which of the following groups of transplant patients currently has the highest rates of long-term survival?

   A. Deceased-donor kidney recipients.
   B. Pancreas recipients.
   C. Living-donor liver recipients.
   D. Heart recipients.
   E. Lung recipients.

The correct response is option C.

Following transplantation, living-donor liver and living-donor kidney recipients experience the highest long-term survival rates (76% alive at 10 years posttransplantation). Recipients of deceased-donor kidneys, livers, and hearts have somewhat lower 10-year survival (61%, 59%, and 53%, respectively) and lung and intestine recipients have the poorest 10-year survival (41% and 26%, respectively) (United Network of Organ Sharing 2009). **(p. 726)**

   United Network of Organ Sharing (UNOS) Web site. Available at: http://www.optn.org. Accessed June 1, 2009.

31.2   The Psychosocial Assessment of Candidates for Transplantation (PACT) is a clinically useful instrument in the psychiatric assessment of organ transplant candidates. In regard to this instrument, which of the following statements is *false*?

   A. It provides an overall numerical score.
   B. It provides a subscale score for psychological health.
   C. It assesses lifestyle factors.
   D. It addresses patient "educability" regarding transplant expectations.
   E. The final rating is determined by an arithmetic mean of the subscale scores.

The correct response is option E.

The PACT was the first published psychosocial structured instrument specifically designed for screening transplant candidates (Olbrisch et al. 1989). It provides an overall score and subscale scores for psychological health (psychopathology, risk for psychopathology, stable personality factors), lifestyle factors (healthy lifestyle, ability to sustain change in lifestyle, adherence, drug and alcohol use), social support (support system stability and availability), and patient educability and understanding of the transplant process. The PACT can be completed in only a few minutes by the consultant following the evaluation but requires scoring by a skilled clinician, without which the instrument's predictive power could be diminished (Presberg et al. 1995). The final rating for candidate acceptability is made by the clinician, with the freedom to weigh individual item ratings variably (Presberg et al. 1995). Thus, a single area, such as alcohol abuse, could be assigned greater weight and could thereby disproportionately influence the final rating. **(p. 729)**

Olbrisch ME, Levenson JL, Hamer R: The PACT: a rating scale for the study of clinical decision making in psychosocial screening of organ transplant candidates. Clin Transplant 3:164–169, 1989

Presberg BA, Levenson JL, Olbrisch ME, et al: Rating scales for the psychosocial evaluation of organ transplant candidates: comparison of the PACT and TERS with bone marrow transplant patients. Psychosomatics 36:458–461, 1995

31.3 Similar to other medically ill populations, transplant recipients experience a significant amount of psychological distress and are at heightened risk of developing psychiatric disorders. Dew et al. (2001) studied the prevalence and risk of psychiatric disorders in 191 heart transplant recipients. Findings from this study included all of the following *except*

  A. The cumulative prevalence of any psychiatric disorder was 38%.
  B. Women were at higher risk than men for posttransplant psychiatric disorders.
  C. Major depression was the most common psychiatric disorder after transplantation.
  D. The cumulative prevalence of posttraumatic stress disorder (PTSD) was 17%.
  E. The incidence of transplant-associated PTSD was the same in each of the 3 years studied.

The correct response is option E.

In a prospective study of 191 heart transplant recipients, the cumulative prevalence rates for psychiatric disorders during the 3 years posttransplantation were 38% for any disorder, including 25% with major depression, 21% with adjustment disorders, and 17% with PTSD (Dew et al. 2001). PTSD related to transplant was limited almost exclusively to the first year after transplantation. In this group of heart recipients, there was a clustering of cases of major depression in the first year, and the cumulative rate of major depression was greater than the rate of any anxiety disorders. Factors that increased the cumulative risk for psychiatric disorders included a pretransplant psychiatric history, a longer period of hospitalization, female gender, greater impairments in physical functioning, and fewer social supports (Dew et al. 2001). These risk factors were additive, and therefore the cumulative risk of a psychiatric disorder increased with the number of risk factors. **(p. 730)**

Dew MA, Kormos RL, DiMartini AF, et al: Prevalence and risk of depression and anxiety-related disorders during the first three years after heart transplantation. Psychosomatics 42:300–313, 2001

31.4 Several studies have suggested an association between psychiatric disorders and transplant health outcomes, although the results have been mixed. Which of the following statements regarding the Singh et al. (1997) study of wait-listed liver transplant candidates is *true?*

  A. Three-fourths of cases had a Beck Depression Inventory (BDI) score higher than 16, consistent with a diagnosis of major depression.
  B. Higher BDI scores were primarily attributable to greater burden of somatic symptoms.
  C. Depressed candidates who later received transplants had poorer postoperative survival than nondepressed organ recipients.
  D. Survival outcomes for depressed patients were highly influenced by social factors.
  E. Candidates who were depressed (based on BDI scores) had a significantly higher likelihood of death while awaiting transplant.

The correct response is option E.

A study of wait-listed liver transplant candidates found that candidates with BDI scores higher than 10 (64% of patients) were significantly more likely than nondepressed candidates to die while awaiting transplantation (Singh et al. 1997). The higher BDI scores were due more to affective than to somatic symptoms. However, for candidates who reached transplantation, pretransplant depression was not associated with poorer posttransplant survival (Singh et al. 1997). These results were not affected by the severity of and complications from liver disease, or by patients' social support, employment, or education (Singh et al. 1997). **(p. 731)**

Singh N, Gayowski T, Wagener MM, et al: Depression in patients with cirrhosis: impact on outcome. Dig Dis Sci 42:1421–1427, 1997

31.5 Postoperative immunosuppressant medication adherence is a critical issue in transplant medicine. In the adherence study by Dew et al. (2007), which organ transplant type was associated with the highest rates of medication noncompliance?

    A. Lung.
    B. Liver.
    C. Pancreas.
    D. Heart.
    E. Kidney.

The correct response is option E.

In a recent meta-analysis including nearly 150 studies of all organ types, the average nonadherence rates ranged from 1 to 4 cases per 100 patients annually for substance use (including tobacco, alcohol, and illicit drugs), to 19 to 25 cases per 100 patients annually for a variety of areas of nonadherence (e.g., immunosuppressant medication, diet, exercise, and other transplant health care requirements) (Dew et al. 2007). Medication nonadherence was especially high, and clinicians can expect to see 23 nonadherent patients for every 100 individuals seen during a given year of follow-up (Dew et al. 2007). Immunosuppressant nonadherence was highest in kidney recipients (36 cases per 100 patients annually vs. 7–15 cases for other organs) (Dew et al. 2007). **(p. 734)**

Dew MA, DiMartini A, De Vito Dabbs A, et al: Rates and risk factors for nonadherence to the medical regimen after adult solid organ transplantation. Transplantation 83:858–873, 2007

31.6 Personality disorders are an important psychiatric consideration in the evaluation and management of transplant cases. Which of the following personality disorders is considered to present the highest risk for postoperative nonadherence?

    A. Obsessive-compulsive.
    B. Narcissistic.
    C. Avoidant.
    D. Dependent.
    E. Borderline.

The correct response is option E.

Of the personality disorders, borderline personality disorder is considered to represent the highest risk for post-transplant nonadherence (Bunzel and Laederach-Hofmann 2000).

The incidence of personality disorders in transplant populations is similar to that in the general population, ranging from 10% to 26% (Chacko et al. 1996; Dobbels et al. 2000), although in some cohorts estimates have been as high as 33% (in a cohort of heart and lung transplant recipients) (Stilley et al. 2005) or even 57% (predominantly in those with a history of substance abuse) (Stilley et al. 1997). However, the identification of personality disorders depends on the definition and measurement methods used. Unfortunately, studies investigating personality disorders and transplantation outcomes have not distinguished among the various personality disorder types (perhaps because of the low prevalence of each type), which makes generalizations difficult. Nevertheless, case reports of patients with severe character pathology demonstrate the extent of adherence problems that can arise from these disorders, resulting in significant morbidity and recipient death (Surman and

Purtilo 1992; Weitzner et al. 1999). The disturbances in interpersonal relationships that can occur with personality disorders also can decrease the likelihood that patients will have stable and reliable social supports during the pre- and posttransplant phases (Yates et al. 1998). (p. 739)

Bunzel B, Laederach-Hofmann K: Solid organ transplantation: are there predictors for posttransplant noncompliance? A literature overview. Transplantation 70:711–716, 2000

Chacko RC, Harper RG, Gotto J, et al: Psychiatric interview and psychometric predictors of cardiac transplant survival. Am J Psychiatry 153:1607–1612, 1996

Dobbels F, Put C, Vanhaecke J: Personality disorders: a challenge for transplantation. Prog Transplant 10:226–232, 2000

Stilley CS, Miller DJ, Tarter RE: Measuring psychological distress in candidates of liver transplantation: a pilot study. J Clin Psychol 53:459–464, 1997

Stilley CS, Dew MA, Pilkonis P, et al: Personality characteristics among cardiothoracic transplant recipients. Gen Hosp Psychiatry 27:113–118, 2005

Surman OS, Purtilo R: Reevaluation of organ transplantation criteria: allocation of scarce resources to borderline candidates. Psychosomatics 33:202–212, 1992

Weitzner MA, Lehninger F, Sullivan D, et al: Borderline personality disorder and bone marrow transplantation: ethical considerations and review. Psycho-Oncology 8:46–54, 1999

Yates WR, LaBrecque DR, Pfab D: Personality disorder as a contraindication for liver transplantation in alcoholic cirrhosis. Psychosomatics 39:501–511, 1998

31.7   Patients with psychosis pose a particular challenge in management before, during, and after transplantation. In the study of transplant recipients with psychotic disorders by Coffman and Crone (2002), risk factors for nonadherence included all of the following *except*

A. Family history of schizophrenia.
B. Antisocial personality features.
C. Borderline personality features.
D. Negative symptoms.
E. Positive symptoms.

The correct response is option D.

Although chronic and active psychosis is thought by many to be incompatible with successful transplantation, case reports of carefully selected patients with psychosis demonstrate that such patients can successfully undergo transplantation and survive after the procedure (DiMartini and Twillman 1994; Krahn et al. 1998). A survey of transplant psychiatrists at national and international transplant programs identified only 35 cases of pretransplant psychotic disorders in transplant recipients from 12 transplant centers (Coffman and Crone 2002), suggesting that such patients are highly underrepresented among transplant recipients. Results of this survey confirmed previously expressed stipulations that patients with psychotic disorders be carefully screened before acceptance. Candidates should have demonstrated good adherence to both medical and psychiatric follow-up requirements; possess adequate social supports, especially in-residence support; and be capable of establishing a working relationship with the transplant team. In this survey (Coffman and Crone 2002), risk factors for problems with adherence after transplantation included antisocial or borderline personality disorder features, a history of assault, living alone, positive psychotic symptoms, and a family history of schizophrenia. (p. 740)

Coffman K, Crone C: Rational guidelines for transplantation in patients with psychotic disorders. Current Opinion in Organ Transplantation 7:385–388, 2002

DiMartini A, Twillman R: Organ transplantation in paranoid schizophrenia. Psychosomatics 35:159–161, 1994

Krahn LE, Santoscoy G, Van Loon JA: A schizophrenic patient's attempt to resume dialysis following renal transplantation. Psychosomatics 39:470–473, 1998

31.8   The immunosuppressant tacrolimus is associated with neuropsychiatric side effects that may limit patients' adherence to posttransplant medication regimens. An uncommon side effect of tacrolimus, seen primarily with high plasma levels, is

   A. Tremulousness.
   B. Headache.
   C. Insomnia.
   D. Anxiety.
   E. Delirium.

The correct response is option E.

Tacrolimus (FK506, Prograf), a macrolide produced by *Streptomyces tsukubaensis,* is used as primary immunosuppressive therapy, as rescue therapy for patients who fail to respond to cyclosporine, and as treatment for graft-versus-host disease. It is more potent and possibly less toxic than cyclosporine, although the neuropsychiatric side effects appear to be similar (DiMartini et al. 1991; Freise et al. 1991). As with cyclosporine, neuropsychiatric side effects are more common with intravenous administration and diminish with oral administration and dosage reduction. Common symptoms include tremulousness, headache, restlessness, insomnia, vivid dreams, hyperesthesias, anxiety, and agitation (Fung et al. 1991). Cognitive impairment, coma, seizures, dysarthria, and delirium occur less often (8.4%) and are associated with higher plasma levels (DiMartini et al. 1997; Fung et al. 1991). **(p. 749)**

   DiMartini A, Pajer K, Trzepacz P, et al: Psychiatric morbidity in liver transplant patients. Transplant Proc 23:3179–3180, 1991
   DiMartini AF, Trzepacz PT, Pager K, et al: Neuropsychiatric side effects of FK506 vs. cyclosporine A: first-week postoperative findings. Psychosomatics 38:565–569, 1997
   Freise CE, Rowley H, Lake J, et al: Similar clinical presentation of neurotoxicity following FK 506 and cyclosporine in a liver transplant recipient. Transplant Proc 23:3173–3174, 1991
   Fung JJ, Alessiani M, Abu-Elmagd K, et al: Adverse effects associated with the use of FK 506. Transplant Proc 23:3105–3108, 1991

Chapter 32

Neurology and Neurosurgery

Select the single best response for each question.

32.1   Partial occlusion of which of the following arteries may produce uni- or bilateral pyramidal signs and ipsilateral cranial nerve palsies?

    A.   Middle cerebral artery.
    B.   Internal carotid artery.
    C.   Basilar artery.
    D.   Anterior cerebral artery.
    E.   Posterior cerebral artery.

The correct response is option C.

Vertebrobasilar strokes (*basilar artery* occlusion) can be extremely diverse in their manifestations. Total occlusion of the basilar artery is usually rapidly fatal. Partial occlusions of the basilar artery typically affect the brain stem, with a combination of uni- or bilateral pyramidal signs and ipsilateral cranial nerve palsies.

The classical presentation of *middle cerebral artery* infarction is contralateral hemiparesis and sensory loss of a cortical type. These are often accompanied by hemianopsia if the optic radiation is affected. If the lesion is in the dominant hemisphere, then aphasia may be expected, whereas a lesion in the nondominant hemisphere may be accompanied by neglect, inattention, or perceptual disturbance.

Internal carotid artery occlusion can be entirely asymptomatic, but much depends on the collateral circulation. The clinical picture is often that of middle cerebral artery infarction. However, in some situations, cognitive and behavioral symptoms are predominant.

Infarctions affecting the distribution of the *anterior cerebral artery* will lead to contralateral hemiparesis affecting the leg more severely than the arm. A grasp reflex and motor dysphasia may be present. Cognitive changes resembling a global dementia may occur, with incontinence.

Posterior cerebral artery infarction presents with a contralateral hemianopsia sometimes accompanied by visual hallucinations, visual agnosias, or spatial disorientation. Transient confusion may obscure the detection of hemianopsia. Dense amnestic symptoms occur if the hippocampus and other limbic structures are involved bilaterally. **(p. 760)**

32.2   A number of behavioral changes may occur following a stroke. A behavioral syndrome characterized by partial or complete unawareness of a deficit is termed

    A.   Affective dysprosodia.
    B.   Anosognosia.
    C.   Global aphasia.
    D.   Apathy.
    E.   Catastrophic reaction.

The correct response is option B.

Anosognosia refers to partial or complete unawareness of a deficit. It may coexist with depression (Starkstein et al. 1990), a finding that both implicates separate neural systems for different aspects of emotions (Damasio 1994) and suggests that depression after stroke cannot be explained solely as a psychological reaction to disability (Ramasubbu 1994). Anosognosia for hemiplegia is perhaps the most often described form of the condition, but anosognosia can occur with reference to any function and is commonly associated with visual and language dysfunction.

Affective dysprosodia is impairment of the production and comprehension of those language components that communicate inner emotional states in speech. These components include stresses, pauses, cadence, accent, melody, and intonation. Affective dysprosodia is not associated with an actual deficit in the ability to experience emotions; rather, it is associated with a deficit in the ability to communicate or recognize emotions in the speech of others.

Global aphasia leads to the abolition of all linguistic faculties. Consequently, the physician must draw inferences about mental state from the patient's behavior and nonverbal communication. Some accounts associate Broca's aphasia with intense emotional frustration that may be secondary to problems in social interaction (Carota et al. 2000). Wernicke's aphasia has been characterized by a lack of insight accompanied by irritability and rage, with recovered patients reporting that they believed the examiner was being deliberately incomprehensible (Lazar et al. 2000).

Apathy is common after stroke—affecting up to 25% of patients—and appears to be distinct from depression (Brodaty et al. 2005). Patients with apathy show little spontaneous action or speech; their responses may be delayed, short, slow, or absent (Fisher 1995). Apathy is frequently associated with hypophonia, perseveration, grasp reflex, compulsive motor manipulations, cognitive deficit, and older age.

Catastrophic reactions manifest as disruptive emotional behavior precipitated when a patient finds a task unsolvable (Goldstein 1939). The sudden, dramatic appearance of such marked self-directed and stereotypical anger or frustration can be startling for both staff and relatives. This symptom is often associated with aphasia, and it has been suggested that damage to language areas is a critical part of the etiology (Carota et al. 2001). **(pp. 761, 763)**

Brodaty H, Sachdev PS, Withall A, et al: Frequency and clinical, neuropsychological and neuroimaging correlates of apathy following stroke—the Sydney Stroke Study. Psychol Med 35:1707–1716, 2005

Carota A, Nicola A, Aybek S, et al: Aphasia-related emotional behaviors in acute stroke. Neurology 54:A244, 2000

Carota A, Rossetti OA, Karapanayiotides T, et al: Catastrophic reaction in acute stroke: a reflex behavior in aphasic patients. Neurology 57:1902–1906, 2001

Damasio AR: Emotion, Reason and the Human Brain. New York, GP Putnam & Sons, 1994

Fisher CM: Abulia, in Stroke Syndromes. Edited by Bogousslavsky J, Caplan L. Cambridge, England, Cambridge University Press, 1995, pp 182–187

Goldstein K: The Organism: A Holistic Approach to Biology Derived From Pathological Data in Man. New York, American Books, 1939

Lazar RM, Marshall RS, Prell GD, et al: The experience of Wernicke's aphasia. Neurology 55:1222–1224, 2000

Ramasubbu R: Denial of illness and depression in stroke (letter). Stroke 25:226–227, 1994

Starkstein SE, Berthier MI, Fedoroff P, et al: Anosognosia and major depression in 2 patients with cerebrovascular lesions. Neurology 40:1380–1382, 1990

32.3 In both Parkinson's disease (PD) and multiple sclerosis (MS), approximately 50% of patients have

    A. Bradykinesia.
    B. Optic neuritis.
    C. Tremor.
    D. Sensory loss.
    E. Depression.

The correct response is option E.

Depression is a common symptom in PD, with a prevalence of around 40%–50%. Timing of onset shows a bimodal distribution, with peaks during early and late stages of the disease (Cummings and Masterman 1999). Several large-scale studies have demonstrated that depression is one of the major determinants of quality of life in PD (Global Parkinson's Disease Survey Steering Committee 2002; Peto et al. 1995). The extent to which depression is caused by brain pathology as opposed to a psychological reaction to disability is unknown.

Mood disorders are common in MS, with more than half of patients reporting depressive symptoms. Depression may be a direct physiologically mediated consequence of the disease, a psychological reaction to the illness, a complication of pharmacotherapy, or coincidental. It is important to distinguish depression from the fatigue and pain that are commonly associated with MS. As in stroke, there has been an attempt to separate out a "biological" depression from a "psychological reactive" depression (Patten and Metz 1997) and to link symptoms to the site of the brain lesions (Fassbender et al. 1998; Honer et al. 1987; Pujol et al. 1997). **(pp. 765, 767)**

Cummings JL, Masterman DL: Depression in patients with Parkinson's disease. Int J Geriatr Psychiatry 14:711–718, 1999

Fassbender K, Schmidt R, Mossner R, et al: Mood disorders and dysfunction of the hypothalamic-pituitary-adrenal axis in multiple sclerosis: association with cerebral inflammation. Arch Neurol 55:66–72, 1998

Global Parkinson's Disease Survey Steering Committee: Factors impacting on quality of life in Parkinson's disease: results from an international survey. Mov Disord 17:60–67, 2002

Honer WG, Hurwitz T, Li DKB, et al: Temporal lobe involvement in multiple sclerosis patients with psychiatric disorders. Arch Neurol 44:187–190, 1987

Patten SB, Metz LM: Depression in multiple sclerosis. Psychother Psychosom 66:286–292, 1997

Peto V, Jenkinson C, Fitzpatrick R, et al: The development and validation of a short measure of functioning and well being for individuals with Parkinson's disease. Qual Life Res 4:241–248, 1995

Pujol J, Bello J, Deus J, et al: Lesions in the left arcuate fasciculus region and depressive symptoms in multiple sclerosis. Neurology 49:1105–1110, 1997

32.4 Which of the following neuropsychiatric disorders is dominantly inherited?

   A. Wilson's disease.
   B. Leukodystrophies.
   C. Wernicke-Korsakoff syndrome.
   D. Huntington's disease.
   E. Creutzfeldt-Jakob disease.

The correct response is option D.

Huntington's disease, also known as Huntington's chorea, first described in 1872 by George Huntington, is a dominantly inherited disorder that causes a combination of progressive motor, cognitive, psychiatric, and behavioral dysfunction.

Wilson's disease is a very rare, autosomal recessive, progressive degenerative brain disease caused by a disorder of copper metabolism, producing personality change, cognitive decline, extrapyramidal signs, and cirrhosis of the liver.

Leukodystrophies—recessively inherited or X-linked disorders of myelination—can be accompanied by neuropsychiatric syndromes, usually with associated neurological features.

Wernicke-Korsakoff syndrome results from thiamine depletion, and any cause of such depletion can lead to the syndrome—including, for example, hyperemesis gravidarum and gastric bypass surgery. However, the overwhelming majority of cases are associated with chronic alcohol abuse, which results in both decreased intake and decreased absorption of thiamine.

The transmissible spongiform encephalopathies are a group of rare dementias caused by an accumulation of abnormal prion protein within the brain. One recently described disorder, variant Creutzfeldt-Jakob disease, is thought to result from infection of humans by consumption of beef products from cattle with bovine spongiform encephalopathy (Will et al. 1996). **(pp. 768–771)**

> Will RG, Ironside JW, Zeidler M, et al: A new variant of Creutzfeldt-Jakob disease in the UK. Lancet 347:921–925, 1996

32.5   Which of the following neuropsychiatric disorders is a rare complication of childhood measles?

   A. Subacute sclerosing panencephalitis.
   B. Progressive multifocal leukodystrophy.
   C. Limbic encephalitis.
   D. Hashimoto's encephalopathy.
   E. Whipple's disease.

The correct response is option A.

Subacute sclerosing panencephalitis (SSPE) is a rare complication of childhood measles in which intraneuronal persistence of a defective form of the virus in the central nervous system (CNS) results in a continuing immune response, with high levels of measles antibody in the cerebrospinal fluid (CSF).

Progressive multifocal leukodystrophy is caused by activation of JC papovavirus within the CNS in an immunocompromised patient. The resulting demyelination gives rise to pyramidal signs, visual impairment, and a subcortical dementia, usually with progression to death within months (Lishman 1997; Richardson 1961).

Limbic encephalitis is an autoimmune-mediated inflammation centered on the limbic system. It can have a range of psychiatric and neurological presentations, including focal seizures, memory impairment, confusion, and alterations of mood, personality, and behavior (Schott 2006).

Hashimoto's encephalopathy, a severe encephalopathic illness manifesting in the presence of high serum anti-thyroid antibody concentrations, responds dramatically to steroids. Seizures, psychosis, confusion, stroke-like episodes, and raised CSF protein, often with normal magnetic resonance imaging findings, are the common features.

Whipple's disease is rare but important, because it is treatable. Infection with *Tropheryma whippelii* typically causes a multisystem disorder with prominent steatorrhea, weight loss, and abdominal pain (Fenollar et al. 2007; Fleming et al. 1988). CNS involvement is common, and neurological and psychiatric symptoms and signs occur in the absence of systemic features (Brown et al. 1990; Louis et al. 1996). **(p. 772)**

> Brown AP, Lane JC, Murayama S, et al: Whipple's disease presenting with isolated neurological symptoms: case report. J Neurosurg 73:623–627, 1990
>
> Fenollar F, Puéchal X, Raoult D: Whipple's disease. N Engl J Med 356:55–66, 2007
>
> Fleming JL, Wiesner RH, Shorter RG: Whipple's disease: clinical, biochemical, and histopathological features and assessment of treatment in 29 patients. Mayo Clin Proc 63:539–551, 1988
>
> Lishman WA: Organic Psychiatry: The Psychological Consequences of Cerebral Disorder, 3rd Edition. Oxford, UK, Blackwell Science, 1997
>
> Louis ED, Lynch T, Kaufmann P, et al: Diagnostic guidelines in central nervous system Whipple's disease. Ann Neurol 40:561–568, 1996
>
> Richardson EP: Progressive multifocal leukoencephalopathy. N Engl J Med 265:815–823, 1961
>
> Schott JM: Limbic encephalitis: a clinician's guide. Practical Neurology 6:143–153, 2006

32.6 A patient with history of seizures is referred to you for psychiatric evaluation. The patient describing an aura at the onset of seizures that involves a dream-like state, flashbacks, and déjà vu. On the basis of this description, your working diagnosis is

    A. Simple partial seizure.
    B. Tonic-clonic seizure.
    C. Complex partial seizure.
    D. Simple absence seizure.
    E. Complex absence seizure.

The correct response is option C.

In a *complex partial seizure*, the patient frequently experiences an aura at the onset of the seizure. The aura is a simple partial seizure lasting seconds to minutes. The content of the aura will depend on the location of the abnormal discharge within the brain. Thus, it may contain motor, sensory, visceral, or psychic elements. These can include hallucinations; intense affective symptoms such as fear, depression, panic, or depersonalization; and cognitive symptoms such as aphasia. Distortions of memory can include dreamy states, flashbacks, and distortions of familiarity with events (déjà vu or jamais vu). Occasionally, rapid recollection of episodes from earlier life experiences occurs (panoramic vision).

The clinical features of *simple partial seizures* depend on the brain region activated. Although the initial area is relatively localized, it is common for the abnormal activity to spread to adjacent areas, producing a progression of seizure pattern. If the activity originates in the motor cortex, there will be jerking movements in the contralateral body part. This can cause progressive jerking in contiguous regions (known as "Jacksonian march"). Activity in the supplementary motor cortex causes head turning with arm extension on the same side—the classic "fencer's posture." Seizures originating in the parietal lobe can cause tingling or numbness in a bodily region or more complex sensory experiences such as a sense of absence on one side of the body, asomatognosia. Seizures of the occipital lobe are associated with visual symptoms, which are usually elementary (e.g., simple flashing lights).

Tonic-clonic seizures are the most dramatic manifestation of epilepsy and are characterized by motor activity and sudden loss of consciousness. In a typical seizure, a patient has no warning. The seizure begins with sudden loss of consciousness and a tonic phase during which there are sustained muscle contractions lasting 10–20 seconds. This is followed by a clonic phase of repetitive muscle contractions that last approximately 30 seconds.

Absence seizures are well-defined clinical and electroencephalogram events. The essential feature is an abrupt, brief episode of decreased awareness that occurs without any warning, aura, or postictal symptoms. At the onset there is a disruption of activity. A *simple* absence seizure is characterized by only an alteration in consciousness. The patient remains mobile, breathing is unaffected, and there is no cyanosis or pallor and no loss of postural tone or motor activity. The ending is abrupt, and the patient resumes previous activity immediately, often unaware that a seizure has taken place. An attack usually lasts around 15 seconds. A *complex* absence seizure involves additional symptoms such as loss or increase of postural tone, minor clonic movements of the face or extremities, minor automatisms, or autonomic symptoms such as pallor, flushing, tachycardia, piloerection, mydriasis, and urinary incontinence. **(pp. 773–774)**

Chapter 33

Obstetrics and Gynecology

Select the single best response for each question.

33.1   Which of the following medications for bipolar disorder has been associated with polycystic ovarian syndrome?

    A. Lithium.
    B. Lamotrigine.
    C. Olanzapine.
    D. Valproic acid.
    E. Carbamazepine.

The correct response is option D.

Valproic acid has been associated with polycystic ovarian syndrome.

Psychiatric illness may impact fertility directly through mechanisms related to chronic stress, altered immune responses, and hormonal changes, as well as indirectly through changes in behavior such as smoking, alcohol, poor nutrition, and lack of exercise. It is also important to consider the impact of psychotropic medications on fertility. For example, selective serotonin reuptake inhibitors have been shown to be associated with a small but increased risk of early miscarriage, valproic acid is associated with polycystic ovarian syndrome, and many antipsychotic medications are associated with anovulation due to hyperprolactinemia (Joffe 2007). **(p. 799)**

> Joffe H: Reproductive biology and psychotropic treatments in premenopausal women with bipolar disorder. J Clin Psychiatry 68 (suppl 9):10–15, 2007

33.2   The psychosomatic medicine consultant working with OB/GYN patients must be particularly attentive to the potential for drug–drug interactions between psychiatric medications and contraceptive agents. Due to the inhibition of glucuronidation, oral contraceptives may increase serum levels of which of the following?

    A. Tricyclic antidepressants.
    B. Selective serotonin reuptake inhibitors.
    C. Lithium.
    D. Benzodiazepines.
    E. Valproate and lamotrigine.

The correct response is option E.

Levels of valproate and lamotrigine can be increased by oral contraceptives (likely via inhibition of glucuronidation).

The major pathway of metabolism for both the estrogen and progesterone components of hormonal contraception is through the liver by cytochrome P450 (CYP) 3A4 (Oesterheld et al. 2008). Medications that induce CYP3A4, thus reducing the efficacy of hormonal contraception, include phenobarbital, oxcarbazepine, carbamazepine, topiramate (at dosages >200 mg/day), modafinil, and St. John's wort. Oral contraceptives can also inhibit the oxidation of various psychiatric medications via CYP1A2, 2B6, 2C19, and 3A4. Importantly, this can result in increased levels of benzodiazepines and tricyclic antidepressants. **(p. 801)**

Oesterheld JR, Cozza K, Sandson NB: Oral contraceptives. Psychosomatics 49:168–175, 2008

33.3   Which of the following statements regarding the behavioral consequences of elective sterilization is *true?*

   A. Postsurgical regret is seen in fewer than 2% of cases.
   B. Women younger than 30 years are less likely than older women to experience postsurgical regret.
   C. Marital conflict over the surgical procedure does not increase the risk of postsurgical regret.
   D. Death of a child has been associated with postsurgical regret.
   E. Sexual satisfaction typically increases postoperatively.

The correct response is option D.

Death of a child has been associated with poststerilization regret, and a survey of women in India identified having few or no male children as a risk factor for regret (Machado et al. 2005; Malhotra et al. 2007).

   The occurrence of postsurgical regret ranges from 5% to 20%. A systematic review of 19 studies found that age was a significant risk factor for postsurgical regret, with women who were sterilized when younger than age 30 more than twice as likely to experience regret as women older than 30 years (Curtis et al. 2006). Other risk factors include marital conflict over the procedure, and subsequent changes in marital partnerships (Jamieson et al. 2002). Sexual satisfaction does not appear to be affected (Peterson 2008). **(p. 801)**

   Curtis KM, Mohllajee AP, Peterson HB: Regret following female sterilization at a young age: a systematic review. Contraception 73:205–210, 2006
   Jamieson DJ, Kaufman SC, Costello C, et al: A comparison of women's regret after vasectomy versus tubal sterilization. US Collaborative Review of Sterilization Working Group. Obstet Gynecol 99:1073–1079, 2002
   Machado KM, Ludermir AB, da Costa AM: Changes in family structure and regret following tubal sterilization. Cad Saude Publica 21:1768–1777, 2005
   Malhotra N, Chanana C, Garg P: Post-sterilization regrets in Indian women. Indian J Med Sci 61:186–191, 2007
   Peterson HB: Sterilization. Obstet Gynecol 111:189–203, 2008

33.4   Endometriosis is a painful and life-limiting condition that often requires comprehensive multidisciplinary management. Gonadotropin-releasing hormone (GnRH) agonists are commonly used to treat endometriosis but are known to cause depression. Which of the following antidepressants appears to be particularly helpful in treatment of GnRH agonist–associated mood symptoms?

   A. Monoamine oxidase inhibitors (MAOIs).
   B. Tricyclic antidepressants (TCAs).
   C. Bupropion.
   D. Trazodone.
   E. Selective serotonin reuptake inhibitors (SSRIs).

The correct response is option E.

Depression occurs commonly in cases where endometriosis is accompanied by chronic pain, dyspareunia, or infertility. In addition, GnRH agonists are often used to treat endometriosis, and depressive symptoms may be associated with this treatment. SSRI antidepressants appear to be significantly helpful in the treatment of mood symptoms during the course of GnRH agonists (Warnock et al. 2000). Psychotherapy and antidepressants also may be helpful in addressing other psychological issues and symptoms in women with endometriosis. **(p. 806)**

   Warnock JK, Bundren JC, Morris DW: Depressive mood symptoms associated with ovarian suppression. Fertil Steril 74:984–986, 2000

33.5   Which of the following statements regarding pseudocyesis is *false?*

    A. In pseudocyesis, the patient ceases to menstruate.
    B. Patients with pseudocyesis show increased abdominal girth.
    C. Classical pseudocyesis occurs in women with schizophrenia-spectrum illness.
    D. Patients with pseudocyesis typically refuse psychiatric care for their symptoms.
    E. In pseudocyesis, the cervix may show physical changes associated with pregnancy.

The correct response is option C.

At the other end of the spectrum from the patient who does not realize she is pregnant is the patient who is convinced she is pregnant when she is not. This condition, referred to as *pseudocyesis*, is a fascinating example of psychobiological interplay. The patient ceases to have menstrual periods. Her abdomen grows, and her cervix may show signs of pregnancy. Some patients with the delusion that they are pregnant are psychotic, but that is not the case in classical pseudocyesis. Patients with pseudocyesis are a heterogeneous group, and they have no other signs or symptoms of frank psychiatric disorder (Rosch et al. 2002). **(p. 809)**

> Rosch DS, Sajatovic M, Sivec H: Behavioral characteristics in delusional pregnancy: a matched control group study. Int J Psychiatry Med 32:295–303, 2002

33.6   Postpartum psychosis may affect women with no prior history of psychiatric illness. Which of the following statements regarding postpartum psychosis is *false?*

    A. The usual period of onset is between 3 and 14 days postpartum.
    B. Because of the risks of suicide and/or infanticide, psychiatric hospitalization for observation is warranted.
    C. Most episodes of postpartum psychosis likely represent bipolar disorder.
    D. The rate of postpartum relapse in bipolar disorder is 30%–50%.
    E. The incidence of postpartum psychosis has tripled in the past 100 years among many cultures.

The correct response is option E.

The overall incidence of postpartum psychosis is estimated at 0.1%–0.2% and appears to have been stable for more than a century and among cultures.

Postpartum psychosis is characterized by extreme agitation, delirium, confusion, sleeplessness, and hallucinations and/or delusions. Onset can be sudden and usually occurs between days 3 and 14 postpartum, with 90% of episodes occurring within 4 weeks of delivery (Harlow et al. 2007). A Swedish population-based study found that 40% of women who were hospitalized for psychosis or bipolar disorder during pregnancy were rehospitalized in the postpartum period (Harlow et al. 2007). Only a fraction of these women will go on to attempt suicide or infanticide, but the risk and the stakes are high enough to warrant considering postpartum psychosis as a medical emergency and hospitalizing the patient, at least for a period of observation.

Many experts believe that most episodes of postpartum psychosis represent bipolar disorder (Attia et al. 1999; Chaudron and Pies 2003). The risk of postpartum relapse of bipolar disorder is 30%–50%; these relapses can be acute and severe. **(pp. 811–812)**

> Attia A, Downey J, Oberman M: Postpartum psychoses, in Postpartum Mood Disorders. Edited by Miller L. Washington, DC, American Psychiatric Press, 1999, pp 99–117
> Chaudron LH, Pies RW: The relationship between postpartum psychosis and bipolar disorder: a review. J Clin Psychiatry 64:1284–1292, 2003
> Harlow BL, Vitonis AF, Sparen P, et al: Incidence of hospitalization for postpartum psychotic and bipolar episodes in women with and without prior prepregnancy or prenatal psychiatric hospitalizations. Arch Gen Psychiatry 64:42–48, 2007

33.7 Although study findings have not been unanimous, which of the following selective serotonin reuptake inhibitors (SSRIs) has most often been associated with fetal heart defects when used in pregnancy?

    A. Fluoxetine.
    B. Fluvoxamine.
    C. Sertraline.
    D. Paroxetine.
    E. Citalopram.

The correct response is option D.

Previous meta-analyses of data examining potential relationships between antidepressant exposure and neonatal/fetal outcomes have been largely reassuring (Addis et al. 2000; Einarson and Einarson 2005). More recently, however, there has been renewal of the controversy regarding the safety of antidepressant use during pregnancy. Paroxetine has been shown in some (Wurst et al. 2010) but not all (Einarson et al. 2008) studies to be associated with heart defects.

Two large prospective databases on antidepressant use in pregnancy were recently published. The Danish database of 493,113 children born between 1996 and 2003 included 1,370 mothers who had had two or more prescriptions of an SSRI filled during the period 28 days before through 112 days after the beginning of gestation (Pedersen et al. 2009). After researchers controlled for maternal age, mental status, and smoking, SSRI use showed no association with overall fetal major malformations. However, an increase in cardiac septal defects was observed. Both sertraline and citalopram were associated with an increase in septal defects, and exposure to more than one type of SSRI was associated with the greatest increase in septal defects.

The Swedish Medical Birth Registry included 14,821 women who used antidepressant medication in pregnancy from 1995 to 2007 (Reis and Källén 2010). Atrial septal and ventricular septal defects were more frequent in infants exposed in utero to tricyclic antidepressants and paroxetine. Paroxetine use was also associated with fetal hypospadias. Although the investigators controlled for maternal age, smoking, and some other drug use, it was not possible to dissociate outcomes from the effects of depression, other comorbidities or exposure, or ascertainment bias. **(pp. 812–813)**

Addis A, Koren G: Safety of fluoxetine during the first trimester of pregnancy: a meta-analytical review of epidemiological studies. Psychol Med 30:89–94, 2000

Einarson A, Pistelli A, DeSantis M, et al: Evaluation of the risk of congenital cardiovascular defects associated with use of paroxetine during pregnancy. Am J Psychiatry 165:749–752, 2008

Einarson TR, Einarson A: Newer antidepressants in pregnancy and rates of major malformations: a meta-analysis of prospective comparative studies. Pharmacoepidemiol Drug Saf 14:823–827, 2005

Pedersen LH, Henriksen TB, Vestergaard M, et al: Selective serotonin reuptake inhibitors in pregnancy and congenital malformations: population based cohort study. BMJ 339:b3569, 2009

Reis M, Källén B: Delivery outcome after maternal use of antidepressant drugs in pregnancy: an update using Swedish data. Psychol Med 5:1–11, 2010

Wurst KE, Poole C, Ephross SA, et al: First trimester paroxetine use and the prevalence of congenital, specifically cardiac, defects: a meta-analysis of epidemiological studies. Birth Defects Res A Clin Mol Teratol 88:159–170, 2010

33.8 According to a recent Cochrane Database meta-analysis of premenstrual dysphoric disorder (PMDD) treatment, which of the following tricyclic antidepressants (TCAs) (along with several selective serotonin reuptake inhibitors [SSRIs]) is effective for PMDD?

    A. Nortriptyline.
    B. Doxepin.
    C. Clomipramine.
    D. Imipramine.
    E. Desipramine.

The correct response is option C.

Like other disorders in the mood spectrum, PMDD is well treated with SSRIs. As of this writing, fluoxetine, sertraline, and paroxetine have received FDA indications for PMDD. For reasons still poorly understood, although SSRIs generally require 2–4 weeks for therapeutic effectiveness in depression, they are reported to be effective for PMDD when used only in the premenstrual phase (Halbreich et al. 2002). Perhaps because of the lack of continued administration, there is no discontinuation syndrome when they are used in this manner. A recent Cochrane Database meta-analysis confirmed effectiveness of either luteal-phase or continuous dosing of the SSRIs fluoxetine, paroxetine, sertraline, fluvoxamine, and citalopram and the highly serotonergic TCA clomipramine (Brown et al. 2009). **(p. 816)**

Brown J, O'Brien PM, Marjoribanks J, et al: Selective serotonin reuptake inhibitors for premenstrual syndrome. Cochrane Database Syst Rev (2):CD001396, 2009

Halbreich U, Bergeron R, Yonkers KA, et al: Efficacy of intermittent, luteal phase sertraline treatment of premenstrual dysphoric disorder. Obstet Gynecol 100:1219–1229, 2002

Chapter 34

Pediatrics

Select the single best response for each question.

34.1 In Piaget's stages of cognitive development, preoperational children are in what age range?

   A. Birth to 2 years.
   B. 2–7 years.
   C. 7–11 years.
   D. 11–14 years.
   E. 14–17 years.

The correct response is option B.

Children's conceptions of their bodies vary widely and are obviously influenced by experiences with illness. In general, however, children appear to follow a developmental path of understanding their bodies that roughly corresponds to Piaget's stages of cognitive development.

Sensorimotor children (birth to approximately 2 years) are largely preverbal and do not have the capacity to create narratives to explain their experiences.

Preoperational children (approximately 2–7 years) understand through perception, but they are able to use words and some very basic concepts of cause and effect. They tend to be most aware of parts of the body they can directly sense, such as bones and heart (which they can feel) and blood (which they have seen come out of their bodies).

Concrete operational children (approximately 7–11 years) are able to apply logic to their perceptions in a more integrative manner. However, the logic is quite literal or concrete and allows for only one cause for an effect.

Formal operational children (≥11 years) are able to use a level of abstract reasoning that allows discussion of systems rather than simple organs and can incorporate multiple causation of illness. **(p. 827)**

34.2 Which of the following statements concerning the diagnosis and clinical course of delirium in hospitalized children is *false*?

   A. Delirium is less frequently diagnosed in children than in adults.
   B. The Glasgow Coma Scale is less effective in predicting prognosis for children than for adults.
   C. Critically ill children who develop delirium are sometimes misdiagnosed as psychotic.
   D. The Delirium Rating Scale does not appear to be applicable to children.
   E. Unlike the case for adults, Delirium Rating Scale scores for children do not predict length of hospital stay.

The correct response is option D.

Pediatric delirium has received little research attention (Turkel et al. 2003) and is less often diagnosed in pediatrics than on the adult units (Manos and Wu 1997), especially among the younger pediatric patients (Schieveld et al. 2007). Critically ill children can develop delirium, with a hyperactive, hypoactive, mixed, or veiled presentation (Karnik et al. 2007; Schieveld et al. 2007). As in adults, it sometimes may present with what are interpreted to be psychotic symptoms (Webster and Holroyd 2000). The consultation request also may be put in terms of a request for an assessment of unexplained lethargy, depression, or confusion.

In adults, delirium has been found to be the strongest predictor of length of stay in the hospital, after studies have controlled for severity of illness, age, gender, race, and medication (Ely et al. 2001).

A recent evaluation of the widely used Delirium Rating Scale found that it does appear to be applicable to children, with scores comparable to those of adults. However, the rating score or diagnosis of delirium in a child may not have the same implications that it has in adults. The scores for children, unlike those for adults, did not predict length of hospital stay or mortality (Turkel et al. 2003). Similarly, the Glasgow Coma Scale appears to be less effective in predicting prognosis for children than for adults (Lieh-Lai et al. 1992). **(p. 831)**

Ely EW, Gautam S, Margolin R, et al: The impact of delirium in the intensive care unit on hospital length of stay. Intensive Care Med 27:1892–1900, 2001

Karnik NS, Joshi SV, Paterno C, et al: Subtypes of pediatric delirium: a treatment algorithm. Psychosomatics 48:253–257, 2007

Lieh-Lai MW, Theodorou AA, Sarnaik AP, et al: Limitations of the Glasgow Coma Scale in predicting outcome in children with traumatic brain injury. J Pediatr 120(2 pt 1):195–199, 1992

Manos PJ, Wu R: The duration of delirium in medical and postoperative patients referred for psychiatric consultation. Ann Clin Psychiatry 9:219–226, 1997

Schieveld JN, Leroy PL, van Os J, et al: Pediatric delirium in critical illness: phenomenology, clinical correlates and treatment response in 40 cases in the pediatric intensive care unit. Intensive Care Med 33:1033–1040, 2007

Turkel SB, Braslow K, Tavare CJ, et al: The Delirium Rating Scale in children and adolescents. Psychosomatics 44:126–129, 2003

Webster R, Holroyd S: Prevalence of psychotic symptoms in delirium. Psychosomatics 41:519–522, 2000

34.3 The only literature review to date on children and adolescent patients who falsified illness revealed which of the following?

    A. Most patients were male.
    B. The mean age was 8 years.
    C. The average duration of falsification prior to detection was 5–6 months.
    D. Few children admitted to their deceptions when confronted.
    E. One of the most commonly falsified conditions was fever.

The correct response is option E.

Libow (2000) conducted the only literature review to date for cases of child and adolescent patients who falsified illness. She identified 42 published cases in which patients had a mean age of 13.9 (range = 8–18 years). Most patients were female (71%), with the gender imbalance greater among older children. Patients engaged in false symptom reporting and induction, including active injections, bruising, and ingestions. The most commonly falsified or induced conditions were fevers, ketoacidosis, purpura, and infections. The average duration of the falsifications before detection was about 16 months. Many admitted to their deceptions when confronted, and some had positive outcomes at follow-up. The children were described as bland, depressed, and fascinated with health care. **(p. 832)**

Libow JA: Child and adolescent illness falsification. Pediatrics 105:336–342, 2000

34.4 Autism spectrum disorders

    A. Affect about 1 of every 1,000 children.
    B. Rarely occur in children with fragile X syndrome.
    C. Occur more frequently in males.

D. Are characterized by impairment in communication.
E. Occur more frequently in Caucasians.

The correct response is option C.

Autistic spectrum disorders such as autism or Asperger's disorder are neurodevelopmental disorders characterized by impairment in communication (verbal and/or nonverbal) and social interactions. Autistic spectrum disorders occur in all racial, ethnic, and socioeconomic groups but are four times more likely to occur in males than in females. In 2006, the Centers for Disease Control and Prevention (CDC) reported that among 8-year-old children in the United States, about 1 in 110 has an autistic spectrum disorder (Centers for Disease Control and Prevention 2009). These disorders occur more often than expected among those who have fragile X syndrome, tuberous sclerosis, congenital rubella syndrome, and untreated phenylketonuria, as well as among those who were prenatally exposed to thalidomide. **(pp. 834–835)**

Centers for Disease Control and Prevention: Prevalence of autism spectrum disorders—Autism and Developmental Disabilities Monitoring Network, United States, 2006. Autism and Developmental Disabilities Monitoring Network Surveillance Year 2006 Principal Investigators. MMWR Surveill Summ 58(10):1–20, 2009

34.5   The most common comorbid psychiatric disorder among children with asthma is

A. Depression.
B. Bipolar disorder.
C. Hypochondriasis.
D. An anxiety disorder.
E. Somatization disorder.

The correct response is option D.

Comorbid psychiatric disorders may reduce asthma treatment compliance, impair daily functioning, or have a direct effect on autonomic reactions and pulmonary function (Norrish et al. 1977). The literature contains some contradictory findings about the prevalence and type of comorbid psychiatric problems, but it appears that internalizing disorders are more common and that more than one-third of asthmatic children have anxiety disorders. Additionally, those with moderate to severe asthma appear to be at a higher risk for anxiety disorders than do those with mild disease. Kean et al. (2006) found that adolescents who have experienced a life-threatening asthma event, and their parents, have high levels of posttraumatic stress symptoms, with 20% and 29% meeting DSM criteria for posttraumatic stress disorder, respectively. Although depression has been less consistently identified as a comorbid psychiatric disorder among pediatric asthma patients, the literature suggests that depression, along with other psychosocial problems, may be a risk factor for death in children with asthma. **(p. 838)**

Kean EM, Kelsay K, Wamboldt F, et al: Posttraumatic stress in adolescents with asthma and their parents. J Am Acad Child Adolesc Psychiatry 45:78–86, 2006
Norrish M, Tooley M, Godfry S: Clinical, physiological, and psychological study of asthmatic children attending a hospital clinic. Arch Dis Child 52:912–917, 1977

Chapter 35

Physical Medicine and Rehabilitation

Select the single best response for each question.

35.1 According to the definition established by the American Congress of Rehabilitation Medicine, a diagnosis of mild traumatic brain injury (TBI) may be made if an injury acutely manifests one or more of a set of four features. Which of the following is *not* one of these four defining features?

   A. Loss of consciousness of 30 minutes or less.
   B. Posttraumatic amnesia of 24 hours or less.
   C. Altered mental state at the time of trauma.
   D. After 30 minutes, an initial Glasgow Coma Scale (GCS) score of 13–15.
   E. "Mild" abnormalities on neuroimaging.

The correct response is option E.

The American Congress of Rehabilitation Medicine has put forth a definition of mild TBI that is widely used, requiring at least one of the following: 1) loss of consciousness (LOC) of 30 minutes or less, with an initial GCS score of 13–15; 2) posttraumatic amnesia of 24 hours or less; 3) presence of any alteration of mental state at the time of the injury (e.g., feeling dazed, disoriented, or confused); and 4) presence of a focal neurological deficit (Kay et al. 1993). Patients with a GCS score of 13–15 who have imaging evidence of intracranial pathology have outcomes more similar to those of moderate TBI and are often classified as having "complicated mild" injuries (see Williams et al. 1990). **(p. 858)**

> Kay T, Harrington DE, Adams R, et al: Definition of mild traumatic brain injury. Mild Traumatic Brain Injury Committee of the Head Injury Interdisciplinary Special Interest Group of the American Congress of Rehabilitation Medicine. J Head Trauma Rehabil 8:86–87, 1993
> Williams DH, Levin HS, Eisenberg HM: Mild head injury classification. Neurosurgery 27:422–428, 1990

35.2 In contrast to post–traumatic brain injury (TBI) depression, post-TBI bipolar disorder appears to be a much less frequent complication of TBI. In the study by Jorge et al. (1993), post-TBI mania was associated with which of the following?

   A. Basopolar temporal lesions.
   B. More severe TBI.
   C. More intellectual impairment.
   D. Posttraumatic epilepsy.
   E. Personal history of psychiatric illness.

The correct response is option A.

Jorge et al. (1993) noted that mania after TBI was significantly related to basopolar temporal lesions but was not associated with type or severity of TBI, degree of physical or intellectual impairment, family or personal history of psychiatric illness, or posttraumatic epilepsy. **(p. 862)**

> Jorge RE, Robinson RG, Starkstein SE, et al: Secondary mania following traumatic brain injury. Am J Psychiatry 150:916–921, 1993

35.3 In the Hibbard et al. (1998) study of mood, anxiety, and substance use disorders following traumatic brain injury (TBI), which of the following was found to be the most common anxiety disorder, with a rate of 14%?

   A. Posttraumatic stress disorder.
   B. Acute stress disorder.
   C. Panic disorder with agoraphobia.
   D. Panic disorder without agoraphobia.
   E. Obsessive-compulsive disorder.

The correct response is option E.

In their assessment of the incidence, comorbidity, and patterns of resolution of DSM-IV (American Psychiatric Association 1994) mood, anxiety, and substance use disorders following TBI, Hibbard et al. (1998) administered the Structured Clinical Interview for DSM-IV to 100 patients with TBI who were randomly selected from a larger quality-of-life study. They reported rates of 14% for obsessive-compulsive disorder, 11% for panic disorder, 7% for phobias, and 8% for generalized anxiety disorder after injury. **(p. 863)**

American Psychiatric Association: Diagnostic and Statistical Manual of Mental Disorders, 4th Edition. Washington, DC, American Psychiatric Association, 1994

Hibbard MR, Uysal S, Kepler K, et al: Axis I psychopathology in individuals with traumatic brain injury. J Head Trauma Rehabil 13:24–39, 1998

35.4 Aggressive behavior in individuals with traumatic brain injury (TBI) typically has several characteristic features. Descriptive terms for post-TBI aggression include all of the following *except*

   A. Nonreflective.
   B. Nonpurposeful.
   C. Reactive.
   D. Periodic.
   E. Ego-syntonic.

The correct response is option E.

Although aggression may be a symptom of many disorders, several features are characteristic of aggression after TBI (Yudofsky et al. 1990). Such behavior is typically *nonreflective*, occurring without any premeditation or planning, and *nonpurposeful*, achieving no particular goals for the individual. It is also *reactive*, triggered by a stimulus, but often a stimulus that would not normally provoke a strong reaction. Aggression after TBI is *periodic*, occurring at intervals with relatively calm behavior in between, and *explosive*, occurring without a prodromal buildup. Finally, it is *ego-dystonic*, creating a great deal of distress for the patient. **(p. 864)**

Yudofsky SC, Silver JM, Hales RE: Pharmacologic management of aggression in the elderly. J Clin Psychiatry 51:22–28, 1990

35.5 Postconcussive syndrome, a somewhat ambiguous and controversial construct, overlaps phenomenologically with several psychiatric disorders, including depression. Which of the following symptoms is characteristic of depression but not of postconcussive syndrome?

   A. Psychomotor changes.
   B. Depressed mood.
   C. Irritability.
   D. Sleep disturbance.
   E. Poor concentration.

The correct response is option A.

Because postconcussive symptoms are not specific to traumatic brain injury, it is important to consider their differential diagnosis. Alexander (1995) and Mittenberg and Strauman (2000) noted that postconcussive syndrome has significant overlap with psychiatric disorders. Both major depression and postconcussive syndrome have symptoms of depressed mood, irritability, sleep disturbance, fatigue, and difficulty with concentration. However, unlike major depression, postconcussive syndrome does not include symptoms of changes in appetite, psychomotor changes, or suicidal ideation. **(p. 867)**

Alexander MP: Mild traumatic brain injury: pathophysiology, natural history, and clinical management. Neurology 45:1253–1260, 1995

Mittenberg W, Strauman S: Diagnosis of mild head injury and the postconcussion syndrome. J Head Trauma Rehabil 15:783–791, 2000

35.6 In addition to traumatic brain injury, spinal cord injury (SCI) is associated with much psychiatric comorbidity. Which region of the spinal cord is the most common site of SCI?

  A. High cervical.
  B. Midcervical.
  C. High thoracic.
  D. Low thoracic.
  E. Lumbar.

The correct response is option B.

The midcervical region is the most common site of SCI.

Tetraplegia (or quadriplegia) denotes SCI that affects all four limbs, whereas *paraplegia* denotes injuries that affect only the lower extremities. SCI usually is described in terms of the level and the completeness of injury. The level of injury refers to the most caudal segment with normal motor or sensory function. Neurological level of injury may vary on the right and the left side, and segments also may be partially innervated. More than half of all injuries (54%) result in tetraplegia, whereas 46% are classified as resulting in paraplegia. **(p. 872)**

35.7 Because some symptoms of mood disorder in spinal cord injury (SCI) may actually be due to the SCI itself, diagnosis of depression can be challenging. Which of the following symptoms in an SCI patient is more specific for a mood disorder?

  A. Weight loss.
  B. Altered appetite.
  C. Sleep disturbance.
  D. Reduced energy.
  E. Worthlessness and self-blame.

The correct response is option E.

Core symptoms of depression in people with SCI are worthlessness or self-blame, depressed mood, and suicidal ideation (Frank et al. 1992). The patient's own experience and interpretation of the negative symptoms can aid the diagnostic process (Elliott and Frank 1996). **(pp. 876–877)**

Elliott TR, Frank RG: Depression following spinal cord injury. Arch Phys Med Rehabil 77:816–823, 1996

Frank RG, Chaney JM, Clay DL, et al: Dysphoria: a major symptom factor in persons with disability or chronic illness. Psychiatry Res 43:231–241, 1992

35.8   Many of the medications used to treat fatigue in spinal cord injury act on the dopamine system via various mechanisms. Which of the following medications has been associated with seizures at usual doses and therefore must be used with caution in seizure-prone patients?

   A. Methylphenidate.
   B. Dextroamphetamine.
   C. Bromocriptine.
   D. Amantadine.
   E. Modafinil.

The correct response is option D.

Amantadine has been associated with an increased risk of seizures (T. Gualtieri et al. 1989), but methylphenidate, dextroamphetamine, and bromocriptine do not appear to lower seizure threshold at typical doses. Bupropion (Marin et al. 1995) and dopamine agonists such as amantadine (Green et al. 2004; Kraus et al. 2005; Sawyer et al. 2008), bromocriptine (McDowell et al. 1998; Powell et al. 1996), and levodopa/carbidopa (Lal et al. 1988) have been used for apathy states, fatigue, and cognitive impairment. Bupropion's stimulating properties may be of particular benefit in the fatigued or apathetic depressed patient.

Methylphenidate and dextroamphetamine are generally safe at standard dosages (e.g., methylphenidate 10–30 mg/day in divided doses) (Alban et al. 2004) and have been used successfully to enhance participation in rehabilitation (C. T. Gualtieri and Evans 1988).

Modafinil has been efficacious in treating fatigue in patients with multiple sclerosis (Rammahan et al. 2000; Terzoudi et al. 2000; Zifko et al. 2002) and excessive daytime sleepiness in patients with traumatic brain injury (Teitelman 2001). **(p. 879)**

Alban JP, Hopson MM, Ly V, et al: Effect of methylphenidate on vital signs and adverse effects in adults with traumatic brain injury. Am J Phys Med Rehabil 83:131–137, 2004

Green LB, Hornyak JE, Hurvitz EA: Amantadine in pediatric patients with traumatic brain injury: a retrospective, case-controlled study. Am J Phys Med Rehabil 83:893–897, 2004

Gualtieri CT, Evans RW: Stimulant treatment for the neurobehavioural sequelae of traumatic brain injury. Brain Inj 2:273–290, 1988

Gualtieri T, Chandler M, Coons TB, et al: Amantadine: a new clinical profile for traumatic brain injury. Clin Neuropharmacol 12:258–270, 1989

Kraus MF, Smith GS, Butters M, et al: Effects of the dopaminergic agent and NMDA receptor antagonist amantadine on cognitive function, cerebral glucose metabolism and D2 receptor availability in chronic traumatic brain injury: a study using positron emission tomography (PET). Brain Inj 19:471–479, 2005

Lal S, Merbitz CP, Grip JC: Modification of function in head-injured patients with Sinemet. Brain Inj 2:225–233, 1988

Marin RS, Fogel BS, Hawkins J, et al: Apathy: a treatable syndrome. J Neuropsychiatry Clin Neurosci 7:23–30, 1995

McDowell S, Whyte J, D'Esposito M: Differential effect of a dopaminergic agonist on prefrontal function in traumatic brain injury patients. Brain 121:1155–1164, 1998

Powell JH, al-Adawi S, Morgan J, et al: Motivational deficits after brain injury: effects of bromocriptine in 11 patients. J Neurol Neurosurg Psychiatry 60:416–421, 1996

Rammahan KW, Rosenberg JH, Pollak CP, et al: Modafinil: efficacy for the treatment of fatigue in patients with multiple sclerosis (abstract). Neurology 54 (suppl 3):24, 2000

Sawyer E, Mauro LS, Ohlinger MJ: Amantadine enhancement of arousal and cognition after traumatic brain injury. Ann Pharmacother 42:247–252, 2008

Teitelman E: Off-label uses of modafinil (letter). Am J Psychiatry 158:8, 2001

Terzoudi M, Gavrielidou P, Heilakos G, et al: Fatigue in multiple sclerosis: evaluation of a new pharmacological approach (abstract). Neurology 54 (suppl 3):A61–A62, 2000

Zifko UA, Rupp M, Schwarz S, et al: Modafinil in treatment of fatigue in multiple sclerosis: results of an open-label study. J Neurol 249:983–987, 2002

C h a p t e r   3 6

Pain

Select the single best response for each question.

36.1 A pain sensation characterized by an increased reaction to a stimulus, especially a repetitive stimulus, is called

    A. Hyperesthesia.
    B. Allodynia.
    C. Hyperpathia.
    D. Nociception.
    E. Paresthesia.

The correct response is option C.

Hyperpathia is pain characterized by an increased reaction to a stimulus, especially a repetitive stimulus, and an increased pain threshold. *Hyperesthesia* is increased sensitivity to stimulation that excludes the special senses. *Allodynia* is pain from a stimulus that does not normally provoke pain. *Nociception* is detection of tissue damage by transducers in skin and deeper structures and the central propagation of this information via A delta and C fibers in the peripheral nerves. *Paresthesia* is an abnormal sensation, spontaneous or evoked, that is not unpleasant. **(p. 902 [Table 36–1])**

36.2 A strong relationship exists between pain and depression. Which of the following statements concerning this relationship is *false?*

    A. Physical symptoms are common in patients suffering from depression.
    B. Depression in patients with chronic pain is associated with greater pain intensity.
    C. Depression is the strongest predictor of suicidal ideation in patients with chronic pain.
    D. Individuals with chronic physical complaints have higher rates of lifetime major depression.
    E. Pain intensity and duration is a better predictor of disability than depression.

The correct response is option E.

Depression is a better predictor of disability than pain intensity and duration.

Physical symptoms are common in patients with major depression. Approximately 60% of patients with depression report pain symptoms at diagnosis. In the World Health Organization's data from 14 countries on 5 continents, 69% (range: 45%–95%) of patients with depression presented with only somatic symptoms, of which pain complaints were most common (Simon et al. 1999).

Depression in patients with chronic pain is associated with greater pain intensity, more pain persistence, application for early retirement, and greater interference from pain including more pain behaviors observed by others (Hasenbring et al. 1994).

Patients with chronic pain syndromes, such as migraine, chronic abdominal pain, and orthopedic pain syndromes, have increased rates of suicidal ideation, suicide attempts, and suicide completion (Magni et al. 1998). The decrease in self-efficacy experienced by patients with chronic pain is highly associated with depressive symptoms that result in feelings of hopelessness (Rahman et al. 2008). Although other psychosocial variables play a role, depression is the most consistent and strongest predictor of suicidal ideation and behaviors in patients with chronic pain (Braden and Sullivan 2008).

Individuals with chronic physical complaints have higher rates of lifetime major depression. The prevalence of major depression in patients with chronic low back pain is more than three times the rate in the general population (Sullivan et al. 1992). Among patients presenting to chronic pain clinics, one-third to more than one-half meet criteria for current major depression (Dersh et al. 2002). **(pp. 904–905)**

Braden JB, Sullivan MD: Suicidal thoughts and behavior among adults with self-reported pain conditions in the National Comorbidity Survey Replication. J Pain 9:1106–1115, 2008

Dersh J, Polatin PB, Gatchel RJ: Chronic pain and psychopathology: research findings and theoretical considerations. Psychosom Med 64:773–786, 2002

Hasenbring M, Marienfeld G, Kuhlendahl D, et al: Risk factors of chronicity in lumbar disc patients: a prospective investigation of biologic, psychologic, and social predictors of therapy outcome. Spine 19:2759–2765, 1994

Magni G, Rigatti-Luchini S, Fracca F, et al: Suicidality in chronic abdominal pain: an analysis of the Hispanic Health and Nutrition Examination Survey (HHANES). Pain 76:137–144, 1998

Rahman A, Reed E, Underwood M, et al: Factors affecting self-efficacy and pain intensity in patients with chronic musculoskeletal pain seen in a specialist rheumatology pain clinic. Rheumatology (Oxford) 47:1803–1808, 2008

Simon GE, VonKorff M, Piccinelli M, et al: An international study of the relation between somatic symptoms and depression. N Engl J Med 341:1329–1335, 1999

Sullivan MJ, Reesor K, Mikail S, et al: The treatment of depression in chronic low back pain: review and recommendations. Pain 50:5–13, 1992

36.3 Which of the following is one of the most significant predictors of failure to return to work in patients with chronic low back pain?

    A. Fear–avoidance beliefs.
    B. Physical therapy.
    C. General fears of physical activity.
    D. Disease status.
    E. Physical impairment.

The correct response is option A.

Fear–avoidance beliefs were one of the most significant predictors of failure to return to work in patients with chronic low back pain (Waddell et al. 1993). Operant conditioning reinforces disability if the avoidance provides any short-term benefits such as reducing anticipatory anxiety or relieving the patient of unwanted responsibilities. In patients with chronic low back pain, improvements in disability following physical therapy were associated with decreases in pain, psychological distress, and fear–avoidance beliefs but not specific physical deficits (Mannion et al. 2001). Decreasing work-specific fears was a more important outcome than addressing general fears of physical activity in predicting improved physical capability for work (Vowles and Gross 2003).

Pain-related cognitions like catastrophizing and fear–avoidance beliefs predict poor coping and adjustment to chronic pain better than objective factors such as disease status, physical impairment, or occupational descriptions (Hasenbring et al. 2001). High levels of catastrophizing and fear of injury prospectively predicted disability due to new-onset low back pain 6 months later (Picavet et al. 2002). Catastrophizing has been shown to be a predictor of suicidal ideation independent of depressive symptoms and pain severity (Edwards et al. 2006). **(pp. 905–906)**

Edwards RR, Smith MT, Kudel I, et al: Pain-related catastrophizing as a risk factor for suicidal ideation in chronic pain. Pain 126:272–279, 2006

Hasenbring M, Hallner D, Klasen B: Psychological mechanisms in the transition from acute to chronic pain: over- or underrated? [in German]. Schmerz 15:442–447, 2001

Mannion AF, Junge A, Taimela S, et al: Active therapy for chronic low back pain, part 3: factors influencing self-rated disability and its change following therapy. Spine (Phila Pa 1976) 26:920–929, 2001

Picavet HS, Vlaeyen JW, Schouten JS: Pain catastrophizing and kinesiophobia: predictors of chronic low back pain. Am J Epidemiol 156:1028–1034, 2002

Vowles KE, Gross RT: Work-related beliefs about injury and physical capability for work in individuals with chronic pain. Pain 101:291–298, 2003

Waddell G, Newton M, Henderson I, et al: A fear-avoidance beliefs questionnaire (FABQ) and the role of fear-avoidance beliefs in chronic low back pain and disability. Pain 52:157–168, 1993

36.4 You are evaluating a 40-year-old woman for depression. She complains of frequent, unilateral, pulsating headaches with associated nausea and photophobia. She also describes a visual prodromal symptom of scintillating scotoma. You conclude that the probable diagnosis is

    A. Tension headache.
    B. Classic migraine.
    C. Chronic daily headache.
    D. Common migraine.
    E. Complicated migraine.

The correct response is option B.

Common migraine is a unilateral pulsatile headache, which may be associated with other symptoms such as nausea, vomiting, photophobia, and phonophobia. The classic form of migraine adds visual prodromal symptoms such as scintillating scotomata. Complicated migraine includes focal neurological signs such as cranial nerve palsies and is often described by the name of the primary deficit (e.g., hemiplegic, vestibular, or basilar migraine).

Chronic daily headache affects about 5% of the population and is composed of constant (transformed) migraine, medication-overuse headache, chronic tension-type headaches, new-onset daily persistent headache, and hemicrania continua (Dodick 2006).

Chronic tension-type headaches typically manifest as daily pain that is difficult to manage and unresponsive to many treatments. **(pp. 907–908)**

Dodick DW: Clinical practice: chronic daily headache. N Engl J Med 354:158–165, 2006

36.5 In the patient described above, you also diagnose bipolar II disorder. You want to prescribe a medication that will treat her hypomanic and depressive symptoms as well as decrease the frequency of her headaches. Which of the following might be a good choice?

    A. Sertraline.
    B. Aripiprazole.
    C. Lithium.
    D. Valproate.
    E. Bupropion.

The correct response is option D.

Placebo-controlled clinical trials support use of nonsteroidal anti-inflammatory drugs and triptans for acute treatment of migraine attacks with propranolol, metoprolol, flunarizine, valproate, and topiramate recommended as the best prophylactic agents (Evers et al. 2006; Mulleners and Chronicle 2008). In general, calcium channel blockers, beta-blockers, antidepressants, and anticonvulsants are the classes of choice for more refractory migraine (Evers et al. 2006; Silberstein 2008). **(p. 907)**

Evers S, Afra J, Frese A, et al: EFNS guideline on the drug treatment of migraine—a report of an EFNS task force. Eur J Neurol 13:560–572, 2006

Mulleners WM, Chronicle EP: Anticonvulsants in migraine prophylaxis: a Cochrane review. Cephalalgia 28:585–597, 2008

Silberstein SD: Treatment recommendations for migraine. Nat Clin Pract Neurol 4:482–489, 2008

36.6   Which of the following synthetic opioid analgesics is highly lipophilic and may be used transdermally?

    A. Morphine.
    B. Oxycodone.
    C. Methadone.
    D. Fentanyl.
    E. Hydrocodone.

The correct response is option D.

Clinically available opioids include naturally occurring compounds (morphine and codeine), semisynthetic derivatives (hydromorphone, oxymorphone, hydrocodone, oxycodone, dihydrocodeine, and buprenorphine), and synthetic opioid analgesics (meperidine, fentanyl, methadone, tramadol, pentazocine, and propoxyphene).

Fentanyl is highly lipophilic with affinity for neuronal tissues, which allows for transdermal or transmucosal delivery. The duration of action of transdermal preparations is up to 72 hours, but interindividual variability is considerable.

Morphine, because of its hydrophilicity, has poor oral bioavailability (22%–48%) and delayed central nervous system absorption and onset of action. This delay prolongs the analgesic effect of morphine relative to its plasma half-life, which decreases the potential for accumulation and toxicity with repeated dosing. Morphine is a more effective epidural spinal analgesic than oxycodone.

Oxycodone is an opiate analgesic with high oral bioavailability (>60%), a faster onset of action, and more predictable plasma levels compared with morphine. Oxycodone, in comparison to morphine, has similar analgesic efficacy, but releases less histamine and causes fewer hallucinations (Riley et al. 2008).

Methadone warrants special consideration in the treatment of chronic pain because of its stigma, low cost, high bioavailability, rapid onset of action, slow hepatic clearance, multiple receptor affinities, lack of neurotoxic metabolites, and incomplete cross-tolerance with other opioids.

Hydrocodone is similar to oxycodone, with rapid oral absorption and onset of analgesia. Hydrocodone is metabolized by *N*-demethylation to hydromorphone, which has properties similar to morphine except for lower rates of side effects. **(p. 911)**

Riley J, Eisenberg E, Muller-Schwefe G, et al: Oxycodone: a review of its use in the management of pain. Curr Med Res Opin 24:175–192, 2008

36.7   Which of the following antidepressant classes have been shown to be most effective in the treatment of both depression and fibromyalgia?

    A. Monoamine oxidase inhibitors (MAOIs).
    B. Selective serotonin reuptake inhibitors (SSRIs).
    C. Serotonin–norepinephrine reuptake inhibitors (SNRIs).
    D. Tricyclic antidepressants (TCAs).
    E. None of the above.

The correct response is option D.

Meta-analyses of randomized controlled trials concluded that TCAs are the most effective agents for neuropathic pain and for headache syndromes. A recent meta-analysis of fibromyalgia treatment trials found positive but diminishing effects comparing classes of antidepressants: TCAs > MAOIs > SSRIs = SNRIs (Hauser et al.

2009). TCAs have been shown to effectively treat central poststroke pain, postherpetic neuralgia, many painful polyneuropathies, and postmastectomy pain syndrome, but not spinal cord injury pain, phantom limb pain, or painful HIV neuropathy. **(p. 912)**

Hauser W, Bernardy K, Uceyler N, et al: Treatment of fibromyalgia syndrome with antidepressants: a meta-analysis. JAMA 301:198–209, 2009

Chapter 37

Medical Toxicology

Select the single best response for each question.

37.1   Acetaminophen overdose is a common means of attempted (and often completed) suicide. Prompt emergency management of this ingestion can significantly improve clinical outcomes. Which of the following statements regarding the metabolism of acetaminophen is *true*?

    A. Following ingestion, 70% of the drug is metabolized to the glucuronide conjugate.
    B. The glucuronide conjugate is directly hepatotoxic.
    C. *N*-acetyl-*p*-benzoquinone imine (NAPQI) is produced solely through the cytochrome P450 (CYP) 3A4 system.
    D. Glutathione depletion leads to systemic toxicity.
    E. *N*-acetylcysteine (NAC) directly neutralizes NAPQI.

The correct response is option D.

Hepatotoxicity is the primary concern and the target for medical intervention. Following oral ingestion, approximately 94% of the drug is metabolized to the glucuronide or sulfate conjugate and about 2% is excreted unchanged in the urine. Neither the parent drug, nor the conjugated forms are hepatotoxic. The remaining 4%, however, is metabolized primarily through CYP2E1 and, to some extent, CYP3A4, to form a toxic metabolite, NAPQI. After therapeutic dosing, any NAPQI formed is conjugated with normal hepatic stores of glutathione (GSH) to produce the nontoxic mercapturic acid, which is excreted in the urine. In the setting of a significant overdose, CYP2E1 metabolizes more acetaminophen, large amounts of NAPQI are formed, and the pool of GSH is rapidly depleted. Direct effects of excess NAPQI and liver failure can impact the function of other organ systems including kidneys, pancreas, and central nervous system.

Coagulation status declines and transaminase levels can exceed 10,000 IU/L before metabolic acidosis, jaundice, and encephalopathy herald fulminant hepatic failure. Hence, it is vital to quickly identify patients with significant acetaminophen overdose, and institute the antidote NAC without delay. NAC repletes GSH stores to detoxify NAPQI and works as an antioxidant to prevent evolving toxicity until nondamaging metabolic pathways clear the parent drug. **(pp. 934–935)**

37.2   Neuropsychiatric findings associated with strychnine poisoning include all of the following *except*

    A. Nystagmus.
    B. Hyporeflexia.
    C. Muscle contraction.
    D. Hyperthermia.
    E. *Risus sardonicus.*

The correct response is option B.

Strychnine toxicity causes rapid, widespread peripheral manifestations of neural excitation including nystagmus, hyperreflexia, and severe generalized painful skeletal muscle contraction, often resulting in hyperthermia, rhabdomyolysis, renal failure, tonic respiratory paralysis, and death.

The myoclonus, *risus sardonicus*, and opisthotonic posturing of strychnine toxicity may be mistaken for seizures. The differential diagnosis also includes tetanus, serotonin syndrome, neuroleptic malignant syndrome, stimulant toxicity, and drug-induced dystonia. Patients have both metabolic and respiratory acidosis, as well as myoglobinuria and elevated levels of creatine phosphokinase and serum aminotransferases. **(p. 937)**

37.3   Physical signs of chronic organophosphate toxicity include all of the following *except*

    A. Pupillary mydriasis.
    B. Nausea.
    C. Diaphoresis.
    D. Diarrhea.
    E. Weakness.

The correct response is option A.

Chronic organophosphate toxicity usually arises from work-related exposure. Symptoms include blurry vision with miosis, nausea, diarrhea, diaphoresis, weakness, and other neurological complaints (Clark 2006). **(p. 938)**

> Clark RF: Insecticides: organic phosphorous compounds and carbamates, in Goldfrank's Toxicologic Emergencies, 8th Edition. Edited by Flomenbaum NE, Goldfrank LR, Hoffman RS, et al. New York, McGraw-Hill, 2006, pp 1497–1512

37.4   A patient presents with depression, irritability, paranoid ideation, and cognitive impairment accompanied with alopecia, nail dystrophy, chorea, and ophthalmoplegia. Neuroimaging reveals cerebral and brain stem edema. Which metal is implicated in this toxicity state?

    A. Manganese.
    B. Lead.
    C. Thallium.
    D. Mercury.
    E. Arsenic.

The correct response is option C.

Chronic thallium toxicity should be suspected in patients when neuropsychiatric complaints (e.g., depression, irritability, paranoia, memory loss, confusion) are accompanied by alopecia, nail dystrophy, painful neuropathy, and gastrointestinal disturbances (Bank 1980). Chorea and ophthalmoplegia are sometimes observed. Central nervous system pathology includes cerebral and brain stem edema. Psychiatric symptoms may persist long after resolution of other toxic sequelae (Rusyniak et al. 2002). **(pp. 940–941)**

> Bank WJ: Thallium, in Experimental and Clinical Neurotoxicology. Edited by Spencer PS, Schaumberg HH. Baltimore, MD, Williams & Wilkins, 1980, pp 570–577
> Rusyniak DE, Furbee RB, Kirk MA: Thallium and arsenic poisoning in a small Midwestern town. Ann Emerg Med 39:307–311, 2002

37.5 A patient presents with personality changes consisting of shyness and social withdrawal paradoxically accompanied by episodic "flushed face" irritability. He also exhibits anxiety and cognitive impairment. This clinical picture suggests chronic exposure to which of the following?

    A. Manganese.
    B. Lead.
    C. Thallium.
    D. Mercury.
    E. Arsenic.

The correct response is option D.

Mercury is found in pharmaceuticals, folk medicines, laboratory and agricultural chemicals, industrial devices, and substituted alkyl compounds that accumulate in the bodies of large carnivorous fish. Toxicity from the metallic form of mercury is mediated through inhalational exposure, whereas organic mercury and its salts cause poisoning via ingestion.

Acute inhalation can cause severe chemical pneumonitis. Acute ingestion of mercury salts produces hemorrhagic gastroenteritis. It is more chronic exposure that gives rise to neuropsychiatric symptoms. Chronic inhalation can lead to a singular combination of personality changes with shyness and withdrawal alternating with explosive, flushed-face irritability. This syndrome is known as *erethism*. Volatile mercury was once used to prepare fur for hats; erethism is the condition referenced when labeling someone "mad as a hatter" (Brown 2002). **(p. 941)**

> Brown JS: Environmental and Chemical Toxins and Psychiatric Illness. Washington, DC, American Psychiatric Publishing, 2002

37.6 A delirium patient exhibits aimless picking movements, vivid visual hallucinations, tachycardia, dry mouth, flushed skin, and mydriasis. Which of the following delirium etiologies is suggested by this presentation?

    A. Anticholinergic toxicity.
    B. Cholinergic toxicity.
    C. Opioid toxicity.
    D. Benzodiazepine withdrawal.
    E. Stimulant overdose.

The correct response is option A.

Anticholinergic toxicity in the central nervous system (CNS) causes delirium, frequently with mumbling speech and carphology or floccillation—aimless "picking movements" of the fingers. Vivid visual hallucinosis and undressing behavior are not uncommon. Peripheral anticholinergic syndrome signs include tachycardia, dry mouth, flushed skin, temperature elevation, mydriasis, ileus, and urinary retention. The duration and severity of CNS manifestations typically exceed peripheral effects (Tune 2001). **(p. 943)**

> Tune LE: Anticholinergic effects of medication in elderly patients. J Clin Psychiatry 62 (suppl 21):11–14, 2001

37.7 Which of the following is contraindicated in the treatment of stimulant toxicity?

    A. Benzodiazepines.
    B. Beta-blockers.
    C. Hydralazine.
    D. Nitroprusside.
    E. Phentolamine.

The correct response is option B.

No specific antidotes for sympathomimetic toxicity exist, but benzodiazepines are the cornerstone of treatment because they attenuate catecholamine release, reduce hypertension, prevent seizures, and provide helpful sedation. Beta-blockers are contraindicated because they would leave alpha-adrenergic stimulation unopposed; thus, direct vasodilators such as hydralazine, nitroprusside, or phentolamine are preferred for treatment of severe hypertension that does not respond to benzodiazepines. **(p. 945)**

Chapter 38

Psychopharmacology

Select the single best response for each question.

38.1   Drug–drug interactions are either pharmacodynamic or pharmacokinetic in nature. Examples of pharmacokinetic interactions include all of the following *except*

   A. Altered absorption.
   B. Altered pharmacological response.
   C. Altered distribution.
   D. Altered metabolism.
   E. Altered excretion.

The correct response is option B.

Drug–drug interactions are pharmacodynamic or pharmacokinetic in nature. Pharmacodynamic interactions involve alterations in the pharmacological response to a drug, which may be additive, synergistic, or antagonistic. These interactions may occur directly, by altering drug binding to the receptor site, or indirectly through other mechanisms. Pharmacokinetic interactions include altered absorption, distribution, metabolism, or excretion and often change the drug concentration in tissues. **(pp. 958, 960)**

38.2   Which of the following is *not* a clinical feature of serotonin syndrome?

   A. Hypertension.
   B. Tachycardia.
   C. Hypotension.
   D. Bradycardia.
   E. Hyperreflexia.

The correct response is option D.

Bradycardia is not a clinical feature of serotonin syndrome. Autonomic nervous system features include hypertension, hypotension, tachycardia, diaphoresis, shivering, sialorrhea, mydriasis, tachypnea, and pupillary dilation. **(p. 970 [Table 38–3])**

38.3   Which of the following medications is a serotonin agonist (i.e., stimulates serotonin receptors)?

   A. Venlafaxine.
   B. Tramadol.
   C. Buspirone.
   D. Moclobemide.
   E. Amphetamine.

The correct response is option C.

Serotonin agonists include buspirone, triptans, ergo alkaloids, trazodone, and nefazodone. **(p. 970 [Table 38–4])**

38.4 The nurse on the psychiatric inpatient unit calls you to evaluate one of your patients who has developed acute symptoms suggestive of either serotonin syndrome or neuroleptic malignant syndrome. The patient was recently started on fluoxetine, olanzapine, trazodone, and as-needed intramuscular haloperidol. Which of the following signs or symptoms is more indicative of serotonin syndrome than of neuroleptic malignant syndrome?

    A. Spontaneous or inducible clonus.
    B. Tachycardia.
    C. Elevated body temperature.
    D. Elevated creatine phosphokinase.
    E. Diaphoresis.

The correct response is option A.

Spontaneous or inducible clonus is indicative of serotonin syndrome. **(pp. 969–971, 976–977 [Tables 38–5 and 38–6])**

38.5 The most common electrocardiogram finding in patients taking lithium is

    A. PR interval prolongation.
    B. Increased heart rate.
    C. Shortened QT interval.
    D. T wave depression.
    E. Prolonged QRS interval.

The correct response is option D.

Lithium causes benign reversible repolarization electrocardiographic changes in 20%–30% of patients (Mitchell and Mackenzie 1982), including T wave depression and inversion. Other cardiovascular effects of lithium include decreased heart rate, prolonged QT interval, and arrhythmias (Burggraf 1997; van Noord et al. 2009). **(p. 973)**

> Burggraf GW: Are psychotropic drugs at therapeutic levels a concern for cardiologists? Can J Cardiol 13:75–80, 1997
>
> Mitchell JE, Mackenzie TB: Cardiac effects of lithium therapy in man: a review. J Clin Psychiatry 43:47–51, 1982
>
> van Noord C, Straus SM, Sturkenboom MC, et al: Psychotropic drugs associated with corrected QT interval prolongation. J Clin Psychopharmacol 29:9–15, 2009

38.6 Weight gain is a common and problematic side effect of mood stabilizers. Which of the following mood stabilizers is associated with the *greatest* amount of weight gain?

    A. Gabapentin.
    B. Carbamazepine.
    C. Topiramate.
    D. Lamotrigine.
    E. Valproate.

The correct response is option E.

Weight gain is a common factor in noncompliance (Mendlewicz et al. 1999). Weight gain is especially a problem with valproate, with an average weight gain of more than 8% of baseline body weight (Chengappa et al. 2002). Gabapentin causes a 1% weight gain (Wang et al. 2002). Although carbamazepine is also reported to cause weight gain, the incidence is less than with valproate (Corman et al. 1997). Lamotrigine has little effect on weight (Biton et al. 2001), whereas topiramate causes a weight loss of about 0.7% of body weight (Chengappa et al. 2002). **(p. 975)**

Biton V, Mirza W, Montouris G, et al: Weight change associated with valproate and lamotrigine monotherapy in patients with epilepsy. Neurology 56:172–177, 2001

Chengappa KN, Chalasani L, Brar JS, et al: Changes in body weight and body mass index among psychiatric patients receiving lithium, valproate, or topiramate: an open-label, nonrandomized chart review. Clin Ther 24:1576–1584, 2002

Corman CL, Leung NM, Guberman AH: Weight gain in epileptic patients during treatment with valproic acid: a retrospective study. Can J Neurol Sci 24:240–244, 1997

Mendlewicz J, Souery D, Rivelli SK: Short-term and long-term treatment for bipolar patients: beyond the guidelines. J Affect Disord 55:79–85, 1999

Wang PW, Santosa C, Schumacher M, et al: Gabapentin augmentation therapy in bipolar depression. Bipolar Disord 4:296–301, 2002

38.7   Which of the following atypical antipsychotics is associated with the *lowest* risk of extrapyramidal symptoms?

    A. Ziprasidone.
    B. Quetiapine.
    C. Aripiprazole.
    D. Risperidone.
    E. Asenapine.

The correct response is option B.

Acute extrapyramidal symptoms—akathisia, akinesia, and dystonia—occur in as many as 50%–75% of patients who take typical antipsychotics (Collaborative Working Group on Clinical Trial Evaluations 1998). High-potency typical antipsychotics are associated with higher rates of extrapyramidal symptoms than are low-potency agents. Among the currently available atypical antipsychotics, the hierarchy of extrapyramidal symptom risk (greater to lesser) is ziprasidone > aripiprazole > risperidone = paliperidone (estimated) > asenapine (estimated) > iloperidone (estimated) > olanzapine > quetiapine > clozapine (Citrome 2009; Gao et al. 2008; Tandon 2002; Weber and McCormack 2009). **(p. 976)**

Citrome L: Iloperidone for schizophrenia: a review of the efficacy and safety profile for this newly commercialised second-generation antipsychotic. Int J Clin Pract 63:1237–1248, 2009

Collaborative Working Group on Clinical Trial Evaluations: Assessment of EPS and tardive dyskinesia in clinical trials. J Clin Psychiatry 59 (suppl 12):23–27, 1998

Gao K, Kemp DE, Ganocy SJ, et al: Antipsychotic-induced extrapyramidal side effects in bipolar disorder and schizophrenia: a systematic review. J Clin Psychopharmacol 28:203–209, 2008

Tandon R: Safety and tolerability: how do newer generation "atypical" antipsychotics compare? Psychiatr Q 73:297–311, 2002

Weber J, McCormack PL: Asenapine. CNS Drugs 23:781–792, 2009

38.8   You believe that your patient with bipolar disorder would benefit from an atypical antipsychotic medication. Because she has a history of cardiac arrhythmias, you want to select the agent with the lowest mean QTc interval prolongation. Which of the following medications fits this profile?

    A. Quetiapine.
    B. Paliperidone.
    C. Ziprasidone.
    D. Aripiprazole.
    E. Risperidone.

The correct response is option D.

A number of antipsychotics may be associated with QTc interval prolongation and risk for torsade de pointes. Ziprasidone, thioridazine, and droperidol carry a "black box" warning regarding dose-related QTc prolongation and risk for sudden death. Mean QTc interval prolongation (greatest to least) for antipsychotics is thioridazine (36 msec) > ziprasidone (21 msec) > quetiapine (15 msec) > paliperidone (12 msec) = risperidone (10 msec) = asenapine (estimated) = iloperidone (9 msec) > olanzapine (6 msec) > haloperidol (5 msec) > aripiprazole (<1 msec) (Citrome 2009; Janssen 2010; Otsuka 2002; Pfizer 2010; Weber and McCormack 2009). **(pp. 977–978)**

Citrome L: Iloperidone for schizophrenia: a review of the efficacy and safety profile for this newly commercialised second-generation antipsychotic. Int J Clin Pract 63:1237–1248, 2009

Janssen: Invega (paliperidone) home page. 2010. Available at: http://www.invega.com. Accessed May 14, 2010.

Otsuka: Abilify (aripiprazole) Tablets, Application No. 21-436, Drug Approval Package, Medical review(s). Food and Drug Administration Center for Drug Evaluation and Research, November 15, 2002. Available at: http://www.accessdata.fda.gov/drugsatfda_docs/nda/2002/21-436_Abilify_medr_P2.pdf. Accessed May 14, 2010.

Pfizer: Geodon (ziprasidone) home page. 2010. Available at: http://www.geodon.com. Accessed May 14, 2010.

Weber J, McCormack PL: Asenapine. CNS Drugs 23:781–792, 2009

38.9   Which of the following nonbenzodiazepine sedatives is a melatonin agonist?

    A. Eszopiclone.
    B. Zopiclone.
    C. Ramelteon.
    D. Zolidem.
    E. Zaleplon.

The correct response is option C.

Ramelteon, a melatonin agonist U.S. Food and Drug Administration approved for insomnia, demonstrated efficacy for insomnia with no next-morning residual effects, an adverse-effect profile similar to that of placebo, and no withdrawal symptoms upon discontinuation in a 6-month controlled clinical trial (Mayer et al. 2009).

Eszopiclone, zopiclone, zolpidem, and zaleplon are very well tolerated short-half-life hypnotics with very few dose-related adverse effects. Adverse effects of eszopiclone and zopiclone include bitter taste, dry mouth, difficulty arising in the morning, sleepiness, nausea, and nightmares (Allain et al. 1991; Najib 2006). Clinical trials of zaleplon report adverse effects comparable to those seen with placebo (Hedner et al. 2000). Zolpidem's adverse effects include central nervous system (dizziness, drowsiness, and headache) and gastrointestinal effects (nausea) (Krystal et al. 2008). **(p. 981)**

Allain H, Delahaye C, Le Coz F, et al: Postmarketing surveillance of zopiclone in insomnia: analysis of 20,513 cases. Sleep 14:408–413, 1991

Hedner J, Yaeche R, Emilien G, et al: Zaleplon shortens subjective sleep latency and improves subjective sleep quality in elderly patients with insomnia. The Zaleplon Clinical Investigator Study Group. Int J Geriatr Psychiatry 15:704–712, 2000

Krystal AD, Erman M, Zammit GK, et al: Long-term efficacy and safety of zolpidem extended-release 12.5 mg, administered 3 to 7 nights per week for 24 weeks, in patients with chronic primary insomnia: a 6-month, randomized, double-blind, placebo-controlled, parallel-group, multicenter study. Sleep 31:79–90, 2008

Mayer G, Wang-Weigand S, Roth-Schechter B, et al: Efficacy and safety of 6-month nightly ramelteon administration in adults with chronic primary insomnia. Sleep 32:351–360, 2009

Najib J: Eszopiclone, a nonbenzodiazepine sedative-hypnotic agent for the treatment of transient and chronic insomnia. Clin Ther 28:491–516, 2006

Chapter 39

Psychotherapy

Select the single best response for each question.

39.1 In a recent systematic review by Jacobsen and Jim (2008), psychosocial interventions for mood and anxiety disorders were shown to be of clinical benefit in patients with cancer. Which of the following statements regarding this study is *false*?

   A. All of the reviewed studies involved adult cancer patients.
   B. Counseling was associated with improved functional ability.
   C. Counseling was associated with enhanced quality of life.
   D. Counseling was associated with fewer symptoms of depression.
   E. The reviewed studies typically had good methodological rigor, allowing for meaningful meta-analysis.

The correct response is option E.

A recent systematic review of psychosocial interventions for anxiety and depression in adult cancer patients concluded that interventions involving counseling can be currently recommended for improving patients' general functional ability or quality of life, degree of depression, and interpersonal relationships (Jacobsen and Jim 2008). However, the review noted the general poor methodological quality of many studies. **(p. 1024)**

> Jacobsen PB, Jim HS: Psychosocial interventions for anxiety and depression in adult cancer patients: achievements and challenges. CA Cancer J Clin 58:214–230, 2008

39.2 Interpersonal therapy (IPT) includes several elements that are highly relevant to the general medical setting and to patients who have emotional difficulties secondary to physical illness. During the first phase of IPA treatment, problem areas in the patient's interpersonal relationships are identified and sorted into four groups. Which of the following is *not* one of IPT's four defined problem areas?

   A. Grief.
   B. Role transition.
   C. Role disputes.
   D. Interpersonal deficits.
   E. Effects of childhood relationships.

The correct response is option E.

Interpersonal therapy (IPT), a psychotherapy model developed as a time-limited treatment for depression (Klerman et al. 1984), bases its treatment approach on the assumption that there is a relationship between the onset or recurrence of a depressive episode and a person's social and interpersonal relationships at the time. There are three stages of development in IPT when it is used to treat depression. In the first phase, depression is diagnosed and explained to the patient so there is a clear understanding of the nature of the condition and its symptoms. An interpersonal inventory is compiled that lists all the patient's relationships, and the main problem areas are identified. Problem areas are classified into four groups: grief, role transition, role disputes, and interpersonal deficits. **(pp. 1025–1026)**

Klerman G, Weissman M, Rounsaville B, et al: Interpersonal Psychotherapy of Depression. New York, Basic Books, 1984

39.3   Psychodynamic Interpersonal Therapy (PIT) is another psychotherapy model with applicability to psychosomatic medicine practice. Which of the following statements regarding PIT is *false?*

   A. Another term for PIT is "Conversational Model" Therapy.
   B. PIT combines elements of psychodynamic and interpersonal therapies.
   C. PIT places less emphasis on the patient–therapist relationship than does interpersonal therapy (IPT).
   D. PIT makes less use of transference interpretations than does conventional psychodynamic psychotherapy.
   E. In PIT, human existence is regarded as being essentially relational, and man is regarded as a "creature of the between."

The correct response is option C.

PIT, also known as "Conversational Model" Therapy, was developed by Hobson (1985), a psychiatrist and psychotherapist. PIT combines elements of psychodynamic and interpersonal therapies. It places greater emphasis on the patient–therapist relationship as a tool for resolving interpersonal issues than IPT, and there is less emphasis on the interpretation of transference than in psychodynamic therapies. One of the central tenets of PIT is the importance of human experience and an individual's sense of self within a personal relationship. Human existence is regarded as being essentially relational, and man is regarded as a "creature of the between." This applies even to people who live a solitary existence. **(p. 1026)**

Hobson RF: Forms of Feeling. London, Tavistock, 1985

39.4   Key features of Psychodynamic Interpersonal Therapy (PIT) include all of the following *except*

   A. The therapist endeavors to know about the patient rather than merely 'getting to know" the patient.
   B. The patient's problems are assumed to arise from relationship disturbances.
   C. The therapist uses a "tentative, encouraging, supportive" approach.
   D. The therapist seeks to link the patient's distress to specific interpersonal problems.
   E. The therapist helps the patient test solutions in the "here and now."

The correct response is option A.

In PIT, the therapeutic emphasis is on getting to know someone, rather than knowing about them.
   Key features of the model include 1) the assumption that the patient's problems arise from or are exacerbated by disturbances of significant personal relationships; 2) a tentative, encouraging, supportive approach from the therapist, who seeks to develop deeper understanding with the patient through negotiation, exploration of feelings, and use of metaphor; 3) the linkage of the patient's distress to specific interpersonal problems; and 4) the use of the therapeutic relationship to address problems and test out solutions in the "here and now." **(p. 1026)**

39.5   Cognitive-behavioral therapy (CBT) has applicability to the experience of psychiatric symptoms in systemic illness. Which of the following is *not* one of the components of multidimensional "illness representations" according to Leventhal et al. (1997)?

   A. Identity.
   B. Perceived consequences.
   C. Timeline.
   D. Control/cure.
   E. Symbolism of the specific illness.

The correct response is option E.

Sensky (2004) has described in detail how CBT has been adapted for use in people with physical illnesses. Crucial to the development of any treatment intervention is an understanding of the patient's model of his or her illness, and a useful model or framework for doing this has been developed by Moss-Morris et al. (2002) in relation to illness perception. This concept was originally developed by Leventhal et al. (1997). Within Leventhal's model, illness representations are considered to be multidimensional, comprising five main components: identity, perceived consequences, timeline, perceived cause, and control/cure). **(p. 1027; Table 39–1)**

Leventhal H, Benyamini Y, Brownlee S: Illness representations: theoretical foundations, in Perceptions of Health and Illness: Current Research and Applications. Edited by Petrie KJ, Weinman J. Amsterdam, The Netherlands, Harwood Academic Publishers, 1997, pp 19–45

Moss-Morris R, Weinman J, Petrie KJ: The Revised Illness Perception Questionnaire (IPQ-R). Psychol Health 17:1–16, 2002

Sensky T: Cognitive therapy with medical patients, in Cognitive-Behavior Therapy. Edited by Wright JH (Review of Psychiatry Series, Vol 23; Oldham JM and Riba MB, series eds). Washington, DC, American Psychiatric Publishing, 2004, pp 83–121

39.6   In a recent review of mindfulness-based therapies by Arias et al. (2006), the strongest evidence for efficacy of these therapies was found for which of the following disorders?

   A. Mood disorders.
   B. Anxiety disorders.
   C. Autoimmune illness.
   D. Epilepsy.
   E. Psychiatric symptoms in cancer.

The correct response is option D.

Mindfulness-based therapies have been used to treat a wide range of stress disorders, including chronic pain (Kabat-Zinn et al. 1987), fibromyalgia (Kaplan et al. 1993; Sephton et al. 2007), mood symptoms in cancer (Carlsson et al. 2003; Smith et al. 2005), and depression (Teasdale et al. 2000). A recent systematic review of meditation techniques for medical illness identified 20 randomized controlled trials with a total of 958 subjects (Arias et al. 2006). The reviewers concluded that the strongest evidence for efficacy was found for epilepsy, symptoms of premenstrual syndrome, and menopausal symptoms. Benefit was also demonstrated for mood and anxiety disorders, autoimmune illness, and emotional disturbance in neoplastic disease. **(p. 1029)**

Arias AJ, Steinberg K, Banga A, et al: Systematic review of the efficacy of meditation techniques as treatments for medical illness. J Altern Complement Med 12:817–832, 2006

Carlson LE, Speca M, Patel KD, et al: Mindfulness-based stress reduction in relation to quality of life, mood, symptoms of stress, and immune parameters in breast and prostate cancer outpatients. Psychosom Med 65:571–581, 2003

Kabat-Zinn J, Lipworth L, Burney R, et al: Four-year follow-up of a meditation-based program for the self-regulation of chronic pain: treatment outcomes and compliance. The Clinical Journal of Pain 2:159–173, 1987

Kaplan KH, Goldenberg DL, Galvin-Nadeau M: The impact of a meditation-based stress reduction program on fibromyalgia. Gen Hosp Psychiatry 15:284–298, 1993

Sephton SE, Salmon P, Weissbecker I, et al: Mindfulness meditation alleviates depressive symptoms in women with fibromyalgia: results of a randomized clinical trial. Arthritis Rheum (Arthritis Care Res) 57:77–85, 2007

Smith JE, Richardson J, Hoffman C, et al: Mindfulness-Based Stress Reduction as supportive therapy in cancer care: a systematic review. J Adv Nurse 52:315–327, 2005

Teasdale JD, Segal ZV, Williams JMG: Prevention of relapse/recurrence in major depression by mindfulness-based cognitive therapy. J Consult Clin Psychol 68:615–623, 2000

39.7 Although psychological treatments can be offered as stand-alone treatments, they are increasingly delivered as part of a stepped-care model offering five different intensities of treatment, sequentially graded according to the severity of the clinical problem. Which of these five steps involves use of brief psychotherapy (e.g., cognitive-behavioral therapy [CBT], counseling, interpersonal therapy) for 6–8 sessions, with consideration of antidepressants?

  A. Step 1.
  B. Step 2.
  C. Step 3.
  D. Step 4.
  E. Step 5.

The correct response is option C.

The stepped care model involves five different intensities of treatment that are offered the patient or client according to the severity or complexity of his or her problems. Most patients start at the bottom of the model and progress to the next step only if their symptoms do not improve.

- Step 1 involves watchful waiting, as many patients who present with symptoms will find their symptoms resolve spontaneously without requiring any help.
- Step 2 usually involves some form of guided self-help and may include computerized CBT, psychoeducation, or help from voluntary organizations. Exercise may also be recommended or even prescribed if such treatment is available from a relevant health service organization.
- Step 3 involves brief psychological therapy (CBT, counseling, interpersonal therapies) for 6–8 sessions. Antidepressants may be prescribed if there is a previous history of moderate to severe depression.
- Step 4 involves depression case management, and the patient may be assigned a case manager or key worker. Medication and more intensive psychological treatments may be offered, with care coordinated by the case manager working with the patient's primary care physician.
- Step 5 is for patients who have not responded to the previous 4 steps. Step 5 may involve crisis intervention services, inpatient treatment, or even more intensive multicomponent treatment packages.

(pp. 1029–1030)

Chapter 40

Electroconvulsive Therapy

Select the single best response for each question.

40.1   If the electrical stimulus in electroconvulsive therapy (ECT) is not of sufficient intensity to cause a seizure, there have been reports of prolonged asystole requiring resuscitation. Premedication with which of the following classes of medications is recommended to decrease the likelihood of this occurrence?

   A. Beta-blockers.
   B. Antihypertensive agents.
   C. Antimuscarinic agents.
   D. Alpha-adrenergic agents.
   E. Cholinergic agents.

The correct response is option C.

After the electrical stimulus, there is a vagally (i.e., parasympathetically) mediated short-lived bradycardia, occasionally with asystole of several seconds. If the electrical stimulus is strong enough to cause a seizure, this initial parasympathetic phase is rapidly replaced by a sympathetically mediated tachycardia and rise in blood pressure during the seizure.

   If the electrical stimulus is not of sufficient intensity to cause a seizure, then the initial parasympathetic effects will not be offset by the sympathetic phase. Thus, there have been rare reports of prolonged asystole requiring resuscitation, especially in patients who have not been given antimuscarinic premedication or who received beta-blockers. For this reason, the use of antimuscarinic premedication is encouraged in ECT. This is especially true at the first treatment session, when a stimulus dose titration is performed to determine seizure threshold, and subconvulsive stimuli are likely. **(pp. 1043–1044)**

40.2   The most common dysrhythmia in electroconvulsive therapy (ECT) patients is

   A. Atrial fibrillation.
   B. Ventricular fibrillation.
   C. Ventricular tachycardia.
   D. Atrial tachycardia.
   E. Bundle branch block.

The correct response is option A.

The most common dysrhythmia in ECT patients is atrial fibrillation. There are several reports of patients in atrial fibrillation who safely received ECT (Petrides and Fink 1996). Occasionally, such patients will convert to sinus rhythm during ECT or convert back to atrial fibrillation if already converted before ECT to sinus rhythm. Atrial fibrillation newly identified before ECT should be assessed by a cardiologist for optimal management, including the decision whether to choose rate control or cardioversion. Therapeutic anticoagulation should be maintained throughout the course of ECT if the patient is already anticoagulated. Close and meticulous monitoring of the patient's hemodynamic status, oxygenation, and electrocardiographic changes in response to treatment is critically important during ECT. Electrocardiographic rhythm should be inspected before each treatment. The patient without history of atrial fibrillation who develops this rhythm during ECT obviously should have a cardiac evaluation before treatment is resumed. **(p. 1045)**

> Petrides G, Fink M: Atrial fibrillation, anticoagulation, and electroconvulsive therapy. Convuls Ther 12:91–98, 1996

40.3 A blood pressure concern in electroconvulsive therapy (ECT) is the management of blood pressure spikes that occur during treatments. Which of the following medication classes is recommended to reduce these spikes?

    A. Alpha-blocker.
    B. Beta-blocker.
    C. Angiotensin-converting enzyme inhibitor.
    D. Angiotensin II receptor blocker.
    E. Thiazide diuretic.

The correct response is option B.

A blood pressure concern in ECT is the management of blood pressure spikes that occur during ECT treatments. If the anesthesiologist is concerned about a patient's blood pressure at the time of a treatment, intravenous beta blockade can effectively dampen the rise in pressure during the seizure. Furthermore, Albin et al. (2007) found that no sustained rise in blood pressure occurs in hypertensive patients during a course of ECT treatment. With the availability of short-acting antihypertensive agents (e.g., esmolol or labetalol), high blood pressure generally can be managed rapidly and effectively during the treatments. **(p. 1046)**

> Albin SM, Stevens SR, Rasmussen KG: Blood pressure before and after electroconvulsive therapy in hypertensive and nonhypertensive patients. J ECT 23:9–10, 2007

40.4 You are asked to evaluate a patient with Alzheimer's disease and agitated depression who has failed to respond to medication. You decide to refer the patient for a course of electroconvulsive therapy (ECT). Prudence dictates that you

    A. Use bitemporal electrode placement.
    B. Use thrice-weekly treatments.
    C. Premedicate with a cognitive-enhancing agent.
    D. Use twice-weekly scheduling.
    E. Administer modafinil before each treatment.

The correct response is option D.

Prudent advice for the ECT practitioner treating patients with dementia is to use unilateral electrode placement and twice-weekly scheduling. If improvement seems to lag from what is expected, then more aggressive treatment (i.e., bitemporal electrode placement or thrice-weekly treatments) can be given. Dementia patients with either depression or agitation who are referred for ECT may improve, but if maintenance treatments are not administered, rapid relapse tends to occur. Furthermore, the frequency of maintenance treatments often needs to be no less than every other week or even weekly to maintain the gains of the index course. This often leads to ongoing worsening of cognition, a side effect that obviously needs to be weighed against improvements in mood and behavior. **(pp. 1047–1048)**

40.5 Electroconvulsive therapy (ECT) should be avoided, if possible, in patients with which of the following conditions?

 A. Parkinson's disease.
 B. Chronic obstructive pulmonary disease.
 C. Diabetes.
 D. Chronic pain.
 E. Recent stroke.

The correct response is option E.

Prudent advice for the ECT practitioner is not to use ECT in patients with recent stroke if possible.

Some reports indicate safe use of ECT in patients with a variety of intracranial masses (Kohler and Burock 2001; Patkar et al. 2000; Perry et al. 2007; Rasmussen and Flemming 2006; Rasmussen et al. 2007). Presence of any central nervous system tumor may lead to an increased risk for neurological complications caused by ECT. In the absence of focal neurological signs, brain edema, mass effect, or papilledema, the risks likely are relatively small. In the presence of such findings, ECT should be considered only when no other reasonable option exists and after consultation with a neurosurgeon or neurologist to discuss strategies to reduce the increase in intracranial pressure that accompanies seizures.

Several case reports and series indicate that ECT is effective for treating depression and even the motor manifestations in patients with Parkinson's disease (Rasmussen and Abrams 1991, 1992; Rasmussen et al. 2002). Common side effects of ECT in patients with Parkinson's disease include delirium and treatment-emergent dyskinesias (Douyon et al. 1989).

Large case series attest to the safe use of ECT in patients with asthma (Mueller et al. 2006) and chronic obstructive pulmonary disease (Schak et al. 2008). Patients who are using inhalers should do so in the morning shortly before treatment.

Single ECT treatments cause a brief approximately 8%–10% rise in blood sugar immediately after treatment in both diabetic and nondiabetic patients (Rasmussen and Ryan 2005; Rasmussen et al. 2006). However, very little change occurs in blood sugar control over a course of treatments (Netzel et al. 2002). Diabetic patients should have blood glucose levels monitored closely during the ECT course, including fingerstick checks before treatment.

Chronic pain syndromes are quite common in psychiatric patients. When the pain symptom is clearly secondary to a melancholic or psychotic depression, the ECT clinician can be optimistic about resolution of the pain symptoms along with other psychiatric symptoms. **(pp. 1048–1050)**

Douyon R, Serby M, Klutchko B, et al: ECT and Parkinson's disease revisited: a "naturalistic" study. Am J Psychiatry 146:1451–1455, 1989

Kohler CG, Burock M: ECT for psychotic depression associated with a brain tumor (letter). Am J Psychiatry 158:2089, 2001

Mueller PS, Schak K, Barnes RD, et al: The safety of electroconvulsive therapy in patients with asthma. Neth J Med 64:417–421, 2006

Netzel PJ, Mueller PS, Rummans TA, et al: Safety, efficacy, and effects on glycemic control of electroconvulsive therapy in insulin-requiring type 2 diabetic patients. J ECT 18:16–21, 2002

Patkar AA, Hill KP, Weinstein SP, et al: ECT in the presence of brain tumor and increased intracranial pressure: evaluation and reduction of risk. J ECT 16:189–197, 2000

Perry CL, Lindell EP, Rasmussen KG: ECT in patients with arachnoid cysts. J ECT 23:36–37, 2007

Rasmussen K, Abrams R: Treatment of Parkinson's disease with electroconvulsive therapy. Psychiatr Clin North Am 14:925–933, 1991

Rasmussen KG, Abrams R: The role of electroconvulsive therapy in Parkinson's disease, in Parkinson's Disease: Neurobehavioral Aspects. Edited by Huber S, Cummings J. New York, Oxford University Press, 1992, pp 255–270

Rasmussen KG, Flemming KD: Electroconvulsive therapy in patients with cavernous hemangiomas. J ECT 22:272–273, 2006

Rasmussen KG, Ryan DA: The effect of electroconvulsive therapy treatments on blood sugar in nondiabetic patients. J ECT 21:232–234, 2005

Rasmussen KG, Rummans TA, Richardson JR: Electroconvulsive therapy in the medically ill. Psychiatr Clin North Am 25:177–194, 2002

Rasmussen KG, Ryan DA, Mueller PS: Blood glucose before and after ECT treatments in type 2 diabetic patients. J ECT 22:124–126, 2006

Rasmussen KG, Perry CL, Sutor B, et al: ECT in patients with intracranial masses. J Neuropsychiatry Clin Neurosci 19:191–193, 2007

Schak KM, Mueller PS, Barnes RD, et al: The safety of ECT in patients with chronic obstructive pulmonary disease. Psychosomatics 49:208–211, 2008

Chapter 41

Palliative Care

Select the single best response for each question.

41.1 Which of the following is *not* a typical sign of anxiety in a terminally ill patient?

   A. Tension.
   B. Restlessness.
   C. Excessive somnolence.
   D. Autonomic hyperactivity.
   E. Rumination.

The correct response is option C.

Excessive somnolence is not a sign of anxiety in a terminally ill patient.

   The terminally ill patient presents with a complex mixture of physical and psychological symptoms in the context of a frightening reality, making the identification of anxious symptoms requiring treatment challenging. Patients with anxiety complain of tension or restlessness, or they exhibit jitteriness, autonomic hyperactivity, vigilance, insomnia, distractibility, shortness of breath, numbness, apprehension, worry, or rumination. Often the physical or somatic manifestations of anxiety overshadow the psychological or cognitive ones and are the symptoms that the patient most often presents (Holland 1989). **(p. 1057)**

   Holland JC: Anxiety and cancer: the patient and the family. J Clin Psychiatry 50 (suppl):20–25, 1989

41.2 The differential diagnosis of anxiety disorder versus delirium in a terminally ill patient may be difficult, as many symptoms overlap between the two conditions. Which of the following symptoms is more suggestive of delirium than of anxiety disorder?

   A. Disturbed level of consciousness.
   B. Impaired concentration.
   C. Cognitive impairment.
   D. Fluctuation of symptoms over time.
   E. All of the above.

The correct response is option E.

Delirium can present with anxiety and restlessness in palliative care settings. Disturbance in level of consciousness, impaired concentration, cognitive impairment, altered perception, and fluctuation of symptoms are important diagnostic indicators of delirium as opposed to a diagnosis of anxiety disorder (Roth and Massie 2009). **(p. 1058)**

   Roth AJ, Massie MJ: Anxiety in palliative care, in Handbook of Psychiatry in Palliative Medicine, 2nd Edition. Edited by Chochinov HM, Breitbart W. New York, Oxford University Press, 2009, pp 69–80

41.3 Treatment of anxiety disorders in terminally ill patients may require modification of usual psychopharmacological practices. For example, many terminally ill patients can no longer reliably take oral medications. Which of the following benzodiazepines can be administered rectally?

    A. Oxazepam.
    B. Midazolam.
    C. Alprazolam.
    D. Diazepam.
    E. Temazepam.

The correct response is option D.

Dying patients can be administered diazepam rectally when no other route is available, with dosages equivalent to those used in oral regimens. Rectal diazepam (Twycross and Lack 1984) has been used widely in palliative care to control anxiety, restlessness, and agitation associated with the final days of life.

For patients who feel persistently anxious, the first-line antianxiety drugs are the benzodiazepines. For patients with severely compromised hepatic function, the use of shorter-acting benzodiazepines such as lorazepam, oxazepam, or temazepam is preferred, since these drugs are metabolized by conjugation with glucuronic acid and have no active metabolites (Roth and Massie 2009). **(p. 1059)**

Roth AJ, Massie MJ: Anxiety in palliative care, in Handbook of Psychiatry in Palliative Medicine, 2nd Edition. Edited by Chochinov HM, Breitbart W. New York, Oxford University Press, 2009, pp 69–80

Twycross RG, Lack SA: Therapeutics in Terminal Disease. London, Pitman, 1984, pp 99–103

41.4 Terminally ill patients can present with a vexing combination of persistent anxiety, insomnia, and profound anorexia. Which of the following antidepressants is most appropriate for management of this constellation of symptoms?

    A. Mirtazapine.
    B. Bupropion.
    C. Citalopram.
    D. Fluoxetine.
    E. None of the above.

The correct response is option A.

Sedating antidepressants such as mirtazapine or trazodone may help patients with persistent anxiety, insomnia, and anorexia. Selective serotonin reuptake inhibitors are also effective in the management of anxiety disorders (Roth and Massie 2009). The utility of antidepressants and buspirone for anxiety disorders is often limited in the dying patient because these agents require weeks to achieve a therapeutic effect. **(p. 1059)**

Roth AJ, Massie MJ: Anxiety in palliative care, in Handbook of Psychiatry in Palliative Medicine, 2nd Edition. Edited by Chochinov HM, Breitbart W. New York, Oxford University Press, 2009, pp 69–80

41.5 In regard to the use of psychostimulants in palliative care, which of the following statements is *true?*

    A. Psychostimulants can cause anorexia at therapeutic doses.
    B. Psychostimulants can cause insomnia at therapeutic doses.
    C. Psychostimulants should not be used in terminally ill patients with a substance abuse history.
    D. Psychostimulants reduce sedation associated with opioid use.
    E. Psychostimulants do not provide adjuvant analgesic affects.

The correct response is option D.

Stimulants have been shown to reduce sedation secondary to opioid analgesics and provide adjuvant analgesic effects (Bruera et al. 1987).

Psychostimulants are particularly helpful in the treatment of depression in the terminally ill because they have a rapid onset of action and energizing effects and typically do not cause anorexia, weight loss, or insomnia at therapeutic doses (Candy et al. 2008; Pessin et al. 2008; Potash and Breitbart 2002). In fact, at low doses, stimulants may actually increase appetite. Abuse is almost always an irrelevant concern in the terminally ill, and stimulants should not be withheld on the basis of a patient's prior history of substance abuse. **(pp. 1061–1062)**

> Bruera E, Chadwick S, Brenneis C, et al: Methylphenidate associated with narcotics for the treatment of cancer pain. Cancer Treat Rep 71:67–70, 1987
> Candy M, Jones L, Williams R, et al: Psychostimulants for depression. Cochrane Database Syst Rev (2):CD006722, 2008
> Pessin H, Alici-Evcimen Y, Apostolatos A, et al: Diagnosis, assessment and treatment of depression in palliative care, in Psychosocial Issues in Palliative Care, 2nd Edition. Edited by Lloyd-Williams M. New York, Oxford University Press, 2008, pp 129–160
> Potash M, Breitbart W: Affective disorders in advanced cancer. Hematol Oncol Clin North Am 16:671–700, 2002

41.6 Delirium in a terminally ill patient can be a very distressing experience for the patient and family members. In the Breitbart et al. (2002) study of delirium in the terminally ill,

    A. Twenty-five percent of patients recalled their delirium experience after recovery.
    B. More severe perceptual disturbances were associated with more recall of delirium symptoms.
    C. The most significant predictor of distress for patients was motor hyperactivity during delirium.
    D. Patients with hypoactive delirium were more distressed than hyperactive patients.
    E. Spouse distress was predicted by the patient's Karnofsky Performance Status.

The correct response is option E.

Spouse distress was predicted by the patients' Karnofsky Performance Status (the lower the Karnofsky score, the worse the spouse distress).

In a study of terminally ill cancer patients, Breitbart et al. (2002) found that 54% of patients recalled their delirium experience after recovery from delirium. Factors predicting delirium recall included the degree of short-term memory impairment, delirium severity, and the presence of perceptual disturbances (the more severe, the less likely recall). The most significant factor predicting distress for patients was the presence of delusions. Patients with hypoactive delirium were just as distressed as patients with hyperactive delirium. **(p. 1065)**

> Breitbart W, Gibson C, Tremblay A: The delirium experience: delirium recall and delirium-related distress in hospitalized patients with cancer, their spouses/caregivers, and their nurses. Psychosomatics 43:183–194, 2002

41.7 Bereavement is an important aspect of palliative care, and an understanding of the terms used to describe various aspects of grief and mourning is helpful. Which of the following is defined as "a pathological outcome involving psychological, social, or physical morbidity"?

    A. Bereavement.
    B. Grief.
    C. Mourning.
    D. Disenfranchised grief.
    E. Complicated grief.

The correct response is option E.

Complicated grief represents a pathological outcome involving psychological, social, or physical morbidity (Rando 1983).

Bereavement is the state of loss resulting from death (Parkes 1998). *Grief* is the emotional response associated with loss (Stroebe et al. 1993). *Mourning* is the process of adaptation, including the cultural and social rituals prescribed as accompaniments (Raphael 1983). *Disenfranchised grief* represents the hidden sorrow of the marginalized patient, for whom there is less social permission to express many dimensions of loss (Doka 2000). **(p. 1073)**

Doka K: Disenfranchised grief, in Disenfranchised Grief: Recognizing Hidden Sorrow. Edited by Doka K. Lexington, MA, Lexington Books, 2000, pp 3–11

Parkes C: Bereavement: Studies of Grief in Adult Life, 3rd Edition. Madison, CT, International Universities Press, 1998

Rando T: Treatment of Complicated Mourning. Champaign, IL, Research Press, 1983

Raphael B: The Anatomy of Bereavement. London, Hutchinson, 1983

Stroebe M, Stroebe W, Hansson R (ed): Handbook of Bereavement. Cambridge, UK, Cambridge University Press, 1993